Peter Lehmann Publishing

Peter Lehmann (ed.)

Coming off Psychiatric Drugs

Successful Withdrawal from Neuroleptics,
Antidepressants, Lithium, Carbamazepine and
Tranquilizers

With prefaces by Judi Chamberlin, Pirkko Lahti and Loren R. Mosher

Contributions by Karl Bach Jensen, Regina Bellion, Carola Bock,
Wilma Boevink, Michael Chmela, Bert Gölden, Ilse Gold, Gábor Gombos,
Katalin Gombos, Maths Jesperson, Klaus John, Manuela Kälin,
Kerstin Kempker, Leo P. Koehne, Jan Kuypers, Elke Laskowski,
Peter Lehmann, Ulrich Lindner, Iris Marmotte, Constanze Meyer,
Harald Müller, Eiko Nagano, Mary Nettle, Una M. Parker, Nada Rath,
Erwin Redig, Hannelore Reetz, Roland A. Richter, Marc Rufer,
Jasna Russo, Lynne Setter, Martin Urban, Wolfgang Voelzke, David Webb,
Gerda Wozart, Josef Zehentbauer and Katherine Zurcher

Translations by Chie Ishii, Mary Murphy, Ivanka Popovic
and Christina White

Peter Lehmann Publishing   Berlin · Eugene · Shrewsbury

Originally published in 1998 in Berlin, Germany, under the title "Psychopharmaka absetzen. Erfolgreiches Absetzen von Neuroleptika, Antidepressiva, Lithium, Carbamazepin und Tranquilizern," 2., revised edition in 2002. Some chapters have not been translated for the English edition, one chapter has been added. The explanations in italic brackets and footnotes are by the editor.

Published by Peter Lehmann Publishing
Switchboard address: Zabel-Krüger-Damm 183, 13469 Berlin, Germany
Tel. +49 30 85963706 · Fax +49 30 4039 8752
Branch offices: Eugene, Oregon (USA) / Shrewsbury, Shropshire (United Kingdom). Please send all postal mail direct to our Berlin switchboard.
E-mail: pl@peter-lehmann-publishing.com
Internet: www.peter-lehmann-publishing.com

Coming off psychiatric drugs: Successful withdrawal from neuroleptics, antidepressants, lithium, carbamazepine and tranquilizers

ISBN 0-9545428-0-0 (British edition)
British Library Cataloguing in Publication Data. A catalogue record for this book is available from the British Library.

ISBN 1-891408-98-4 (American edition)

Cover design by Wolfram Pfreundschuh, Munich
Printed by Fuldaer Verlagsagentur GmbH, Fulda, Germany

Contents

Counterweights

To Withdraw with Professional Help

Better Sometimes than Forever

Professional Acting

The Time After

Closing Words

Appendix

Note about Liability

Psychiatric drugs are more dangerous than many (ex-)users and survivors of psychiatry and even physicians realize. Psychiatric drugs can cause serious adverse effects. Psychiatric drugs can also produce powerful physical dependence. For example, their withdrawal can cause sleeplessness, rebound and withdrawal psychoses, withdrawal-emergent tardive syndromes, return of base line psychological and emotional problems and even life-threatening withdrawal reactions (see pp. 25–38). Especially when psychiatric drugs have been taken for prolonged periods of time, experienced clinical supervision may be advisable or even necessary during the withdrawal process.

The problems which led to administration of psychiatric drugs may return when you stop taking them. Decisions to withdraw from psychotropic drugs should be made in a critical and responsible way. It is important to have a safe and supportive environment in which to undertake withdrawal (see pp. 311–321) and to consider the possibility that you may experience so-called relapse or worsening of your condition. Withdrawal may not work for everyone. Sometimes the difficulty of withdrawal or the base line psychological and emotional problems seem insurmountable, so people may decide to maintain on lower amounts of drugs or fewer drugs. Many psychiatrists do not support withdrawal and are convinced that people with psychiatric diagnoses like "schizophrenia," "psychosis," "manic depression" or "major depression" need psychiatric drugs or maintenance electroshock "therapy" for the rest of their lives.

We do not provide medical advice. Although this is the first book to describe positive experiences of coming off psychiatric drugs, it is not intended as a substitute for professional help. Should you have any health care-related questions, please call or see your physician or other health care provider promptly. The publisher, editor, authors and suppliers are not responsible if

Peter Lehmann

Prefaces

Much of the conventional wisdom about psychiatric drugs is wrong. Psychiatrists and the pharmaceutical industry have successfully convinced much of the public, through the media, that psychiatric drugs are "safe" and "effective" in "treating" "mental illnesses." Let us look at each of these words in turn:

Safe—generally accepted to mean that they cause no harm, despite many known negative effects such as movement disorders, changes in brain activity, weight gain, restlessness, sudden death from neuroleptic malignant syndrome and many others.

Effective—generally accepted to mean that they reverse or cure the symptoms for which they are prescribed, despite the fact that much research has shown they have a generally sedating effect that masks not only the targeted behavior, but all activities.

Treating—generally accepted to mean that the prescribed agents have specific effects on specific disease processes.

Mental illnesses—generally accepted to mean that there are specific clinical entities known as "schizophrenia," "bi-polar disorder" etc., despite the fact that there are no known structural or chemical changes in the body that can distinguish people who have these so-called illnesses from those who do not.

How is it that these myths have been so successfully accepted as fact? For one thing, those promoting the drugs are authority figures, doctors and scientists who are generally accepted to be presenting value-free experimental results. Another factor, perhaps even more significant, is that those who are given the drugs and who are the ones who have spoken out about their negative effects, are automatically discredited by having been labelled mentally ill. The diagnosis of mental illness carries with it a host of associations, particularly that the person so labelled has impaired judgment and is not a reliable reporter of his or her own experiences.

Nonetheless, it is personal stories which in fact carry enormous weight in the evaluation of the value of these drugs. Reading the eloquent personal testimonials of people who have taken and then discontinued these drugs, some who started with the belief that they were truly lifesaving agents, should be considered along with the positive accounts of researchers and pre-scribers. In psychiatry, it is the experiences, thoughts and feelings of the patient which are considered to be diseased; therefore, these experiences, thoughts and feelings in response to treatment must be taken into account. Of course, many psychiatrists and other believers in the efficacy of psychia-tric drugs can dismiss these accounts by considering them additional "symp-toms," but this, of course, is circular reasoning.

The experiences of people who have taken (or continue to take) psychiatric drugs are enormously varied. Some people find them helpful in dealing with troublesome symptoms, and these people, of course, are unlikely to want to discontinue using them. In fact, within this group, many are willing to toler-ate troublesome unwanted effects because they find the benefits outweigh the negatives. This group of people is not the subject of this book.

Instead, the book focuses on people who, for a wide variety of reasons, have decided that the drugs are not helpful to them, and who have made the decision to discontinue their use. Such a decision carries enormous conse-quences, as the treating physician almost always wants the patient to continue and the physician often has enormous powers (such as involuntary commit-ment) at his or her disposal in order to "persuade" the patient to continue. In-deed, the lack of support a person faces upon a decision to discontinue the use of drugs is often a factor in what is labelled relapse.

As an advocate and activist in the field of mental health and patients' rights (and as a person who discontinued the use of drugs as part of my own per-sonal process of recovery), one of the most common questions I am asked is "how can I discontinue the use of psychiatric drugs?" There is a crying need for information on stopping safely, as well as for supportive structures (such as short-term residential programs and physicians who are willing to consider non-drug approaches) that will enable people who wish to withdraw to do so.

The act of choosing to stop taking psychiatric drugs may be taken for a va-riety of reasons. Often it is that the negative effects are more troubling than the original problems, or it may even be that no positive effects are experienced at all (this was certainly my own experience). Unfortunately, the media image of a person who has stopped taking psychiatric drugs is the one that has captured the popular imagination: a person so deluded that he or she is unable to realize that his or her behavior is abnormal and who then usually goes on to commit some horrendous violent crime. Reading about real people and the complex reasons behind their decisions might be a way to counter this negative and destructive image.

It is often said that psychiatric drugs are given to people labelled mentally ill in order that those around them, such as medical personnel and family members, can feel better. Certainly, being around people who are troubled, especially when they are vocal about what is troubling them, can be wearing and difficult. But simply silencing them is not the answer. Instead, we need to listen carefully to the real experiences that people have so that we can learn the true costs of psychiatric drugs on people's lives.

Judi Chamberlin
Co-Chair, World Network of Users and Survivors of Psychiatry, Director of Education and Training, National Empowerment Center
Arlington, Massachusetts, October 30, 2002

This world wide first book about the issue "Successfully coming down from psychiatric drugs," published in Germany in 1998, primarily addresses individuals who want to withdraw based on their *own* decisions. It also addresses their relatives and therapists. Millions of people are taking psychiatric drugs, for example Haldol[1], Prozac[2] or Zyprexa[3]. To them, detailed accounts of

---

1 Neuroleptic, active ingredient haloperidol, marketed also as Dozic, Haloperidol, Peridol, Serenace

2 Antidepressant, active ingredient fluoxetine, marketed also as Auscap, Deprax, Eufor, Felicium, Fluohexal, Fluox, Fluoxetine, Lovan, Oxactin, Psyqual, Sarafem, Veritina, Zactin

3 Neuroleptic, active ingredient olanzapine

how others came off these substances without once again ending up in the in the doctor's office are of existential interest.

Many of my colleagues in the mental health field spend much of their time developing criteria for the application of psychiatric drugs. Diagnoses like compulsive acts, depression, dermatitis, hyperactivity, hyperemesis gravidarum, insomnia, nocturnal enuresis, psychosis, stuttering, travel sickness etc. can lead to the application of neuroleptics, antidepressants, lithium[1], tranquilizers and other drugs with psychic effects. This development of indications is a responsible task, rich with consequences.

Diagnoses and indications often result in a treatment with psychotropic drugs that can last for a long time. Who can predict whether the drugs—when time arrives—can be withdrawn from easily? From minor tranquilizers, especially the benzodiazepines, we already know the effects of dependency. Withdrawal without therapeutic help and without knowledge about the risks can take a dramatic course. What risks arise from the withdrawal of neuroleptics, antidepressants and lithium.

What factors favor successful withdrawal—successful in the sense that patients do not immediately return to the doctor's exam room, but live free and healthy lives, as all of us would wish? Have we not heard about pharmacogenic withdrawal-problems, receptor-changes, supersensitivity-psychoses, withdrawal-psychoses? Who is able to distinguish relapses from hidden withdrawal problems?

Do we not leave our patients alone with their sorrows and problems, when they—for whatever reasons—decide by themselves to come off their psychotropic drugs? Where can they find support, understanding and good examples, if they turn away from us disappointed (or we from them)?

Peter Lehmann, board-member or the European Network of (ex-)Users and Survivors of Psychiatry and former board-member of Mental Health Europe (the European section of the World Federation for Mental Health), has earned recognition for this difficult task as the first world wide expert to gather experiences from people themselves and their therapists, who have

---

1 Mood stabilizer, marketed also as Camcolit, Camcolith, Cibalith, Eskalith, Li-Liquid, Liskonum, Lithicarb, Lithium, Lithobid, Lithonathe, Lithotabs, Priadel, Quilonum

withdrawn from psychotropic drugs successfully or who have supported their clients to do so. In this manual 28 people from Australia, Austria, Belgium, Denmark, England, Germany, Hungary, Japan, the Netherlands, New Zealand, Serbia & Montenegro, Sweden, Switzerland and the USA write about their experiences with withdrawal. Additionally, eight psychotherapists, physicians, psychiatrists, social workers, psychologists, natural healers and other professionals report on how they helped their clients withdraw. Via the internationality of the authors the book provides a broad picture of different experiences and knowledge.

The book has a provocative message; life-experiences sometimes differ from scientific agreements. The book is based on the personal experiences of (ex-)users and survivors of psychiatry and the few professionals helping people come off psychiatric drugs. So it is a good place to begin the discussion. The book should be available in each medical practice, in each therapeutic ward, and in each patient's library.

Pirkko Lahti
Executive Director of the Finnish Association for Mental Health and President of the World Federation for Mental Health
Helsinki, August 19, 2002

"There is no tyranny so great as that which is practiced for the benefit of the victim"—C.S. Lewis

This volume is devoted to a topic that is the subject of a great deal of misguided thinking these days. We live in the era of a "pill for every ill" but too little attention has been devoted to the pills given specifically to affect our psyches. What does it mean to medicate the soul, the self, and the mind? Webster's dictionary defines psyche in all three ways. Are not these chemicals ("psychotropic drugs") interfering with the very essence of humanity? Should not great care and thought be given to this process? If begun, should it not be continuously monitored? Since all three—soul, self and mind—are at the core of each human being should not he/she determine whether these drugs should be taken based on her/his own subjective experience of them? The answer is, of course, a resounding yes.

Now let's get real. Since there are few objective indicators of the effects of these drugs the patients' own reports are critical. Do the psychiatrists and other physicians prescribing psychotropic drugs listen carefully to each patient's personal experience with a particular one? The answer to the question varies of course but if you speak a different language, are a member of a minority, poor, seen as "very ill" or forcibly incarcerated in a mental hospital the likelihood of being really listened to falls dramatically—although it is not very high for anyone.

Hence, the focus of this book—the stories of persons who were not listened to as they suffered torment of the soul, self and mind from psychotropic drugs—often given against their will, is very important. They are the stories of courageous decisions made against powerful expert doctors (and sometimes families and friends)—and the torment that sometimes ensued. Stopping medications began to restore their brains' physiology to their pre-medication states. Most had never been warned that the drugs would change their brains' physiology (or, worse yet, selectively damage regions of nerve cells in the brain) such that withdrawal reactions would almost certainly occur. Nor were they aware that these withdrawal reactions might be long lasting and might be interpreted as their "getting sick again." They are horror stories of what might happen (but does not have to happen) when attempting to return brains to usual functioning after being awash with "therapeutic" chemicals. Unfortunately, the suffering was usually necessary in order restore soul, self and mind—the essence of humanity.

However, because the drugs were given thoughtlessly, paternalistically and often unnecessarily to fix an unidentifiable "illness" the book is an indictment of physicians. The Hippocratic Oath—to above all do no harm—was regularly disregarded in the rush to "do something." How is it possible to determine whether soul murder might be occurring without reports of patients' experiences with drugs that are aimed directly at the essence of their humanity? Despite their behavior, doctors are only MD's, not MDeity's. They, unlike gods, have to be held accountable for their actions.

This book is a must read for anyone who might consider taking or no longer taking these mind altering legal drugs and perhaps even more so for those able to prescribe them.

Loren R. Mosher MD
Director, Soteria Associates
Clinical Professor of Psychiatry
University of California at San Diego
School of Medicine
August 26, 2002

The point of departure for this book is the moment at which those who are taking psychiatric drugs—the objects of psychiatric treatment—have already made their own decision to quit or to want to quit. This starting point may be alarming to those readers who look upon the consumers of these substances not as subjects with a capacity for individual decision-making but rather as psychologically unsound and, above all, unable to recognize their own illness (or alternately as consumers of pharmaceuticals from whom they can profit).

Psychiatric drugs are substances which are given to influence the psychic condition and the behavior of their patients. This book refers to the treatment of human beings only. Mentioned are neuroleptics, antidepressants, lithium, carbamazepine[1] and tranquilizers. The withdrawal of drugs used to treat epilepsy in the field of neurology is not a subject of this book.

- Neuroleptics (known also as "major tranquilizers") are so-called antipsychotic drugs, which are administered when physicians (mostly general practitioners, pediatricians or psychiatrists) decide to give a diagnoses such as psychosis, schizophrenia, paranoia, hebephrenia and hysteria. Other possible symptoms that lead doctors to prescribe neuroleptics are those sometimes considered psychosomatic in origin: whooping-cough, asthma,

---

1 Mood stabilizer, marketed as Atretol, Carbamazepine, Carbatrol, Epitol, Tegretol, Teril, Timonil

stuttering, disturbances of sleep and behavior in children, travel sickness, pruritus (itching) or vegetative dystonia. In the same way that rebellious or aggressive animals of all sorts are given drugs to calm stress-related reactions, so too are elderly disturbed people treated with neuroleptics.

- Antidepressants are given after diagnoses such as reactive, neurotic or brain-organic depression, restlessness, anxiety disorder or obsessive-compulsive disorder, night-anxiety, panic attacks, phobia (e.g. school-anxiety in children), nocturnal enuresis, insomnia and many others. Unhappy animals might receive antidepressants, too, for instance sad dogs, if they are locked up in the house all day while their master is at work.
- Lithium is administered mostly under diagnoses such as mania or schizo-affective disorder.
- The main psychiatric indication for carbamazepine (as well as the chemically-related oxcarbazepine[1] and valproate[2]) is the diagnosis of affective psychosis, especially when the treating psychiatrist has failed to reach the effect he desires with his normal psychiatric drugs. Carbamazepine, valproate and oxcarbazepine which are administered for the treatment of epilepsy in the field of neurology are not subjects of this book.
- Tranquilizers (sometimes called "minor tranquilizers") are substances which are administered after diagnoses such as a lack of motor impulse, depressed mood, phobia, neurosis, panic attack, sleep disorder. Tranquilizers which are administered for the treatment of epilepsy in the field of neurology, are not a subject of this book.

"Authors wanted on the subject: 'withdrawing from psychiatric drugs.'" This was the call for articles I sent out to relevant groups worldwide in 1995:

"'Coming off Psychiatric Drugs. Successful Withdrawal from Neuroleptics, Antidepressants, Lithium, Carbamazepine and Tranquilizers.' This is the title of a book that will be published in German in 1997/98. A publication in English translation is intended later. We are looking for people who have been prescribed one or several of the above-mentioned psy-

1 Mood stabilizer, marketed as Trileptal
2 Mood stabilizer, marketed as Convulex, Depacon, Depakene, Depakote, Epilim, Sodium Valproate, Valpro, Valproic Acid

chiatric drugs and who have decided to quit taking them. Of particular interest are positive examples that show that it is possible to stop taking these substances without ending up in the treatment-room of a physician or right back in the madhouse again. For that reason I am looking for authors willing to report—in exchange for royalties—about their own experiences on the route to withdrawal and who now live free from psychiatric drugs. I am also looking for reports from people who have successfully helped others to withdraw from psychiatric drugs in the course of their professional life (e.g. user-controlled support centers, natural healers, homeopaths, social workers, psychologists, pastoral workers, physicians, psychiatrists etc.) or in their personal life (e.g. supporting friends, relatives, self-help-groups etc.)."

I received a series of responses from people who were interested in contributing to this book, including people who had been taking psychiatric drugs as well as some professionals whose articles also appear in this book. One psychiatrist withdrew her offer to contribute, fearing (not without reason) that her practice might be flooded with people wishing to stop taking psychiatric drugs. Because I had received no responses from family members of (ex-)users and survivors of psychiatry, I sent my call for articles to the German "Association for Family Members of the Mentally Ill." The reaction was again silence. Is the reason for this perhaps that those family members who have organized themselves into support groups have been inundated in the past years with free lectures and information from the pharmaceutical industry?

In any case, it would be a mistake to reduce the problem of the prolonged use of psychoactive drugs and the possible complications arising from withdrawal to the fault of disinterested or naïve family members, irresponsible doctors, and the profit-oriented pharmaceutical industry. Two authors who had showed initial interest in contributing their experiences with withdrawal later took back their offer because they had "relapsed." One of them reported that she had mistimed her withdrawal to concur with a breakup. The other informed me that she was in a clinic again because she had experienced another psychosis. Did she experience what those in the field call a "withdrawal psychosis," or was she just overwhelmed with the sudden return of old problems that had yet to be worked through?

Throughout my endeavor to address this subject, I've been cautious enough never to urge others to stop taking psychiatric drugs. I was careful to only approach those who had already quit before I sent out my call for articles. Nonetheless, I wonder if I may have been responsible for leading others to quit in an unconsidered and potentially dangerous way just by having published material on the subject.

Ever since the emergence of psychiatric drugs, many people who have taken prescriptions have made their own decision to quit. One can only speculate how many people have attempted to quit after having been exposed to the idea in an uninformed way only to experience a "relapse" and eventually another prolonged administration of the drugs. I think it is safe to say that a great number of attempts to quit would have been more successful if those wishing to quit and those around them had been better informed as to the potential problems that may arise as well as of means for preventing the often-prophesied relapse. With only a few exceptions, many professionals have little considered how they can support their clients who have decided to withdraw. Responses such as turning their backs on clients and leaving them alone with their problems indicate that professionals have little sense of responsibility regarding this subject.

The many different methods of successfully withdrawing from psychiatric drugs cannot be represented in a single book. As the editor of this book, it was important to me that "my" authors, with the exception of the contributing professionals, openly describe the personal path they took as well as the wishes and fears that accompanied them. They were told that there was only one thing they should not do, namely, to tell others what they should do or to offer surefire prescriptions for how to withdraw. Every reader must be aware of the potential problems and the possibilities, of their own personal strengths and weaknesses, and of their individual limitations and desires such that they can find their own means and their own way of reaching their goal. These reports by individuals who have successfully withdrawn are intended to show that it is possible to reach this goal and to live free of psychiatric drugs.

My sincere thanks go to the numerous good people, who have helped with proof-reading and with other preparatory tasks: Bill Spath, Chie Ishii, Christina White, Craig Newnes, David Oaks and MindFreedom Support Coalition International (www.MindFreedom.org), Jeffrey M. Masson, Joey Depew, Laura Ziegler, Marc Rufer, Mary Murphy, Mary Nettle, Myra Manning, Peter Stastny, Ronald J. Bartle, Tricia R. Owsley and Wolfram Pfreundschuh. Without friends and supporters I would have been lost.

Two authors are no longer living: Ilse Gold, who died on September 7, 1998 from breast cancer, which developed after the psychiatric treatment, and Erwin Redig, who quitted his life on June 14, 1999 after repeated violent psychiatric treatment. They had deserved a life of a hundred years.

Peter Lehmann
Berlin, April 14, 2004

Translation from the German by Mary Murphy

Introduction

According to the literature, anyone trying to stop taking psychiatric drugs must reckon with withdrawal problems. Ample evidence is provided for this statement in my book "Schöne neue Psychiatrie" *("Brave New Psychiatry,"* Lehmann 1996b, pp. 356ff.). In this book, "Coming off Psychiatric Drugs," I only provide a summary of the withdrawal symptoms. They may or may not occur.

When one discusses the issue of dependency with psychiatrists, most often their first reflex is to deny the danger of dependency for users of anti-depressants and neuroleptics. For example, the psychiatrists of the German Pharmaceutical Watch Group for Psychiatry have defined dependency as follows:

> "Psychological dependency is understood as the irresistible longing for a medication in order to increase a feeling of well-being or to reduce uncomfortable symptoms. Physical dependence can be established with the appearance of withdrawal symptoms after the reduction or withdrawal of a medication." (Grohmann / Rüther / Schmitz 1994, p. 279)

The risk of further problems developing in addition to the usual withdrawal symptoms, for example a rebound effect or hypersensitivity, should be taken into consideration when deciding whether or not to withdraw. Rebound effects are counter-regulatory adjustment reactions that lead to a temporary pronounced recurrence of the original symptoms.

Rebound effects have a mirroring-effect that make it particularly difficult to recognize withdrawal symptoms as distinct from the original problems. Because a prolonged use of psychoactive drugs raises the probability of various withdrawal problems—in addition to the usual damage of using the drugs—it is wise to consider sooner rather than later whether or not the time has come to limit these risks and to withdraw in a safe manner.

Taking psychoactive drugs can, under certain circumstances, lead to a temporary relief of psychological stress; but at the same time this leads many people slowly into dependency without their knowing it and with the support of the medical establishment. Many people attempt to stop taking psychiatric drugs, for a variety of reasons: lack of "therapeutic" effect; unwanted effects; pregnancy; lack of insight into their "illness." Generally they have been left to cope with withdrawal problems on their own. In popular medical advice books (Curran / Golombok 1985; Neild 1990; Trickett 1991; Gadsby 2000) there is no mention of withdrawal from carbamazepine, lithium, antidepressants or neuroleptics. A few specialist journals published apparently random reports of severe withdrawal symptoms. But until recenly, textbooks and information leaflets aimed at psychiatric drug users and their families still claimed withdrawal symptoms only arose with tranquilizers. In the past few years withdrawal effects of the newer antidepressants have gained some public notoriety. It is even possible to find information about dependence on "atypical" neuroleptics like Zyprexa (Support4Hope 2003). You only have to search long enough in the internet.

Typical withdrawal studies demonstrate quite serious methodological deficiencies, which have also been noticed by doctors: double-blind studies, in other words studies where neither the subject nor the treating physician knows what substance is actually being administered, are as rare as the administration of a placebo to a control group (which is also problematical). Furthermore, there has been a lack of systematic follow up, a lack of information on the duration of hospitalization and of prior treatment as well as of the strength of dose of the psychiatric drug being withdrawn. Also, the period covered by the studies is too short, and finally, what is meant by any "relapse" mentioned is left completely unclear (Andrews / Hall / Snaith 1976). Those being treated were considered "improved" if in the eyes of the administrator of the psychiatric drugs they were not ready to be discharged but caused less trouble on the ward (Glick / Margolis 1962).

As Bertram Karon from the Psychology Department of Michigan State University concluded, the only purpose of some of these studies is simply to justify the prescribing practices of psychiatric drugs (Karon 1989, p. 113). For example, the American psychiatrist Philip May in his "California Study" (May 1968), much quoted among his circle of colleagues, claimed to prove the superiority of neuroleptics, antidepressants and electroshock treatment over psychotherapeutic procedures. However, the report failed to point out that the therapists he used were untrained and unpaid trainees. A further deficit is the fact that in long-term studies only subjects who are motivated to take psychiatric drugs are included (Tegeler / Lehmann / Stockschläder 1980); people who stop taking psychiatric drugs on their own initiative and who live without them do not figure in such studies and their experiences are ignored.

The fact that no distinction is made between withdrawal problems such as receptor changes caused by the treatment, rebound effects or supersensitive reactions and relapse is another serious deficiency. Brigitte Woggon from the Zurich University Psychiatric Hospital, who favors psychiatric drugs, sees problems with the lack of differentiation made, even drugs are abruptly withdrawn, between withdrawal symptoms and the return of the original psychological symptoms:

> "Interestingly, in most studies on withdrawal no position is taken on possible withdrawal symptoms apparently because the studies are not set up to deal with these findings." (Woggon 1979, p. 46)

Nonetheless, doctors continue to refer to their studies and speak with a great deal of pathos of a sudden relapse if the drugs are stopped without their authorization, particularly in the case of lithium, antidepressants and neuroleptics. The situation is somewhat different in the case of carbamazepine and tranquilizers. In contrast to its use in preventing epileptic fits in neurology, carbamazepine is rarely used alone in psychiatry—its claimed antimanic effect is disputed anyway (Lerer et al. 1985)—and there have been practically no withdrawal studies. Partly as a consequence of decisions reached in the law courts on compensation, awarded because patients were insufficiently informed on the risk of dependency associated with tranquilizers, these substances have come to be seen as problematic by orthodox medicine.

Tranquilizers

Taking tranquilizers involves a risk which should not be underestimated. The development of tolerance and rebound phenomena can occur after taking the psychiatric drugs for only a short time and in low dosage. Massive, life-endangering withdrawal symptoms, especially convulsions, can make stopping psychiatric drugs a very dangerous undertaking. Often withdrawal symptoms are so pronounced that withdrawal can only be done under hospital care. After withdrawal, a rebound-like explosion of feelings that had been chemically repressed may be released.

Depression, in some cases long-lasting, as well as anxiety states or hallucinations and deliria may occur during withdrawal. A "fear of rebound" is a generally recognized withdrawal symptom associated with tranquilizers. These symptoms are associated with risks, not least the repeated prescription of psychiatric drugs, becoming a psychiatric "case," and the switch to even more risky psychiatric drugs such as antidepressants or neuroleptics.

Withdrawal symptoms can register in the central nervous system as EEG (electroencephalogram) disturbances, difficulty in concentrating, pressure headaches, generalized pain, nervousness, restlessness, disturbed sleep and disturbed perceptions such as an increased sensitivity to stimuli. According to many doctors, withdrawal symptoms such as insomnia and excitability can be traced to a reactive hyperactivity of receptors which have been chemically altered. Many speak of a "rebound insomnia." Sometimes this phenomenon continues for weeks or months until the molecular mechanisms have settled at a new tolerable level.

Various vegetative symptoms can also often be explained as unhealthy physiological rebound effects. These symptoms may last for weeks, making it difficult to interpret whether they are drug withdrawal symptoms or recurring symptoms of the underlying condition. Weight loss, hot-cold sensations, fever, and heart and circulatory problems often occur (the latter for example as a rapid heart beat, shortness of breath, constriction, a rapid pulse, dizziness and weakness). Breaking out in sweats is an accompanying symptom. Intestinal and stomach disorders are another common withdrawal symptom (diarrhea, nausea, loss of appetite). Stomach cramps also occur. Disorders affecting vision sometimes accompany these symptoms as well.

Withdrawal may also bring muscular and motor disturbances, for example, jitters and shaking, limb pain, back tension, an insecure gait, as well as alternating muscle contractions that may cause jerking and shaking.

Withdrawal symptoms occur at a rate of 30–50% even when withdrawal is gradual.

Especially in the case of benzodiazepine tranquilizers, the approaches to withdrawal studies are mixed. Some include reports on the (problematical) administration of carbamazepine, antidepressants or neuroleptics to suppress withdrawal symptoms, although they seldom include warnings of the additional toxic burden (e.g. Klein et al. 1994). The tranquilizers are frequently replaced on a long-term basis by other psychiatric drugs. All the same, in recent years several authors of such studies have spoken not just in favor of a gradual withdrawal of tranquilizers; they also observed good long-term results in avoiding relapses back to the original unproductive mechanisms of dealing with problems and in avoiding problems of new dependencies (Ashton 1987; Rickels et al. 1988). This was also true of people with varying diagnoses (Golombok et al. 1987) and even in the case of repeated relapses (Crouch / Robson / Hallstrom 1988). Even in the eyes of professionals self-help groups have proven to be effective (Tattersall / Hallstrom 1992), as has psychological support in learning non-psychopharmacological strategies (Ashton 1994) when they encouraged people to persevere, to actively confront the problems caused by the continuous use of tranquilizers (Bish et al. 1996) and when psychotherapeutic support was provided during withdrawal and in the ensuing months (Otto et al. 1993; Kaendler / Volk / Pflug 1996).

Carbamazepine

Withdrawal symptoms associated with carbamazepine appear to be relatively minor. Nonetheless, in the few known controlled studies on withdrawal, a series of psychological, central nervous, vegetative and motor disturbances occurred.

L.A. Demers-Desrosiers and his colleagues from the Montreal Neurological Hospital and Clinic published two case studies of first-time occurrences of psychotic symptoms in two people who had been taking the anti-epileptic drug carbamazepine for three and four years respectively to treat epilepsy and had withdrawn slowly (Demers-Desrosiers / Nestoros / Vaillancourt 1978). The British neurologist John Duncan, together with his colleagues as the Centre for Epilepsy in Chalfont/England, carried out a systematic withdrawal study of the drug carbamazepine. A double-blind study of 24 adults with epilepsy diagnoses was carried out in which some subjects withdrew slowly and some abruptly. According to the 1988 report, although all of them continued taking a second anti-epileptic drug, 23 persons still showed withdrawal symptoms, including paranoia and confusion in one patient, a lack of energy in four patients, depression and/or irritability in five, tension and feelings of depersonalization in two, states of anxiety in three, a weak memory and loss of concentration in two, insomnia and/or headaches in four, loss of appetite in three, muscular pain in five, jerking in four, muscle jitters and/or an insecure gait in two. Some of these disturbances were accompanied by low blood pressure and a racing heartbeat. According to the neurologists, in comparison with the chemically closely-related tricyclic antidepressants, the carbamazepine withdrawal symptoms were not nearly as pronounced as was found in the first study (Duncan / Shorvon / Trimble 1988).

The biggest withdrawal problem, especially in people taking this substance for epileptic attacks or to suppress psychological states—possibly together with neuroleptics or lithium—, lies in the danger of the recurrence or sudden new occurrence of epileptic attacks.

Lithium

In the case of lithium the usual vegetative withdrawal symptoms seem not to occur. However, depending on dose, duration of administration, as well as the patient's physical and psychological state, rebound phenomena and states of confusion can be expected which bring with them the danger of renewed hospitalization. Therefore, a gradual approach is recommended when stopping this psychiatric drug.

In 1979 D.G. Wilkinson, a psychiatrist at Bethlem Royal Hospital in London, was the first to report on withdrawal problems, citing states of confusion (Wilkinson 1979). Other authors have since confirmed Wilkinson's statements: a state of fear increases, irritability and an unstable state as well as the rebound phenomena of mania and psychosis result. Y.D. Lapierre and his colleagues at the Royal Ottawa Hospital took into consideration what they found to be an unexpectedly high "relapse" rate after the withdrawal of lithium and came to the following conclusion:

"Such quick relapses suggest some sort of exaggerated neurochemical or physiological response to abrupt withdrawal. (…) Such rebound pheno-

mena have also been observed after withdrawal from benzodiazepines."
(Lapierre / Gagnon / Kokkinidis 1980, p. 863)

J.R. King and R.P. Hullin from the High Roads Hospital in Ilkley, England found in 1983 that the relatively high number of cases of anxiety states and other withdrawal reactions (irritability and an increase of strong emotions) are obviously withdrawal symptoms and rebound phenomena, and that their occurrence two or three days after withdrawal is characteristic of the delayed reaction typical of withdrawal from medication (King / Hullin 1983). The excessive increase of "relapses" within a few weeks after withdrawal from lithium, which has often been described, was addressed by Janet Lawrence of McLean Hospital in Belmont, Massachusetts, who said:

> "Such withdrawal might trigger psychosis by altering neurotransmitter balance with previously unipolar depressed patients relapsing into depression and bipolar patients into mania. This is of especial interest as it implies that lithium treatment may adversely affect the natural history of the underlying disease in an analogous fashion to the rebound psychosis postulated for antipsychotics by Chouinard and associates." (Lawrence 1985, pp. 873f.)

More recent withdrawal studies with lithium do not show uniform results. In general, it was observed that gradual withdrawal reduces the risk of the recurrence of the same depressive and manic moods which had led to psychiatric treatment and the administration of lithium in the first place (Mander / Loudon 1988; Faedda et al. 1993; Suppes et al. 1993). One study showed that after getting through the first three months following withdrawal, relapses were no more frequent than in those persons who continued to take lithium (Mander 1986). Some psychiatrists expect the occurrence of a withdrawal rebound, in other words an increased risk of relapse with temporarily more severe "symptoms" especially if the psychiatric drugs are stopped abruptly (Hunt / Bruce-Jones / Silverstone 1992; Schou 1993). Others found no such rebound (Sashidharan / McGuire 1983) or at least only a partial one (Klein et al. 1991). The claim that lithium prevents depressive or manic attacks is not undisputed in orthodox medicine ("Lithium" 1969). Publications continue to appear on "individual cases" where the claimed protection provided by lithium proved to be an illusion (Prien et al. 1984), as well as on considerable rates of relapse (Lusznat / Murphy / Nunn 1988) and several cases of suicide including while under the influence of lithium (Schou / Weeke 1988).

Antidepressants

In 1982 Dennis Charney and his colleagues at University of New Haven, Connecticut described the typical reaction to the withdrawal of antidepressants:

> "Symptoms first appeared approximately 48 hours after the last dose and included excessive anxiety, restlessness, and autonomic symptoms such as diaphoresis, diarrhoea, hot and cold flushes, and piloerection *(goose-bumps)*. In addition, the development of hypomanic and manic symptoms has been observed to occur during the first week after cessation of chronic TAD *(tricyclic antidepressants)* treatment." (Charney et al. 1982, p. 377)

When stopping antidepressants, more psychological withdrawal symptoms can be expected, for instance apathy, social withdrawal, a depressed mood, but also panic attacks, aggression, or delirium. Withdrawal psychoses can also occur.

Besides stomach and intestinal tract disturbances, insomnia probably represents the second most common withdrawal problem, according to Steven Dilsaver and John Greden of the University Hospital in Columbus, Ohio. Further symptoms of the central nervous system include headache, restlessness, hyperactivity, insomnia, a dazed state, apparently paradoxical improvements, tiredness, jittering and nervousness as well as disruptive dreams, for example nightmares. According to the German psychiatrists Otto Benkert und Hanns Hippius, severe cramping, which is known to occur particularly with the withdrawal of tranquilizers, can also develop when antidepressants are withdrawn, especially if the dosage had been high:

> "Favorable conditions for the development of severe cramping include beginning with a high dosage, rapidly increasing the dosage, or a rapid withdrawal from a high dosage. A sudden withdrawal from antidepressants after years of use should always be avoided." (Benkert / Hippius 1980, p. 34)

The occurrence of vegetative withdrawal symptoms has been observed in cases of both gradual and abrupt withdrawal. Intestinal tract and stomach disorders, for example diarrhea, stomach ache, tenesmus (painful, lasting cramp-like urges to release the bowels or bladder), and associated nausea, vomiting and loss of appetite, are the most common symptoms. In addition, the following should also be mentioned: cold-sweats, weakness, an increase in libido, a racing heartbeat, abnormal heart rhythms, as well as lowered blood pressure and extreme anxiety associated with physical collapse.

Motor disturbances are a more rare. Some individual reports have noted also muscle pain, Parkinson-like symptoms such as slowed movement, cog wheel phenomenon, as well as restlessness and withdrawal dyskinesia.

In 1984 Dilsaver und Greden provided an overview of the available literature on withdrawal. They reached the conclusion that withdrawal symptoms very frequently appear, that is, in 21% to 55% of adults. Other authors reported a rate of 80% (Dilsaver / Greden 1984).

Withdrawal symptoms that include a worsening of the psychological state must carefully be separated from a return or relapse to the original psychological problems that led to treatment in the first place, according to Janet Lawrence at the McLean Hospital in Belmont, Massachusetts. The two are not easy to distinguish. A "relapse" occurs three to 15 weeks after withdrawal, whereas withdrawal symptoms occur within two weeks and usually subside within a week or two (Lawrence 1985). The problems associated with withdrawal from antidepressants are as old as antidepressants themselves. Already in 1960, the antidepressant pioneer Roland Kuhn wrote that withdrawal symptoms:

> "… can look really bad, under certain circumstances bringing on severe headaches, profuse sweating, tachycardia attacks *(racing heart beat)*, sometimes also vomiting, all of which disappear within a half hour of resuming the medication. This is a phenomenon that looks very similar to the 'withdrawal symptoms' of toxicomania *(drug dependence)*…" (Kuhn 1960, p. 248)

Rudolf Degkwitz, former president of the German Association for Psychiatry and Neurology, compared the withdrawal symptoms of psycholeptics (neuroleptics and antidepressants) with those of alcaloids, the group of substances to which morphine among others, belongs. In addition, sleeping pills are considered addictive, and it is known that withdrawal from them can bring on severe, even life-threatening, cramping. According to Degkwitz:

"The reduction or withdrawal from psycholeptics leads, as described above, to considerable withdrawal symptoms that cannot be distinguished from those symptoms occurring with the withdrawal of alcaloids and sleeping pills." (Degkwitz 1967, p. 161)

The development of tolerance and rebound phenomena even after only short-term usage in moderate doses as well as receptor changes may necessitate a gradual withdrawal. This counteracts the risk of withdrawal symptoms (which can last for several weeks) being confused with the recurrence of the original problems thus leading to renewed prescription of antidepressants and other psychiatric procedures. In those withdrawal studies which deal with antidepressants psychiatrists reported, among other things, relatively good prognoses in the time after withdrawal in older people (Cook et al. 1986), especially if the subjects had been symptom-free for 16 to 20 weeks (Prien / Kupfer 1986). They do not, however, deal with the question of what use that statement is to people who despite or because of antidepressants are suffering from depressive symptoms. Other studies saw higher relapse rates after withdrawing all kinds of antidepressants (Misri / Sivertz 1991; Solyom / Solyom / Ledwidge 1991); but the suspicion that antidepressants lead rather to depression becoming chronic (Irle 1974, pp. 124f.) was not dealt with while the question of how to evaluate the effect of psychotherapy or self-help (which was not offered) was not even posed in the first place

Neuroleptics

Psychiatrists have reported the following psychological withdrawal symptoms: a depressed mood, fear, a desire to run away, and fits of crying. Because a reduced dosage may result in motor disturbances and emotional pain caused by the neuroleptics becoming more pronounced and/or particularly intense (due to the fact that the emotional numbing of the drugs has subsided), a temporary—but nonetheless serious—risk of suicide may arise during withdrawal.

Tension, restlessness, destructiveness, aggression, irritability, and excitability may develop into withdrawal psychoses and delirious states. Fritz Reimer, like Degkwitz a former President of the German Association for Psychiatry and Neurology, concluded the following concerning the possibility of post-withdrawal delirium that may last several days:

> "The ultimate factor in the delirium syndrome is certain to be the psychoactive pharmaceuticals. On the surface, it appears to compare to the withdrawal delirium of the alcoholic." (Reimer 1965, pp. 446f.)

Some psychiatrists deliberately employ withdrawal and its effects to provoke a so-called therapeutic delirium, for example to stimulate those with a "numbed foundation" and to create new target syndromes for the neurolepsy, as they put it (cf. Lehmann 1996a, pp. 125f.).

Tardive dyskinesia, that is, muscle disorders that appear during treatment, withdrawal or thereafter and which are not treatable nor controllable, have in the past been deemed impairments resulting from treatment, and some victims have been successful in obtaining compensation for this. In 1977 George Simpson from the Psychiatric Institute in Orangeburg, New York was the first psychiatrist to warn that:

> "The potential of neuroleptics to produce dyskinesia, a serious complication, in a considerable number or patients would indicate that an attempt should be made to withdraw in every patient." (Simpson 1977, p. 6)

In the same year, Urban Ungerstedt und Tomas Ljungberg at the Karolinska Institute in Stockholm published results of studies in which rats were administered the conventional neuroleptic haloperidol and as a comparison the "atypical" clozapine[1]. They believe that "atypical" neuroleptics modify subtypes of specific dopamine-receptors, produce their supersensitivity and contribute to the risk of new, increasing, or chronically powerful psychoses of organic origin, which can be understood as "counterpart to tardive dyskinesia" (Ungerstedt / Ljungberg 1977, p. 199). Since then, medical journals have steadily published findings on supersensitivity, rebound and withdrawal psychoses (Chouinard et al. 1979, 1984; Chouinard / Jones 1980, 1982; Borison et al. 1988; Ekblom / Eriksson / Lindstroem 1984).

The frequent damage caused by typical neuroleptics like haloperidol arises from changes in dopamine-D_2-metabolism, observable as motor disturban-

---

1 Neuroleptic, marketed as Clopine, Clozapine, Clozaril

ces; the usual damage caused by "atypical" neuroleptics like clozapine, sertindole[1] or quetiapine[2] goes in the direction of changing the metabolism of special subtypes of dopamine-receptors, dopamine-D_1 and -D_4, seen as producing or increasing mid- and long-term psychotic syndromes of organic origin. Frank Tornatore and his colleagues at the University of Southern California School of Pharmacy in Los Angeles warned of the development of supersensitivity psychoses:

> "There is a worsening of the psychosis (delusions, hallucinations, suspiciousness) induced by long-term use of neuroleptic drugs. Typically, those who develop supersensitivity psychosis respond well initially to low or moderate doses of antipsychotics, but with time seem to require larger doses after each relapse and ultimately megadoses to control symptoms." (Tornatore et al. 1987, p. 44)

Supersensitivty should be understood as the result of an increased tolerance to the drugs, as they point out in an additional citation in the German translation of the book four years later: "Thus, a tolerance to the antipsychotic effect seems to develop." (Tornatore et al. 1991, p. 53)

Withdrawal symptoms related to the central nervous system are well known to psychiatrists. In 1960 psychiatrists at the University Clinic in Vienna published their initial observations on the effects of Melleril[3]:

> "What we noticed was that when medication was suddenly withdrawn, even after several months patients experienced insomnia and considerable restlessness as well as occasional states of pronounced excitability." (Hofmann / Kryspin-Exner 1960, p. 900)

Further symptoms in this area include headaches, restlessness, insomnia, nightmares, numbness and taste impairment.

Vegetative withdrawal symptoms that may occur include anorexia (or a lesser loss of appetite), binging, nausea, vomiting, gastritis, diarrhea, stomach

---

1 Neuroleptic, marketed as Serdolect
2 Neuroleptic, marketed as Seroquel
3 Neuroleptic, active ingredient thioridazine, marketed also as Aldazine, Mellaril, Rideril, Thioridazine

ache, colic, pronounced nasal discharge, sebaceous gland discharge, hot flashes, freezing, pronounced sweating, cardiovascular (i.e. heart and circulatory system) problems such as a racing heartbeat, dizziness and physical collapse. The dangers that proceed from the habituation of a vegetative state and a physical dependence on neuroleptics have been shown in a rabbit study by Helma Sommer and Jochen Quandt at the Psychiatric Clinic in Bernburg/Saale. Their observations were based on noted metabolic changes induced by chlorpromazine that caused a circulatory collapse after withdrawal from the neuroleptic, despite the fact that metabolism was in fact returning to normal. For six months, Sommer and Quandt administered neuroleptics to 20 rabbits. The four animals that had received the highest dosage (16.7 mg/kg) died after a brief fit of cramping:

> "At a dosage of 13.3 mg/kg of chlorpromazine, abrupt withdrawal led to a sudden death within 14 days, probably due to irreversibly blocked metabolic processes that stopped functioning (similar observations in human beings have been published in which death followed a brief stage of cramping)." (Sommer / Quandt 1970, p. 487)

Withdrawal from neuroleptics can cause various muscle and motor disturbances. Parkinson-like disorders are common, and muscle jerking or withdrawal dyskinesia and tongue atrophy often increases or is initiated.

Roy Lacoursiere and his colleagues at the Veterans Administration Hospital in Topeka, Kansas, have stated that the rate of withdrawal symptoms of all kinds is as high as 75%. The observed rate will depend on how closely subjects are observed, how well the withdrawal symptoms can be distinguished from the "mental illness," and how well the psychological condition of the subjects before treatment has been documented. Thus it is no surprise that some psychiatrists have published rates of 0% (Lacoursiere / Spohn / Thompson 1976). Up to 80% of patients experienced vegetative and especially stomach and intestinal problems with withdrawal (Greil / Schmidt 1988, 1989). There is very little evidence available on the rate of supersensitivity psychoses. In 1982 the pharmacologist Guy Chouinard and his colleague Barry Jones at the University Clinic in Montreal reported that they had found signs of supersensitivity psychoses among 30% of the 300 patients they studied, many of whom had not necessarily gone through an abrupt withdrawal

(Chouinard / Jones 1982). Degkwitz has repeatedly reported on withdrawal symptoms—not publicly, but in specialized journals:

"We now know that it is extremely difficult, if not impossible, for many of the chronic patients to stop neuroleptics because of the unbearable withdrawal-symptoms." (Degkwitz / Luxenburger 1965, p. 175)

George Brooks, psychiatrist at the Vermont State Hospital in Waterbury said:

"The severity of the withdrawal symptoms may mislead the clinician into thinking that he is observing a relapse of the patient's mental condition." (Brooks 1959, p. 932)

Medical opinion on continued administration of neuroleptics is split. In 1995 Patricia Gilbert and colleagues in the Psychiatric Department of the University of California in San Diego published a meta-analysis in which they looked at 66 studies conducted between 1958 and 1993 on almost 5600 persons. They summed up the problems of the continued administration of neuroleptics for the treating physician:

"The issue of prolonged neuroleptic treatment in a patient with chronic schizophrenia places the clinician on the horns of a dilemma. Since neuroleptic treatment does not cure schizophrenia, a large majority of such patients need long-term treatment. At the same time, prolonged use of these drugs carries a high risk of adverse effects, including TD *(tardive dyskinesia)*. It is therefore recommended that continued prescription of antipsychotic drugs over a long period not be undertaken without adequate justification for both clinical and legal purposes. This may imply attempts at neuroleptic withdrawal. Drug withdrawal, however, is associated with a risk of psychotic relapse. To complicate matters further, a number of patients withdrawn from antipsychotic therapy do not experience relapse, at least over a short period, while some patients maintained on therapy do experience relapse. Thus, the clinician and the patient have to choose between two unwelcome risks: relapse and adverse effects of continued treatment." (Gilbert et al. 1995, p. 173)

Both psychotherapeutic treatment providers and biologically-oriented psychiatrists admit in internal discussions that they do not know whether neuroleptics in individual cases actually help or cause damage. William Carpenter and Carol Tamminga from the Maryland Psychiatric Research Center in Baltimore, who provided the opportunity of a controlled withdrawal, came to the conclusion:

> "Although adverse events, such as suicide, dissatisfied patients or relatives, loss of job, deteriorating course, and brain abnormalities, can all be observed during drug withdrawal, each of these is also commonly encountered in the clinical care of medicated patients!" (Carpenter / Tamminga 1995, p. 193)

Hanfried Helmchen from the University Hospital in Berlin, a psychiatrist who can be seen as a strong supporter of long-term neuroleptic treatment, expressed himself back in the 1980s in a discussion among colleagues in a notably skeptical tone:

> "When looking back on the 25 years since neuroleptics have been made available to us, it can be concluded that indication predicators for a neuroleptic treatment have not been found but are essential. There are clearly patients who remain symptom-free even without neuroleptics, and there are those who continue to display symptoms while gaining no benefit from neuroleptic therapy and who become even more handicapped." (Helmchen 1983)

His colleague Karl Leonhard from the Psychiatric Department of the Humboldt-University in Berlin differentiated what he determined to be "nuclear schizophrenias" versus so-called cycloid psychoses (for example anxiety psychoses, confusion psychoses, happiness psychoses or motility psychoses with a catatonic-like state). Based on this, he considered it malpractice if prescribed neuroleptics are not soon thereafter withdrawn again:

> "Today I unfortunately see very many cases of cycloid psychosis that remain in a toxic, pathological state because of constant medication, but which would be perfectly normal without medication. If one could prevent the development of further phases of psychosis with constant medication, then this practice would be justified, but unfortunately that is not the case. Thus those patients who would be healthy for extended periods, or perhaps forever, are held in a permanently toxic state…" (Leonhard 1980, p. 3)

Several further factors should make people think twice before allowing themselves to be pressured by doctors' and psychiatrists' frequent insistence on a long-term administration of neuroleptics:

- The duration of hospitalization is not shortened when neuroleptics are taken (Hartlage 1965); in fact people are discharged earlier if they take none at all (Epstein / Morgan / Reynolds 1962).
- The state of older people taking neuroleptics is worse in comparison with those who are free of psychiatric drugs (Tune 1992).
- The aim for rapid success—quiescence and management—is also considered by psychotherapists as absolutely misplaced: what is important is personal development as well a change in the kind of family relationships which lead to illness and mental disturbance (Haley 1989).
- Neuroleptics probably suppress "self-healing tendencies" (Ernst 1954, p. 588) and prevent "cure" (Stierlin / Wynne / Wirsching 1985; Harding / Zubin / Strauss 1987). Those who weather their crises without psychotropic drugs have better medium and long-term prognoses (Goldberg / Klerman / Cole 1965; Hogarty / Goldberg / Baltimore Collaborative Study Group 1974; May / Goldberg 1978; Wehde 1991, pp. 44ff.), and are less frequently "psychotic" than those treated with psychiatric drugs and land far less often in psychiatric wards (Young / Meltzer 1980; Heinrichs / Carpenter 1985).
- "Relapses" under neuroleptics result in longer periods of hospitalization than "relapses" which occur when no psychiatric drugs are used (Gardos / Cole 1976).
- Neuroleptics contribute nothing to long-term rehabilitation (Niskanen / Achté 1972), generally inhibit everyday "functioning" (Schooler et al. 1967), and often lead to social deterioration (Müller / Günther / Lohmeyer 1986).

Uninformed, isolated and therefore defenseless individuals are understandably afraid to be sent back to the loony-bin and to be forcibly treated with neuroleptics, so they go on taking neuroleptics at the insistence of "their" psychiatrists or their families. It is particularly important that this group of "users" of psychiatric drugs be exposed to the alternative experiences of others.

Translation from the German by Christina White

The Decision to Withdraw

Ilse Gold
After Discharge

Neuroleptics: Haldol, Sigaperidol

Today, Friday, February 8 1991, I was discharged from the madhouse. The previous 14 days were the most horrific of my life and I'm not in a good state at all right now. I can not rejoice at all at my regained freedom. I'm shaky, confused, restless and heavy, tired but not tired at the same time.

My clearest, but at the same time indefinable, feeling can best be compared with wonder and astonishment. But this feeling gets lost before I become fully aware of it. Very briefly, I'm surprised at the half-finished picture on my easel, and I'm half aware of the astounding idea that only a few weeks ago I had done something out of pure enjoyment, like painting a picture.

I find Gerda's presence uncomfortable. Her presence is a necessary evil, but strangely enough I'm not ashamed of this feeling, although she is my sister. Even though I had reason to be grateful to her in the past, she is the one I have to thank for being locked up for two weeks and pumped full of all kinds of drugs.

And I have to keep taking this Haldol. The asylum physician had given me all sorts of tablets for the next few days until my appointment with the psychiatrist. She had warned me about not taking them because that would be very dangerous. The dose must be reduced very slowly and I could not expect to recover very quickly. In fact, I'm in rather a bad state, and I almost look back with something like trust at this Dr. Hollmann, because so far she has been proven right in her prognosis. So I decide—even if unwillingly—to follow her instructions on taking the pills.

I asked my sister to get me a laxative from the pharmacy. I had become constipated during my stay in the madhouse and suddenly blame all my feelings of illness on this fact. I tell myself that everything will be much better when I can empty my bowels. That will be on Saturday evening when Gerda is leaving, finally! She has to be back at work on Monday, and thank heavens she lives at a relatively safe distance so I can at least have my peace until next weekend. But today is only Friday, and I feel desperately impatient and restless, and I'm wandering back and forth around my flat. I simply can not sit still and read for instance, until Gerda gets back with the pills.

She is barely back before she starts getting on my nerves again. She talks non-stop and keeps giving me unasked for advice: my constipation is caused by the Haldol, she explains and she wants to know why I had done nothing about it in the hospital. I just think: "Hospital! What hospital? I was in a madhouse, you idiot!" On no account should I stop taking the Haldol, I must put that out of my mind, she keeps insisting, although I hadn't said anything of the sort. Now she repeats what I had heard this morning from Dr. Hollmann. If Gerda only knew how much I would hate her for her idiotic chatter if I wasn't so totally lacking in emotions. Her endless droning would be reason enough to throw all these bloody tablets at her feet out of protest and anger. Again, another flutter of surprise that I don't actually do it, that I don't explode and that I am really putting up with her tirade. But the strength of my feelings is not sufficient for real anger, objection and protest and is far too little to repress the fear of "what might happen if…" So I take the pills and swallow them right in front of Gerda. I even resist the desire to offer her some out of nasty generosity.

By now it's evening and we are watching television. I continue to work on a cover I'm knitting, a pretty normal activity for me while watching TV, but I'm incredibly awkward and act as if I had just learned to knit. And I can't seem to sit comfortably and keep moving around in my armchair. I keep having to change the position of my body, and my legs in particular do not feel right wherever they are. Gerda watches me—furtively she thinks, but doesn't dare say anything. I stand up and go into the kitchen because I can't sit still anymore. When I come back straight away I'm asked:

"What's up?"

"What should be up?" is my irritable answer and again I slide around the chair making the leather of the armchair squeak. I don't understand myself what is wrong with me and would love it if someone could explain it to me.

"Why are you perspiring so much?" is the next question from my sister, and after a while, "your forehead is wet."

"I'm not perspiring," I snap at her, "you know I always had greasy skin." She insists that the way I look is not normal and that I'm perspiring. I don't care what she thinks. When I had seen myself in the mirror earlier on, I had thought that I looked dreadful, but right now I'm far more worried about not being able to sit still. And on top of that the feeling of being continually observed is enough to make me puke. She is so self-important in her role as my nurse. I can't stand it anymore, whether it is this restlessness or Gerda's presence, I don't know and that's not the point anyway. I take the consequences and go to bed. That I don't answer when Gerda calls after me and asks whether I'm alright and why am I going to bed so early. This is a small satisfaction for me and about the only pleasant feeling I have had all day.

I'm in the waiting room at the psychiatrist's and I'm quite happy to be alone there, since I'm afraid that anyone could easily see how tortuous I find this waiting. I have already walked up and down several times and looked at all the pictures on the walls and I'm sure that I have had all of the magazines in my hands. However, I'm not nervous and restless out of fear of the psychiatrist and his treatment. In contrast I'm waiting for him as if he were my savior. Every few seconds I look at the clock. The half hour I have waited seem like an eternity and just when I think "this is it, I can't wait anymore," the door opens and I'm called into the consulting room.

I'm asked how I am. "Very well," I answer and tell him how pleased I am to be free of my sister because she has, after all, gone skiing and not cancelled and come to stay with me for a holiday as she had suggested. Proudly, I tell Dr. Niederländer that I succeeded in preventing this. He does not appear particularly pleased about this and for my taste shows far too much interest in where dear Gerda is skiing. I can't satisfy his curiosity because I haven't taken note of the address and why should I anyway. In any case, I'm sure that right now there is a card from Gerda with her address and telephone number on its way to me or is already in my letter box. Nevertheless, I wouldn't dream of contacting her. The most I would do is to occasionally answer the phone in case she calls or the other relatives and friends whom she has doubtless instructed to keep themselves or her up-to-date on my condition.

It was disgusting the day before yesterday—I had barely put the phone down after a long local call when a woman from the telephone company called to find out if I was alright as my sister and brother were worried that something might have happened to me and had called the phone company because my line had been engaged for a long time. Dr. Niederländer interrupted my thoughts by asking me if I had gained some distance to the events which had led to my "psychosis." I made it clear to him that I had not been ill at the time I was committed, even if certain people claimed that I had very serious problems, but that now I had serious problems dealing with the violence I had been subjected to by my sister and the doctors. Dr. Niederländer ignored what I said so I asked him if he knew about the brutal methods used by the police to get me out of my apartment and into the madhouse. Did he know that I had been handcuffed, and that I had been taken away completely naked. (This was because I had been in the shower when they broke into my apartment and I had refused their order to get dressed and accompany them.)

Dr. Niederländer does not appear to be impressed and seems quite uninterested. Yes, he had heard that the situation was quite turbulent, he muttered, and concentrated on the letter from his colleague Dr. Hollmann which I had handed to him. Since I had opened the letter as a matter of course, I know that apart from the strength of the Haldol dose, the letter also intimated that I would probably not be able to work for several weeks.

"Well, I had better prescribe you drops rather than the tablets you taking now. It will allow you to elegantly reduce the dose step-by-step." That makes sense to me and the fact that Dr. Niederländer spoke so automatically of reducing makes me suddenly like him because reducing means of course that I soon won't be taking anything at all. Impatiently and restlessly, I wait for him to calculate how many drops I have to take of the medication he is prescribing for me. He takes ages, arithmetic does not appear to be his strength. And the fact that he does not say anything and does not include me in his ruminations at all changes my positive attitude towards him rapidly. Finally, he is finished and I'm given a sick note and a new appointment. I'm disappointed that I have to return within a few days and that my sick note only lasts until then. So I'm forced to go through the same unpleasant procedure very soon again.

At least he is not too curious about me, I think as I leave the practice, and I go to the nearest pharmacy for my prescription. When I go to pay, all my small change falls out of my purse and scatters across the floor. It is embarrassing how noticeably my hands shake as I pick up the coins (a few customers help me) and how awkward I am. It was the same at home yesterday when I tried to work on the picture, the half-finished tree, I had started. I couldn't hold the brush steady so I gave up fairly quickly and looked for another occupation to rid myself of this continuous and tortuous agitation. But there was no occupation which made me feel better, so I had ended up spending the time from the early afternoon until going to bed early crying quietly and helplessly. That's the state I fell asleep in and the same state I woke up in. It is really quite strange, I fall asleep very easily. Curiously enough this agitation which poisons and prevents almost everything else does not prevent me falling asleep. And when I wake up I do so abruptly, and I'm just as agitated and nervous as the evening before. I miss the half-asleep state of which I have such pleasant memories. That gentle dreaming into a sleeping state and the gently delayed waking up that I always try to drag out as long as possible. Now I wake up suddenly and it is just as tortuous to lie still as it is to sit still later. But it is not as if I wake up in the middle of the night or don't get enough sleep, which makes me nervous. I'm awake punctually before seven every day after nine full hours, which is why I don't understand why I feel so wiped out every morning. I should feel well since nothing occupied me or bothered me enough to stop me falling asleep. But nothing occupies me or bothers when I'm awake, I am capable of occupying myself. Purely mechanical things are best, apart from the fact that I'm very awkward and slow and everything is very strenuous.

On the way to the bus stop I drop in at the baker's. The shop assistant asks me three times before she gives me the sunflower loaf I had asked for. It is not the first time I notice that people have difficulty understanding me when I speak. I myself find my voice strange and unnatural. I'm relieved to get out of the shop. At least the embarrassment of the pharmacy has not been repeated. I almost bump into a colleague from work. I notice the shock and distance with which she observes me as we greet and shake hands. Embarrassment and inhibition on both our parts and the escape through seeming hurry: her husband is waiting in the car and I have to catch my bus.

I'm supposed to take 28 drops every evening. The new medication is called Sigaperidol *(neuroleptic, active ingredient haloperidol)* but it contains the same active ingredient as Haldol. After reading the information leaflet (I read it several times a day!) I finally know how my physical state is described by physicians and scientists. There it is in black and white—and suddenly it clicks!—that I may experience restlessness, problems with my sight and stiff muscles. Dyskinesia (disturbances of movement) and Parkinson-like symptoms can be alleviated by reducing the dose (I don't have to be told twice), and more detailed information can be obtained in the scientific brochure. Dr. Niederländer will surely give it to me when I go the next time.

I shall certainly start with the dose reduction. There is no question of taking more than twenty drops. That is less than the amount prescribed by Dr. Niederländer but is still double the standard therapeutic dose described in the leaflet. Nonetheless, I feel a flutter of fear at my actions since the warnings of the doctors are still ringing in my ears and repeated again and again by Gerda with such absolute dependability that the text had been become almost automatically part of my flesh and blood.

I observe myself very anxiously in those days but notice no difference, I don't feel better or worse and I certainly do not feel well.

Nor does Dr. Niederländer notice any change in me; I say nothing to him during my next consultation of the fact that I am meanwhile only taking a third of the dose he has prescribed for me, and there is no reason for him to be suspicious. The possibility that someone might doubt the correctness of his therapy and not trust him blindly does not occur to him. But now I tell him about my symptoms, the agitation, the shaking and expect that he will confirm my own secret decision by suggesting an improvement to my state by reducing the dose. Way off the mark, Dr. Niederländer reacts completely differently: it is much too early to think of a reduction, and the dose I was taking was a dose suitable for a small child. He explains to me that my shaking and the other symptoms were simply a result of my over-sensitivity. He brushed aside my fears of not being able to cope with my job as a secretary (because my handwriting and typing had become so clumsy and I took far too long) by saying that someone in a different job, a wood cutter for example—would not even notice these symptoms. I find it difficult to follow Dr. Niederländer's train of thought—should I perhaps retrain as a forester? Then I remember that I want to ask him whether he can give me the scientific leaflet about haloperidol.

My request was perhaps not quite proper, because right in the middle of my request this small, slight man past his best years spoke to me very angrily. He abused the pharmaceutical manufacturers who only upset patients with their information and make the work of the doctors more difficult. These people were incompetent and irresponsible. He then asks whether I seriously think I'm capable of understanding scientific information. His already hoarse voice threatens to fail him altogether. "Have you studied? Why do you think I spent so many years studying, so that any Tom, Dick or Harry could come along…?!"

"Yes, why?" went through my head. "Perhaps so you Dr. Smartass can tell me what in your opinion I'm supposed not to understand," I think, but of course do not dream of saying. With Haldol in the bloodstream you barely think (such thoughts), never mind actually saying them out loud. The fact that I can think at all and decide not to return to this quack is the result of the fact that—without the knowledge of the doctor—I had been taking practically no Haldol for the past few days.

I wait silently until he writes me another sick note and I do not contradict him when he writes me a new prescription for haloperidol (I don't need to collect it), and do not say that I have loads of the stuff at home. I suddenly feel superior to this man with whom I can deal, who is not going to give me an injection, this little dwarf. I almost feel sorry for him, not least because he has lost all authority over me with his outburst and his silly arguments. The previous weeks I was already very annoyed when I left the practice and had decided not to tell him any personal details.

This person had actually repeated and commented on things to me from my childhood and my private life which I had never spoken to him about. For example, he passed judgement on my relationships to my siblings and told me that, in contrast to these, I was the only one with a close relationship to my father which is why I had not been able to deal with his death last autumn.

This, and a few small things which had already surprised me before, led me to understand that he had been or still was in contact with my sister. When I questioned him and asked him how he knew these things, which I saw quite differently, he reacted as if he had been caught and swore that he had this information from no one other than me. I didn't bother to contradict him and tell him that he was lying and that our conversations had only consisted of a few scraps and the arrangements for our next appointment, with the latter taking up the most time as he usually spent a great deal of time studying his empty diary.

On my way home I decide that this was my last visit to Dr. Niederländer.

And then I decided not to take one more drop of haloperidol or anything like it, no matter what happened. I had been written sick until Friday which meant that if I did not go back to him or go to another doctor, then I would have to go back to work in few days. I can't risk being committed again because I had not returned to work and not sent in a sick note, they would jump at the chance. It was a piece of luck that I only needed to work for one week and then had holidays, almost five weeks, the whole month of April. For a long time I have been dreaming about spending my holidays in my second home—the south of Spain. In recent years something had always happened to prevent it but this year everything seemed to be perfect—until now. I have to write today to the friends whose apartment I can use but I'm hardly capable of dealing with everyday details, never mind organizing a long journey. Anyway, why travel when I'm in no position to even look forward to it. There is no way that I want my Spanish friends and one-time colleagues to see me in my present state after ten years. Some anger, and in particular self-pity, comes over me. Even my holiday has to be sacrificed to these idiots (and by this I don't mean psychiatric patients). Again I'm crying, also because I have no idea how things are supposed to go on and because I'm afraid.

Translation from the German by Christina White

Peter Lehmann

Relapse into Life

*Neuroleptics: Haldol, Imap, Orap, Semap, Taxilan, Triperidol, Truxal /
Anti-Parkinson drugs: Akineton*

Daytime: 3 x 200 drops Haldol

Akineton retard 2 x 1 tablets

Nighttime: 40 drops Haldol

50 mg Truxal

This is what the instructions on my prescription list looked like on May 24, 1977 at the Winnenden Psychiatric Clinic near Stuttgart, where I was confined from April 6 until June 1, 1977. At the beginning it was Haldol, Truxal[1], Triperidol[2], Orap[3] and Akineton[4] that were violently pumped into my body via infusions or injections or as a "cocktail" in response to typical diagnoses such as "paranoid psychosis" and "hebephrenic schizophrenia."

A vegetative state

According to the hospital's records, my resistance to the psychoactive drugs lessened with time and, consequently, "the illness visibly changed and a stuporous, catatonic condition became predominant."

---

1 Neuroleptic, active ingredient chlorprothixene, apparently not currently marketed in AU, CA, GB, NZ and US

2 Neuroleptic, active ingredient trifluperidol, apparently not currently marketed in AU, CA, GB, NZ and US

3 Neuroleptic, active ingredient pimozide

4 Anti-Parkinson drug, active ingredient biperiden

After my parents had me committed during a moment of crisis in which they were unsure what else to do, at first I strongly resisted being held hostage, stripped down, tied up and psychopharmacologically treated against my will. Unfortunately, as the psychiatric drugs began to take their effect, my resistance weakened. Apathy, symptoms resembling Parkinson's disease, muscle disturbances resembling paralysis, involuntary mouth twitching, a choking sensation, slurred speech, obesity and hair loss set in as I began to believe that I was mentally ill and "needed my medication." I believed this because the corner stone of discussions with my psychiatrist was that without the medication I would experience an "immediate relapse."

Not knowing where to turn as I contemplated the fact that I was 27 years old and already feared becoming a chronic psychiatric patient like so many others, in May 1977 I called my ex-wife from whom I had been divorced just three months ago. She traveled from Berlin, where I also lived at the time, to the south of Germany to meet me, and we made an agreement that I would be out of the hospital by Christmas or she would bring me enough sleeping pills so that I could end the psychiatric torture I was engulfed in.

In Berlin she contacted a long-time friend of mine, Ellen, who arranged a "bed" for me in the University Psychiatric Clinic in Berlin-Charlottenburg located in Nussbaum Allee. I was moved there on June 1. The treatment there differed only in dosage, but the effects remained the same: a half dose of Haldol and a new dosage of Taxilan[1]. (It may be the case that I was lied to about the new dosages and drugs; after employing all possible legal means to gain access to the hospital records and still being denied, there is plenty of room for speculation that illegal steps were taken and lies were told by the hospital.) More and more demoralized and not fit enough to shave myself or even brush my teeth, the hospital director Hanfried Helmchen discharged me on August 10—without consultation and against my will, since I was now convinced that I no longer had the ability to survive on my own.

Because it had been drummed into me in the hospital that I "needed medication," I went to a weekly appointment with the catamnetic psychiatrist

---

1 Neuroleptic, active ingredient perazine, apparently not currently marketed in AU, CA, GB, NZ and US

Adolf Pietzcker for a shot of Imap[1]. The friends with whom I had initially been living soon asked me to leave. Not only did they need the room in which I was staying for the new baby they were expecting any day, but I can imagine that it was not very pleasant to share an apartment with me given my constant involuntary lip-smacking and my apathetic silence. It didn't take long to find an apartment for me in an older building. My old apartment-mates were happy to help me move my belongings which were still stored at their place. After that I was more or less on my own, with the exception of the weekly appointment with the psychiatrist, which constituted the only regularly recurring fixed point in a world that had become absolutely devoid of meaning, hope and joy for me.

Freedom within a community

From morning until evening I lay in bed feeling wretched. I didn't even want to turn on the television. I wasn't even in a position to try to cook something for myself. Once a day I went to a nearby store and got myself a bar of chocolate and a few bottles of beer, and that was all I consumed for weeks. When Ellen came to visit me one day, she was horrified that I had not even put sheets on the mattress. Cornelia, a friend of mine whom I had told about my miserable situation, announced that she would help me to fix up my apartment. But after one attempt at putting up a poster on the wall with me, she resigned.

It was impossible for me to imagine how I was going to get through the winter. How was I going to find coal for the heating, and who was going to keep it lit? Me? I had previously lived in apartments with coal heating, but now the work involved seemed impossible for me to manage. And doing the laundry? How was I going to wash the clothes that were getting dirtier and dirtier? Worse yet was the issue of my paperwork. While I was in the hospital someone had taken care of my health insurance, the rent, my registration as a

---

1 Neuroleptic, active ingredient fluspirilene, apparently not currently marketed in AU, CA, GB, NZ and US

university student and such things. How was I going to do all this by myself when I couldn't even keep up with opening the mail as it arrived?

As earlier in the Nussbaum Allee hospital, I once again considered if and how I could put an end to my vegetative state. In the hospital I often feared I would be transferred to a longstay psychiatric unit. I had heard about the Phönix—a longstay hospital nearby where some people became so desperate that they jumped out of the top-story windows to their deaths. I was in an apartment on my own and not locked up, but even so I often stood at the window and looked out at the street below. I considered whether or not I would meet a certain death if I jumped from the fourth floor. I didn't want to waste-away as a life-long patient who needed someone else's care. It seemed certain to me that my life had been botched up and I would never again experience anything pleasant. I was too scared; however, that if I jumped out the window I might "only" break my back and become wheelchair-bound. This thought—as well as thoughts of how much my mother and my friend Ricci would mourn my death if I succeeded—were the only things that kept me from taking that final step. I also thought of my other friends, but for them it would certainly be a relief if their mentally crippled friend would finally disappear from the face of the earth—I was now only a burden to them.

In the meantime, my mother had suggested I move back to Fellbach. That was a possible solution for me. My mother could wash my laundry, I wouldn't have to manage the coal heating or cooking, and she could take care of my paper work.

My brother announced that he was coming for a visit in October, 1977. Being a dedicated fan of the Stuttgart soccer team, he was coming to Berlin to watch a game. I wanted to clean up my apartment and straighten out my mess, but I wasn't able to. All I was able to manage was to make a hot meal. My brother expected me to show him Berlin's nightlife that evening after dinner. But I could only accompany him to the bar around the corner. By eight o'clock I was so strung out and exhausted I had to go home immediately and collapse into bed. My brother invited me to come and live with him and his wife, and then he headed out for the nightlife on his own.

After his visit I quickly set out to find someone to sublet my apartment so I wouldn't have to pay the rent by myself throughout the winter. Spurred on by the possibility of being able to leave my uncomfortable, cold, and disorderly apartment, I managed to put an ad in the paper. Two people were interested in the place, a man and a woman, and I had to choose. I decided to let Erwin have the apartment, thinking that his car was an asset for future grocery-shopping trips.

Shortly before my departure I met my former girlfriend Brigitte R. in the subway, someone I had met through a personals ad. Though she seemed to show interest in seeing me again, I was afraid to get too close to her because if our contact were perhaps to become intimate, she would notice I was also sexually incompetent. I was certain that I had become impotent. And besides, I had not felt any kind of sexual inclination since my stay at the hospital in Winnenden. The entire time since then I had not had an erection or even a wet dream. I told Brigitte R. I had been in "the clinic" and things were still going quite badly for me. We agreed we would write to each other while I was in Fellbach.

At my last meeting with Adolf Pietzcker, I reported nothing regarding my fears about my sexuality, as this was a subject I had not mentioned during the entire time I was treated by psychiatrists or therapists. But I did tell him about my decision to return to my parents in Fellbach. He said I was to go to a psychiatrist in Fellbach and he gave me a letter to hand to him containing information about my condition. Adolf Pietzcker was concerned that things could take a bad turn again for me if I did not receive "my medication" regularly.

On October 20, 1977 I packed my dirty laundry and the letter for the psychiatrist in Fellbach and headed to my brother's house in Rommelshausen (which is near Fellbach).

The local psychiatrist

I was being sent to another psychiatrist, so I was apparently a psychiatric case. Every once in a while during this period, I tried to think about what exactly was wrong with me that caused me so much suffering. But thinking about this was too difficult. The neurologist and psychiatrist Dr. Becher, on the other hand, seemed to know a lot about it. He read the letter from Pietzcker, asked me a few questions about what I had done before my stay in the hospital and where I lived now, and then he seemed to have all the information he needed. That was the extent of his interest in me as a person. After that, I came to a "consultation" with him every Thursday during which he simply injected an ampoule of Imap into my bottom. Whether or not we ever engaged in any kind of "consultation" I can't say for sure any more. It is possible that occasionally while the shot was being administered a "How are you, then, Mr. Lehmann?" and a "Not better yet." was exchanged.

My parents were worried about me and made sure that I went to the psychiatrist regularly. During the time I lived with my brother, I worked at my father's small printing press doing odd jobs. Thursday afternoons my mother would call me at work and remind me of my appointment. My father was also eager to help and he too made sure I didn't miss my appointment.

The work I did was very simple and quite monotonous. I was happy to have something to do that was intellectually and physically manageable and that diverted my attention away from my self-torturing and depressive thoughts. Given that I was the son of the boss and (supposedly) in a recovery phase, all the workers were very nice to me, as was my father. He could read my every wish just by looking at me; he brought me pretzels and he even let me use his car. I didn't hear a single harsh or nagging word in all those months. I frequently got up late and didn't show up at work until after the lunch break, but even then I was treated with understanding.

The whole time I was apathetic. I had a constant choking sensation, I was nauseated, and I was not thrilled about the idea of having to get through an endless number of such days that—with few exceptions—were all the same and very boring.

The monotony was only broken two evenings a week when there was table tennis training in the Fellbach gymnasium. I suffered a lot on those days because my hand was still paralyzed and I played like a beginner, but at least I got to see my friend Ricci. He otherwise had little time for me because he was preparing for his exams in electrical engineering. Ricci treated me no differently than in the old days. It couldn't have been much fun playing table tennis with me because I could hardly return the ball to him, but he encouraged me. He was convinced that I would be able to play again. He said he knew me too well and that I could not have forgotten how to play; he insisted I try again and again, and he never allowed me to give up.

I became a burden for my sister-in-law Ingrid, who was pregnant at the time. In December 1977 I moved to my parents place. My situation hadn't changed much. Dr. Becher was still giving me injections of Imap. Feeling hollow, desolate and empty, I didn't feel much of anything else. After I had gotten through a torturous day of work, I still had to get through the evening. My mother did her best to help me. She played games with me, tried to cheer me up, went for walks with me, and tried to get me to write my friend Brigitte R. or to take care of things like my insurance, my university registration, my finances etc. I still couldn't control the lip-smacking and the twitch in my hand. I didn't want to be around other people, and I felt I wasn't able to write either. But I was now better able to sit up, and I could watch television. I watched Eduard Zimmermann's "XY Unsolved," Hans Rosenthal's "Dalli dalli" or Wim Thoelke's "Golden Prize"—programs for which you do not have to think too much. Then I imagined that things were perhaps going a little better. I forced myself to read. But after I had tried ten times to get beyond the first page of Simmel's "Es muß nicht immer Kaviar sein" *("It Doesn't Always Have to be Caviar")*, I gave up again. There seemed no reason for me to have high hopes of recovering. I didn't want to poison myself in my mother's apartment, and so I considered going back to Berlin in order to be alone and to put an end to my miserable vegetative state.

An opportunity to withdraw

At some point in the winter of 1977/78, Dr. Becher changed my prescription from Imap to Semap[1]. With the new prescription, I was supposed to take a tablet once a week. This meant the doctor was able to go on his two-week vacation without having to send me to another doctor. I was never told by him what kinds of different effects Semap might have in comparison with Imap, but since I had never heard any of the psychiatrists make a single speci-

---

1 Neuroleptic, active ingredient penfluridol, apparently not currently marketed in AU, CA, GB, NZ and US

fic comment about "their" drugs, it did not occur to me then to wonder about such things.

But because the days were so monotonous and my parents were too preoccupied with their Christmas party preparations to keep tabs on my prescriptions, I forgot to take my pill on the first Thursday. It only occurred to me the next day that I hadn't taken it. I started to panic, thinking that the prophesied relapse could strike at any moment. Then I imagined that something even worse could happen. I thought I would end up back in the hospital at Winnenden—I knew how terrible that was—and then after that they would take me back to my parents again. On the other hand, I began to think that if a relapse hadn't come yet after having forgotten my pills for a day, then why shouldn't I take a risk given that I was surrounded by so many people wishing to help? How would my situation ever change if I continued to be under the influence of psychiatric drugs? How would I ever get through my final exams? So I made a decision on my own to try living without psychiatric drugs. I didn't tell anyone else because I feared they would never understand my seemingly irresponsible decision.

I wondered what might happen. After a few days, the lip-smacking began to subside. With time, my tiredness began to wear off. I tried to read—this time a different book—and it worked. In three days I had read a biography of Mao's widow that was several hundred pages long. Two weeks after I quit the drugs, the lip-smacking disappeared completely. I noticed that my mood was much better.

My mother also noticed I had stopped smacking my lips. She said to me it seemed I was finally feeling better again. At that point, I decided the moment had come for me to tell her I had secretly quit my drugs. She responded with shock and fear. She promptly called the doctor, who had returned from his vacation. He set up an immediate appointment for me. He was as accommodating as ever and even more so, promising my mother that I need not sit in the waiting room and would be seen immediately. He said I should at least show up for the appointment so that he could speak with me. But I refused to go. I said to my mother she would have to kill me first before I would ever willingly go to a psychiatrist again. She was anxious and afraid. When my father came home that evening, he was also horrified—how could I be so irresponsible and not listen to the doctor? Late that night my father came to my bed and told me my mother was unable to sleep and at the very least for her sake I should take "my medication." But I refused again.

The better things went for me, the more my parents got used to my stubborn refusal—particularly because there was no indication that a prophesied relapse would happen. Now the only thing I still suffered from was the near-paralysis in my hand. Four weeks after withdrawing from the drugs, this handicap had not disappeared. I wondered if I would be forced to accept that I had become a cripple. One evening—it was at the end of January in 1978—I was playing table tennis with Ricci as usual with my half-paralyzed hand. Suddenly from one second to the next, in the middle of a stroke, the feeling returned to my hand. I could play again as well as I had earlier. I could move my hand as I always had been able to. The players who had not known me previously and had only seen me play with my lame hand couldn't understand the sudden change in my game. Those who had always been able to beat me now experienced just the opposite. I tried to explain this "wonder" by relaying that I had quit "my medication," but no one other than Ricci understood what I meant. They stared at me uncomprehendingly.

Soon after I had recovered, I decided to return to Berlin and take my exams. I worked a few more weeks at my father's firm, where I earned good money. Just after Easter in 1978—almost exactly one year after I had initially been taken to Winnenden—I drove back to Berlin in the car my parents had given me for Christmas.

Epilog

After I returned to Berlin in the spring of 1978, I took up contact with Sabrina, a friend who had tried so hard to cheer me up while I was in the Nussbaum Allee hospital. She was taking neuroleptics. Feeling desperate because nothing seemed to change in her situation while she was being treated "medically" at a so-called day hospital at the university, she tried to take her life in the summer of 1978. Her attempt was unsuccessful. In the spring of 1979 she visited me accompanied by Laura, who was also taking neuroleptics. A few weeks later I was told that Laura was dead. Her suicide attempt was successful. Laura was an actress, which meant that she was professionally dependent upon a functioning and lively talent for expression and mimicry. Under the influence of neuroleptics, the capacity for expression and mimicry is often extinguished.

Months later Ricci told me my father had tried to convince him that, as my best friend, he should try to talk me into taking "my medication." Ricci—who is truly my best friend—disagreed with my father, arguing that if I am the one who was taking the psychiatric drugs, then I should be the one who knows best if they are good or bad for me.

After several discussions with my parents, their position on psychiatric drugs and psychiatrists has since changed fundamentally. During an interview for a 1980 television film made in the context of my legal proceedings to obtain my psychiatric records, my parents reported they had recently realized how absurd it was to have put me under so much pressure just at the moment when I had come to life again before their very eyes after having stopped the neuroleptics. I watched as my parents insisted that the filmmaker include these self-critical statements in the film. When the film was aired, however, this passage just happened to be missing.

Translation from the German by Christina White

Withdrawal Without Pharmacogenic Problems

Gábor Gombos

How to Deny a Psychiatric Family History

Antidepressants: Amitriptyline, Maprotiline, Trimipramine / Carbamazepine / Tranquilizers: Chlordiazepoxide, Clonazepam, Diazepam, Nitrazepam

First I was treated with tricyclic antidepressant when I was 16. I had to spend my entire school holidays in hospital because of suspected encephalitis, and my mood was rather down. Since my mother was a "well-known manic depression patient' in psychiatric wards, my doctors were afraid that my bad mood was the onset of a severe depression and they put me on trimipramine[1] (100 mg daily). I took it for two months, without any improvement in my mood, so I stopped taking it (I was still in hospital), and I recovered only after I was discharged.

Next time I was in hospital, now in a psychiatric ward, in 1980, after a family and emotional crisis. My stepfather had a stroke, but his brain was damaged. He was paralytic, couldn't speak properly and was aggressive with my mother who was supposed to be his only carer. (I had just begun my university studies 200 km away.) She could not get on with this task alone, broke down and made suicidal attempts. I left the university for home and tried to help my mother, without success. At the same time I learned about the severe

---

1 Antidepressant, marketed as Surmontil, Tripress

side-effects of the antidepressant I took against the supposed encephalitis. I was told to prepare for hormonal disfunctioning affecting even my sexuality. This was too much to cope with, I also broke down. Three of us from the family were in three hospitals, all in psychiatry. My doctors treated me with amitriptyline[1] (150 mg daily). Although the professor of the ward told me that I had real problems to be solved and drugs do not solve them, my doctor gave me the diagnosis of manic depression. After three months I was discharged but still permanently took amitriptyline in a lower dose (100 mg daily).

This continued until 1984 when I began to complain about my sleepless nights. They provided me with a sleep inducing drug, nitrazepam[2] (25 mg). Then I could sleep at night, but was very tired next day and failed in my exams. This breakdown led me again to psychiatry. They changed my antidepressant to maprotiline[3] (100 mg daily) and increased my benzodiazepine dose. Beside nitrazepam they ordered diazepam[4] (20 mg daily) and chlordiazepoxide[5]. After being discharged, the long term treatment consisted of 45 mg maprotiline, 25 mg nitrazepam and carbamazepine. My last hospitalisation took place in 1990. After a long and successless battle with the local authorities. (With my mother I lived in an apartment in a very bad state of repair but had no money to do the renovation.) I was exhausted in despair with suicidal thoughts. As a scientific rescarcher –meanwhile I had passed my exams—I could not afford a proper living, even to heat up our apartment in winter was an unsolvable problem. In the hospital I took maprotiline in injec-

---

1 Antidepressant, marketed as Amitrip, Amitriptyline, Elavil, Emitrip, Endep, Enovil, Lentizol, Serotex, Triptafen, Tryptanol, Tryptizol, Typtanol, component of Etrafon, Limbitrol, Triavil

2 Tranquilizer, marketed as Alodorm, Insoma, Mogadon, Nitrados, Somnite

3 Antidepressant, marketed also as Ludiomil, Maprotiline

4 Tranquilizer, marketed as Antenex, Dialar, Diazemuls, Diazepam, Ducene, Pro-Pam, Rimapam, Stesolid, Tensium, Valclair, Valium, Valpam, Valrelease, Vazepam

5 Tranquilizer, marketed as Chlordiazepoxide, Librelease, Libritabs, Librium, Nova-Pam, Sereen, Tropium; component of Clindex, Clinoxide, Clipoxide, Librax, Lidox, Lidoxide, Limbitrol, Menrium

tion for two months (the top dose was 250 mg daily). Then as a maintenance I took 45 mg maprotiline, 5 mg clonazepam[1] and 25 mg nitrazepam daily.

In the spring of 1993 my mother died. I was so down that had no energy to go either to hospital or even to my GP. I was totally mad, could not sleep, work, leave my home. After a week of starving a friend visited me by chance. He was familiar with my emotional breakdowns. At the time he studied theology and did not believe that my poor condition had anything to do with some disease. He began to feed me, cleaned my home, spent long hours with me every day.

After three weeks I realized that I was without psychiatric drugs and still survived. In a month I became better, could communicate with my friend and others in my neighborhood and spent several hours in my office. This was the time when I decided not to take psychiatric drugs any more. A doctor (who treated my mother for a short time) also supported me in that decision. Instead of drugs I spent much time with friends. I understood that love was missing in my life and began to look for it. A few months later I found it in its perfect form of love and conversation.

After stopping psychiatric drugs I went through several disturbing symptoms. For almost a year I could not sleep properly. In the first two months I did not sleep more than two hours a night. Then gradually this amount increased and now I have no difficulties with sleeping at all. For about two months I had severe symptoms of cold or flu with some fever. Sometimes I had strong vertigo, I could not even sit in a chair. I had to walk around or to sit on the ground. Up to now rarely I have an overwhelming feeling of intensive fear ("panic") but I have learnt to control it. My friends, later my wife and above all prayer has helped a lot to survive these periods without drugs.

In spite of all the inconvenient side-effects I felt much better. My life had a totally new perspective. The very first time I had a perspective. I understood that my mood is a sensitive thermometer that I can learn to use. With the aid of love I was not a servant of my emotions any more. They are helpful tools to show me if there are severe unsolved problems in my life.

---

1 Tranquilizer, marketed as Clonazepam, Klonopin, Paxam, Rivotril

Jasna Russo

What If I Don't Sleep Ever Again?

*Neuroleptics: Moditen / Antidepressants: Flormidal, Ladiomil /
Tranquilizers: Apaurin, Fluzepam*

It is difficult for me to write and think of my past with psychiatric drugs separately from my whole past. I actually still feel strange while I am trying to separate the aspect of psychiatric drugs from the whole story, because I have underestimated their effect for a long time. I learned this underestimation in psychiatry, where there is no talk of drugs whatsoever, except about their necessity, and where every difficulty and deterioration are ascribed to the "illness." I did not believe in the illness and considered myself responsible for everything.

To free oneself of the responsibility for all of ones states and at least partly ascribe them to the drug, to admit that in some of those states there was more chemistry than myself, is certainly liberating, but at the same time crushing and very sad. Many things that have happened in my life I would like to be able to call the past, but I cannot because they are still following me and are too much part of me. I, therefore, feel relief and a certain pride that all these years have given me the right to say that at least Moditen[1], Apaurin *(tranquilizer, active ingredient diazepam)*, Fluzepam[2], Flormidal[3], and Ladiomil *(antidepressant, active ingredient maprotiline)* are in the past for me.

---

1 Neuroleptic, active ingredient fluphenazine, marketed also as Anatensol, Fluphenazine, Modecate, Permitil, Prolixin

2 Tranquilizer, active ingredient flurazepam, marketed as Dalmane, Durapam, Flurazepam

3 Tranquilizer, active ingredient midazolam, marketed as Hypnovel, Midazolam, Rocam, Versed

Those are "medications" that I was prescribed after I was discharged from psychiatric hospital. I know that I consumed them voluntarily and then stopped. I do not know all the things that my body ingested during my stay in psychiatry, nor is it possible to obtain the history of my "illness." They are not accessible to patients in Yugoslavia, not even after many years. I remember the injections after which I could not get up and kept falling back onto the bed. I remember the three additional hormone injections I received after I told my psychiatrist that I was a lesbian. They were allegedly supposed to promote my periods which I stopped getting with the depot injections of Moditen. They did not. I remember the white paper bags that we glued together in work therapy. With these bags full of psychiatric drugs we were discharged home for the weekend. For every free day three bags. They were marked, without a date, only with large letters when they were to be taken, for example Saturday morning, Saturday noon, Saturday evening.

There were six or seven tablets in each bag. I swallowed them without objection in the hope that everything would pass quickly. Back on the ward I remember holding a book in my hand and trying to read. The letters were moving, I could not focus. The ward round was coming and I wanted to give an impression that I was functioning in the hope that they might discharge me. I pretended to be reading. My psychiatrist said: "You need not try. We know that with this therapy you do not see those letters."

I remember how I was trying to write a letter. The handwriting was not my own. It was becoming smaller and smaller. I could not hold the pencil. I remember how I could not remember anything for hours. I remember that I could not remember whole days.

Twice in my life I was committed to a closed psychiatric ward. And twice I stopped taking Moditen. After the first discharge I continued taking tablets for another four months and I cannot remember how I decided to stop. I cannot remember making any decisions in that period. I did not see any sense in anything, not even in my fear that I would go mad. It left me, together with many other feelings and I think that is how I stopped taking Moditen. I was losing contact with everything that was surrounding me, with everyone, with myself. No matter how everything around me seemed, I preferred to have direct contact with it. Carrying Moditen within me, I longed for any kind of feeling, even the most horrible ones. I longed for the wall between me and everything else to break, for the cotton wool that had covered me, distanced and softened everything to disappear, so that the impressions could reach me as impressions again and not only as memories of them. My distance from everything was unbearable, reality alleviated and somehow leveled. The days were endlessly long and I would have done everything then only for it to stop, but I did not have the strength to do anything.

Both times when I stopped taking Moditen the expected moment in which everything would change was missing. Everything was still the same, I felt no change. Moditen was leaving me for months and I did not differentiate what was me and what was that chemistry. I mostly blamed everything on myself and was hurt the most by the memory of the me from before and the belief that I would never be like that again. My life was no longer a life, but a memory of it. I was terribly ashamed of how I felt and how I looked and started wishing I could disappear. And then I tried. I considered for a long time my so far only attempt at suicide, my first decision in that worst and most hopeless time of my life. With the failure of it, that time was finally over. As if all the despair had reached a pinnacle and, therefore, its limits. I woke up connected to an infusion in the toxicological ward of a hospital, and suddenly I was me again and wanted to live.

When I now look at all of this in a broader context, I feel forced to give up to me so dear and necessary illusion how through that act (regardless of how destructive it was) I again became a subject in my own life, how it was a matter of my own desire and how, due to the ambivalence of that desire, I did not kill myself. I don't like to see myself as a victim, nor to use other people's actions to fully explain my own. But more and more in that suicide attempt I see an imminent consequence of the whole psychiatric intervention performed on me, rather than my own authentic desire to die. I just could not take it anymore. I was 21 and besides the diagnosis, the experience of a mental institution and all the other horrors that preceded that, there was another thing that for a long time I did not attribute any special significance to—for the first time I was under the influence of neuroleptics (seven months continuously). I did not know anything about how they weaken all the vital energy, nor did I have any information on them except for my own feeling. I think

I became a subject only later when I refused further psychiatric treatment, which is the most common continuation of every suicide attempt. Because suicides are never seen in connection with the treatment, they are considered further proof of the "mental illness." My psychiatrist supported my suicide in a gentlemanly manner by immediately prescribing me what I requested of him—an unusually large quantity of Apaurin and Fluzepam. He was a little disappointed that I still refused Moditen, but he praised that I finally understood that I needed help and that I started to accept psychiatric drugs.

After that I visited him only one more time, in the same closed ward where I had been. For the first time I was somehow awake and heard what he was telling me very well. He said that a suicide attempt was something normal, that it happens to many patients, that I should understand that I was also one of them. He told me to immediately continue with Moditen and to stop believing that my intelligence would save me in life. It was clear from the findings of the toxicological ward, where I recovered for five days, that if I had not been found and had continued to sleep for about another three hours, I would not be writing this text now. Everything in me rebelled, I decided that it was my life after all and that I would not allow psychiatry to kill me. The nurse unlocked the door for me and told me to think it over again and that that door would always remain open for me.

The fact that the closed ward opened again for me six years later had a large warning effect on me. A warning that the ones I was living with would repeatedly have me committed and a warning that everything I thought I had done in the meantime was, in a sense, an illusion because everything had collapsed again. Among all the other things I was getting Moditen injections and after my discharge I was supposed to get them once a month. I clearly remember the day when I did not go to get another injection. That day my psychiatrist called, said that she usually never did such a thing, but that she was very involved in my case. She did not understand why I was complaining because "Moditen maybe did not even have any effect on me given that I was enduring it and also that the anti-Parkinson drugs were fine as I did not experience any stiffness from them." She offered to personally administer the injection in her office where there would be no males present, only the two of us. I was mostly silent on the phone and finally repeated that I would not come. I ignored all her persuasions, as well as her "scientific" explanations about me and my pathological sensitivity. No matter what she said and reported about it, I only wanted to get that sensitivity back because I considered it the best part of me and essential for life.

The decision to quit Moditen was not difficult. No matter how great my fear of oncoming madness and of psychiatry, life under this "medication" was worse. The absence of Moditen did not in itself solve anything, but it was that necessary condition without which nothing would have started moving. Only when I was completely free of it (several months after the final injection) could I think and feel again. Only then did I slowly get my strength back, as well as ideas about what I could do. Only then did I actually do something. I moved away far from my parents so that all my subsequent problems would catch up with me somewhere else. And so since 1992 no one has had me committed.

The story of these problems is long and will probably never be completely finished. I try to live with it the best I can and I try not to let it overpower and disintegrate me. Moditen was taking this story away from me, making it unclear and transforming it into another one. After all my experiences with and without Moditen, I can state that my problems were more understandable and resolvable in their natural rather than in their "medicated" form. And unfortunately much worse and more real than what the psychiatric reports wanted to say about them.

The two times in psychiatry were not the only two times when I went mad. In the meantime I calmed my madness and my fear of it, as well as my pathological "sensitivity" with sleeping pills. Quitting them was far more difficult than quitting Moditen. Sleeping pills came into my life at the same time as Moditen—before psychiatry I never took them. But as opposed to Moditen, they were my great love. It was difficult to resist the moment at which everything ceased and I sunk into a barbiturated sleep. To resist the moment in which everything drifted away, disappeared and I had several hours of complete rest from myself and from everything, without thoughts, images, memories and presence.

Regardless of the fact that objectively everything was changing, the fear of madness stayed deep inside of me and I would do anything for it not to occur. And as it always began with insomnia, it was crucial and imperative for me to achieve sleep. It seems to me that I was much more dependent on that fear than on the pills. They were always with me, I did not travel anywhere without them, but proportionally to their presence, I used them seldom. Fear was what never abandoned me. Fear was what I had to stop being addicted to, fear had to stop being the major principle.

At that time others helped me a lot. Others who trusted me and were not afraid of me, who were interested in me and to whom I was not unbearable. The fact that someone else beside me was not afraid of the same as I was, left me space to confront my fear, to understand where it was mostly coming from. My last crisis was the first one that passed without sleeping pills. I dared to see what it was that I was at all costs trying to sleep through, what it was that I was trying to forget all of my life. I did not sleep for several nights and due to the exhaustion I was constantly at a boundary. I wanted to cross it, to completely lose contact with reality because I could no longer bear my thoughts and memories. But I did not succeed. I could not even go mad anymore.

Since then (1995) there are no more sleeping pills in my home, in my bag and in me. I do not think that this is the most important fact about how I live and I certainly could not sum myself into a story with a happy end. The problem of memory and oblivion and especially attaining oblivion are still topics in my life. I cannot imagine them disappearing. But the best of all is finally the absence of fear of what comes from within me and what may still come.

Translation from the Serbo-Croatian by Ivanka Popovic

Carola Bock

And Finally I Said it All

Neuroleptics: Orap, Prothazin / Antidepressants: Amitriptyline / Lithium / Carbamazepine: Finlepsin / Anti-Parkinson Drugs: Akineton

I was first hospitalized in July 1988. This was preceded by years of marriage problems and the triple load of a satisfying but strenuous profession, the responsibility of running a household and being the mother of two children—a son and a mildly mentally handicapped daughter. I had also been dogged by health problems—a difficult gallbladder operation as result of bottled-up frustration and repressed anger. My gallbladder was gone but my problems remained. My cup finally spilled over in 1988, resulting in a nervous breakdown: I jumped out of the window of the psychiatric hospital from a height of approximately six to seven meters *(about 20 feet)*. I spent the following year on crutches and could not drive or ride a bicycle. I was mentally at rock bottom and on top of all that there were the psychiatric drugs. My father encouraged me constantly: "Carola," he said, "you can still hear, you can still see and you can still speak, you're lucky!" At that time I was angry with him. But as time passed I came to understand him and today I am happy to have survived my attempt at suicide and to have been able (in my self-help group "Depression and Anxiety") to show others who had taken psychiatric drugs alternative routes towards the light from the depths of their soul.

But allow me to return to my personal story. At times during my stay in the hospital I was given up to 32 tablets per day. After I was discharged at the beginning of 1992 I was under the influence of drugs. These included amitriptyline and Prothazin[1] as well as Orap *(neuroleptic, active ingredient pimozide)*. After I had spent three weeks in the hospital in December 1991, I began very gradually, week for week at the beginning of 1992, to stop taking Orap over a period of three months. From the very first day I started to take Esbericum *(herbal antidepressant, active ingredient hypericin)*. My decision to withdraw had been influenced by the miserable quality of my life: the state one find's oneself in when under the influence of psychiatric drugs, i.e. constantly tired (especially after taking the tablets) with emotions, mental capacity and motor abilities all running at half strength. I had the feeling that I would never again be the woman with the zest for life that I used to be. It was an appalling thought. What kind of life is it when you have go to bed "with the cows" every evening at 7 o'clock. I wanted to take part in life again. I didn't know much about side-effects, but the idea "without this stuff you ended up in cri-

---

1 Neuroleptic, active ingredient promethazine, marketed as Anergan, Avomine, Insomn-Eze, Pentazine, Phenergan, Promethazine; component of Mepergan, Phenergan VC

sis and became ill" had the effect of making me gather all my strength, my energy and my will. I wanted to get out of the mess.

In December 1991 I had spoken to the doctors in the hospital and told them that more than anything else I wanted to stop taking the psychiatric drugs. At this time I was in a different hospital and noticed a different approach in treatment, support and care. I felt looked after and understood. They took time for one-to-one consultations and group discussions and their creative suggestions aroused a response in me. I recognized that taking pills was not the only solution and that it was more important to develop dialogs based on trust in order to pinpoint problems and to try to alleviate and heal mental wounds. Thus I regained the courage to talk openly to the doctors and psychologists about things that were important to me.

This had never been possible in the other hospital despite attempts on my part. The only response I ever got was another pill. Now the doctors advised me to continue taking the tablets in order to avoid a relapse but I objected: I wanted to live life, with its highs and lows, I wanted to feel and to bear unpleasant things that are part of life. O.K. they said, after my discharge I should continue to take Orap for approximately one month, then I should drop one tablet and if I had no problems with the reduced dose, I should drop another one until I finally stopped altogether. However, my outpatient neurologist made me nervous: "Good god, the relapse…," but I stood firm. In view of her warning I had difficulties; who wouldn't with fear breathing down their neck? But I took good care of myself and would have increased the dose again had I had serious problems.

I had no withdrawal symptoms. I felt myself coming alive again and I was happy, almost euphoric, although I knew I needed to keep my feet firmly on the ground. I didn't want to take off as had happened with my second attack in 1990 when I became manic for 14 days before crashing into depression again.

Esbericum had come to my attention after I had seen a fellow patient with a packet of it and read the package insert. I was very impressed with the indications in which I recognized myself and with the lack of side-effects: well, I thought, that sounds positive, it is exactly what you need, no side-effects, purely herbal, exactly my thing since I had never been a pill swallower—if I had a migraine I used a wet cloth on my forehead.

Along with stopping the drugs I began to try to find a solution to the problems which had landed me in the crises in the first place, and I started to take control of my life again and to sort it out—I simply began to take up the fight again. In February 1992 I filed for divorce and I felt stronger and began to recognize what had pushed me into crisis in the first place.

Today I know that I am partly to blame for the states of crises because I acted wrongly and was no angel at all. I often tried to solve my problems the wrong way, too top-heavy, and I had not collected enough experience of life either.

It is wonderful that we are never too old to learn. We must always be prepared to try new approaches and to make a new start every day. Enjoy each day! After I filed for divorce I lived apart from my husband. Then my husband began to talk to me and we talked for hours, days, weeks and finally I said it all, I told him about everything that had upset me throughout the years. I didn't care any more, the divorce was almost complete and I had nothing to lose. But talking brought us onto the same wavelength and I know today just how important talking is—it is far better to have a storm because it clears the air. If you swallow everything and allow yourself to be repressed, if you subject yourself to your partner and bury your self-confidence and allow yourself to be eaten up with criticism, you become mentally ill.

When my son noticed at the beginning of 1992—I had begun cutting back the drugs—that his mother was alive again, that she answered back and established clarity he said: "You're finally fighting again, you're your old self,'" it was extremely encouraging. My daughter too, who needed me, noticed quickly that her mother had come back and that she could talk to her.

Right up to today I still find it best to talk openly about problems immediately. I understand a great deal better today than I used to the things that came together to cause my crises. The psychiatric drugs certainly did not protect me from crises; these happened with and without the drugs. There had always been external problems and they simply had to be solved.

Things are very similar with my daughter. During October 1992 she was in crisis. She was at home and being worn down by unemployment and began to take some psychiatric drugs to calm herself. Prior to 1989 in the former German Democratic Republic she had worked as a seamstress quite normally with other co-workers, but after the wall came down that was no longer possible. From March to June 1993 she was hospitalized for the first time. She was given all kinds of psychiatric drugs including lithium. She was discharged with a diagnosis of "schizoid psychosis" and lithium 1-0-1, Akineton retard 1-0-1, Finlepsin *(mood stabilizer, active ingredient carbamazepine)* 400, Orap forte 4 mg 0-0-1 and 2 tablets Prothazin for nights. She swallowed them all until Christmas 1993 and gained several pounds. I had also put on 50 pounds within three months under the influence of psychiatric drugs, which is why I later attended Weight Watchers for the support of this self-help group in getting back to my normal weight—crazy when you think about it. My daughter had always been somewhat plump but after her discharge from the hospital she was simply gross and I am quite certain that the psychiatric drugs are partially responsible for the four hundred pounds she now weighs.

In December 1993 I was in the Ruhr region and had a telephone conversation with Matthias Seibt, a member of the board of the German Association of (ex-)Users and Survivors of Psychiatry (BPE), and to question him about the pros and cons of lithium. I had joined BPE two months previously and had read his query in the associations newsletter "Who uses lithium?" Matthias Seibt gave me useful information about the effects and risks of this substance, the results of which I had long recognized in my daughter's physical condition. Blood samples had been taken but her thyroid had not been investigated. It was our GP who examined her on my insistence on my return and who discovered the changes. The neurologist who I asked to reduce the dose was somewhat cooperative, but I had the strong impression that I could only tell her what she wanted to hear.

In December 1993, with the full agreement of my daughter (she was by then 23 years of age) I stopped all her psychiatric drugs over a period of six months. I stopped the lithium immediately and the rest gradually. As my daughter is a good sleeper, I first cut out the evening dose of Prothazin, and she continued to sleep well. Then followed Finlepsin and Akineton. Week for week she took a little less ending finally with Orap, again step-by-step. All in all the withdrawal went well and she had no symptoms of withdrawal. She too took Esbericum during the withdrawal period. After she had stopped the lithium and was given a special antidote, her thyroid fortunately recovered in time.

During the following years she went through a number of crises sometimes taking a psychiatric drug (although only for a brief period) and sometimes Esbericum. Because she required a sick note during these crises she had to visit the neurologist. However, I was always involved and made sure that she was not prescribed too much. At her request we lived through her last episode of psychosis—that was the diagnosis when she became aggressive for hours at a time, agitated and jealous as well as exploding with anger—from March to July 1997 without a neurologist and without psychiatric drugs. She does not like the pills or their side-effects, neither does she like the hospital where she never found any peace.

It is not easy to get through these periods without psychiatric drugs, but the "experiment" worked. We, that is her partner and me, were often at the end of our patience and strength and threatened to have her admitted to the hospital or to call the doctor. Since on no account did she want to go to hospital again, the recognition that we were at the end of our tether had the effect of calming her down. In such situations our GP does not favor hospitalization in these phases. When we could no longer deal with my daughter, she always encouraged us to last out. I particularly wanted to prevent her being hospitalized, since once there she would only be pumped full of the all the same old stuff and she would have dealt badly with the hospitalization, and the drugs would have made life very difficult for her after discharge.

Since that episode she has been well and much more balanced than she has ever been. Because I was with her daily while she was in this state and could observe her and talk to her and experience her explosions of anger first hand—she talked about everything which affected her in these states—we talked together, calmed each other or exploded together. Once, for example, she told me that she was possessed by the devil and I gave her a hanger I had in my hand at that moment and told her: "Kill him!" Unfortunately he had just disappeared. I said: "We'll get him." We cried together, we loved her, we lived through everything together. But there were fun times too, not every day was a bad one.

At present she is not taking anything. It must be remembered that she had suffered from a lack of oxygen during her birth. As a result she is mildly mentally handicapped and went to a special school and now works in a sheltered workshop. In the former German Democratic Republic she was a semiskilled worker and worked full-time as a seamstress with satisfactory results.

Because my daughter trusted me she had no qualms about stopping the pills. We had asked her neurologist to reduce her dose and she did so. But she would not have been willing to withdraw the drugs completely and it would not have worked with her. Instead, my daughter had the support of her partner who she was living with and who has also learned a lot from the way we deal with our crises. Furthermore, we always try together to prevent problems becoming too big and try right from the start to sort them out. I also make it clear that she need not put up with everything or to be misused as a scapegoat for other people.

In my opinion it takes a great deal of courage to get through a psychotic episode without psychiatric medication or a neurologist. We succeeded among other things thanks to Dorothea Buck's book "Auf der Spur des Morgensterns" *("On the Trail of the Morning Star"*; Zerchin 1990), which was my companion and support. In addition I had the telephone and written support of a member of the German Association of (ex-)Users and Survivors of Psychiatry from Krefeld. We both talked a great deal about our experience with self-help.

Our GP—we have known each other for almost 20 years—often questions me about my experience and my knowledge, which I really appreciate. She has asked me what she can do in cases of acute crises when she has to respond to an emergency, and she finds the experiment with my daughter very positive. When I went through my crises it was unfortunate that my GP was on holiday.

Solving the problems which lead to crises is far more productive than their chronic suppression with psychiatric drugs. The soul is not an organ which can be healed with the tools of medicine. I have a great deal of respect for all those specialist surgeons who understand their field. But I have grown very suspicious of psychiatrists and when I visit a hospital these days I don't just watch, but instead I encourage patients to point out to the doctors that dose regimens may be too high or I bring their attention to the damaging side-effects and express a desire for one-to-one consultations, or I tell the professionals what I think. I never forget why I tried to kill myself by jumping out of the window in the hospital and not at home—I live on the 13th floor. Today I know the answer to this question because I know why I jumped: it was what happened in the hospital which finally pushed me over the edge.

You can only solve your mental problems yourself. Working together with your family is also important, having to put up with each other and to understand each other (and if that is not possible then at least to respect each other), talking about things as soon as they arise and—especially if one is inclined to get very upset very quickly—a balanced lifestyle. Nowadays, as before my time in contact with psychiatry, I am prepared to push myself to the limit. However, I have become more cautious and more reflective. I do not ever want to be so depressed again and to become suicidal. I simply enjoy life too much.

Translation from the German by Mary Murphy

Jan Kuypers

Don Quixote and the Drug-Free Zone or: What Now, Little Jumping Jack?

Neuroleptics: Etumine, Haldol, Imap, Melleril, Nozinan, Sordinol / Lithium: Maniprex / Tranquilizer: Rohypnol

Representation 1: For the hasty readers

During a period of seven months in 1980-1981 I was pumped full of drugs in a hospital on the Flemish Archipelago Gulag. This was done by the hands of criminals in white coats using physical violence under the pretense of a treatment for mania. What started it all was my free-thinking and my rejection of the delusions of the Catholic faith.

After I was released, I remained in a twilight zone for months. Then I ritually burned the Huxley Soma tablets. The main ingredients of the Caligariesque cabinet of horrors were the neuroleptics Haldol (made in Belgium),

Imap *(neuroleptic, active ingredient fluspirilene)*, Etumine[1], Nozinan[2], Sordinol[3], lithium poison Maniprex and the sleeping pill Rohypnol[4].

"Either you are part of the problem or a part of the solution," said Ulrike Meinhof back then. That's why I decided to bear witness to the public concerning the medical totalitarianism I experienced on my own body. So that no one can later say they hadn't known anything about it.

Representation 2: For Literature Fans

"Ruined by war, dedicated to victory, memorializing peace," is written on the victory gates in Munich. In the context of our subject this would read: "Ruined by chemistry, dedicated to withdrawal, memorializing a drug-free state."

Involuntarily committed

So you're a process engineer responsible for the gold-plating of electrical plugs. You are thirty-eight years old, tobacco and alcohol-free, a family man with two sons aged seven and eleven. The boys' school asks you routinely to vote on what type of religion or world view they should be instructed in. You choose the morality of undogmatic free-thinking. Suddenly all hell breaks loose. They work on you but you insist on your conscientious position. They'll get you one way or another. They'll get you, all right. Without you having done anything evil, you are arrested by three guardians of the law and immediately sent off to a madhouse run by a Catholic charity. You learn the term "involuntarily committed," in Flemish "kollokatie" (that means "an assembly of similar kinds"). You are injected seven months long and then simply set free again. What now, little jumping jack?

---

1 Neuroleptic, active ingredient clot(h)iapine, apparently not currently marketed in AU, CA, GB, NZ and US

2 Neuroleptic, active ingredient methotrimeprazine, marketed also as Levoprome

3 Neuroleptic, active ingredient clopenthixene, apparently not currently marketed in AU, CA, GB, NZ and US

4 Tranquilizer, active ingredient flunitrazepam, marketed also as Hypnodorm

Drug addiction

You are homeless, without money and drug-addicted. So-called cold turkey makes you completely crazy. So you go to a rehab center. On the same day you take off because the guys there belong to a subculture you can't understand and yet you are worse off than them—can't stand, sit, lie, sleep or wake even for a minute. Your soul leaks out like water through a sieve. You ask the fool in the mirror what he's doing there. Involuntarily you go back to the damned madhouse and beg for the same pills or drops that you had previously managed to spit up again in the most creative ways. A seductive inner voice suggests suicide. You consider it and decide for life instead. As a preventative measure you sign in at a psychiatric hospital with a good reputation, you swallow Melleril and for three months, you only get up in order to eat.

One day a very clean cut person with the expression of a grave digger shows up. "Blood letting," she says, and she means it seriously (not in a medical sense but in the financial sense). You take off immediately and go to your father for a crisis session. He doesn't understand why you are constantly grinning and twitching like a monkey with a rash. You need a lawyer—but only the sun comes up for free. Your father rents you a room. You are going mad. For months you stare at the white-washed ceiling, 20 to 22 hours a day and you attempt to comfort yourself with the thought that things could have been worse. You have no idea what to do. Will you kill yourself? You write your wife and kids a 100-page testament, give them courage, and lay yourself down on a primitive cot after getting some things done. You are wondering what else will happen. Nothing happens. After a week you go walking on the streets, purified for the first time in months. There are people who move forward like ants without the least effort. You are invited for a coffee by a charismatic group. Regarding further care, they refer you to a childhood friend who belongs to the same group, a mother of six children, the wife of a teacher at the art academy and living in the opposite part of the country. You find yourself in a real living room again with a stove in the middle. The family is astonished at your shaking, your robotic movements and zombie mimicry. You are lovingly taught to eat, speak, walk, stand, sit and lie down again. But the psychiatric drugs get in the way, and withdrawing gradually is difficult for you.

Ritual

Your childhood friend, a former hippie girl, thinks up a ritual. You proclaim the place a drug-free zone in which you throw the chemicals into the stove one by one and listen to them crackle. With each one you say the magic word "goodbye" and let out a good cry for joy. Eight pairs of hands applaud you. You spare half the cabinet of poisons in case you need to repeat the ritual in the far corner of Belgium, where even your mother-tongue sounds foreign. That place will also become drug-free, just like everything else. It is 1982; there is life after death. So you get on your way down yonder, not yet aware of your future nickname, Don Quixote.

Translation from the German by Christina White

Maths Jesperson
Between Lobotomy and Antidepressants
Neuroleptics

I suffered terribly when I was mad. But there was one good thing in all my misfortune: the timing of my madness. I went mad in 1980/81, and at that time psychiatry had no medicinal methods at its disposal for treating "obsessional neurosis." They simply didn't know what to do with "obsessional neurotics."

My madness was diagnosed by psychiatrists as "obsessional neurosis of the severest degree," incurable. Fifteen years earlier I would have been lobotomized, in other words my thalamus nerve tract would have been cut surgically. But this method was now banned. Fifteen years later it was discovered that antidepressants could have some "positive effects" in treating "obsessional neurosis," but at that time this was not known. What choice did they have at the time except to give me neuroleptics? So they tried for two years to treat me with neuroleptics—psychiatric drugs which have no effect on "obsessional neuroses." Of course, there was no way they could cure me using neuroleptics, no chance at all. It was an amazing discovery for me to realize that people really do exist who believe that they can cure mental problems with chemicals. How stupid! The psychiatrists with these weird ideas must be really crazy.

Instead of curing me, or at least alleviating my suffering, the only effect of the neuroleptics was to increase my suffering. My troubles were doubled: on top of the original torture, I now suffered unbearable side-effects. This was real terror. When I left the asylum two years later my madness was worse than ever. Psychiatry had not helped me, but had made things far worse. The neuroleptics were simply instruments of torture.

When I was discharged from the asylum my psychiatrist gave me lots of neuroleptics and a few prescriptions for more. When I got home I threw all these down the garbage disposal.

At the time I did not know that after a relatively long treatment period of two years one should not stop suddenly but should do so gradually. However, my sudden withdrawal from the neuroleptics had no negative consequences for me.

It was my great fortune that psychiatry had not yet discovered the so-called positive effects of treating "obsessional neuroses" with antidepressants. Otherwise I would probably have accepted these psychiatric drugs because they would have alleviated my sufferings somewhat. But I would not have become healthy and by now would have become chronically ill and permanently dependent on antidepressants. I have described how I freed myself of my "obsessional neurosis" elsewhere (Jesperson 1993).

Madness is no illness to be cured. My madness arose as a means of forcing me into a new life. The torments I suffered at the time were, on the one hand, signals that the state of life at the time was not good and, on the other hand, they were the driving force which pushed me to search for a way out of my unbearable and pointless life situation and to find an authentic life. Without this inner drive I would not have moved. Psychiatric drugs in contrast would have blocked this driving force and my life would have remained one of permanent suffering and madness.

Translation from the German by Mary Murphy

Coming off Step by Step

Wilma Boevink

Monsters from the Past

Antidepressants / Tranquilizers: Lexotanil, Librium, Seresta, Temesta, Valium

The story of how someone stopped taking psychiatric drugs must really begin with how they started taking them in the first place. Withdrawing from such medication does not simply entail freeing oneself physically and mentally from them. You have to find the courage to confess to yourself how things went so far.

Approximately 15 years ago the doctors prescribed antidepressants for me because they could not find any physical explanation for my symptoms. During the time while I was leaving my parents' house and trying to live my own life I suffered from severe loss of hearing, noises in my head and dizziness. No medical diagnostic apparatus could explain the symptoms of my abnormality. The conclusion was therefore drawn that the cause was psychological. In other words: I was diagnosed as crazy.

What the antidepressants were supposed to do in this case has remained a mystery to me until today. They did not help: not against my symptoms, and not against the increasing dejection and loss of courage resulting from these symptoms. The fact is I was becoming more and more negatively affected by the things going on in my head. I withdrew more and more because of the deafness and began to interpret the noises in my head. For instance, I was convinced that there was something in me making me go crazy and driving me to destruction. I did not know what it was exactly but I did know the reason for it. I was to blame for the misery in the world. I was a bad person and because nobody else understood that and did anything about it, I was being punished inside.

I kept the hopelessness and the fear that I felt at the time under control with alcohol. I still remember that at the beginning when the problems were not so great I "only" drank in the evenings. As time went on the amounts grew larger, the drinks stronger and the time of day when I started drinking was getting earlier by the day. In the end I was having alcohol for breakfast. Without it I couldn't function. In the meantime, the antidepressants had been replaced by all kinds of tranquilizers, Valium, Librium *(tranquilizer, active ingredient chlordiazepoxide)*, Seresta[1], Lexotanil[2], Temesta[3]. I was set on the path of tranquilizers when I was brought to the doctor suffering from delirium. He prescribed the tranquilizer on which I became dependent. I was swallowing ever larger numbers of pills and was washing them down with alcohol.

Finally, within my own four walls and starting a training course, I tried to get my life in order. I wanted to function like everyone else and tried to put up with my life. For this purpose I needed intoxication of all kinds, alcohol, hash and pills. The numbing effect was—although it sounds paradoxical—at the same time both survival strategy and destruction. Because it was the intoxication which drew me out of reality and allowed me to withdraw more and more into my own crazy world and isolate me from the world around me.

After three years I was walking around like a zombie. In fact I wasn't going anywhere, I lay in bed all the time. I wasn't eating anymore, I wasn't speaking anymore and I was barely sleeping. The only things I did were drink, swallow pills and bury myself in my crazy world. The only thing I can remember from this time is my fear and the smell of destruction that surrounded me. I was in control of nothing anymore. Today I know that I was persecuted by events from my childhood and that my childish fears blurred my perception of reality. But at the time I was convinced that the inevitable was happening: I was a problem and the problem had to be solved. I knew my fate but could not

1 Tranquilizer, active ingredient oxazepam, marketed as Alepam, Murelax, Oxazepam, Ox-Pam, Serax, Serepax

2 Tranquilizer, active ingredient bromazepam, marketed as Lectopam, Lexotan

3 Tranquilizer, active ingredient lorazepam, marketed also as Alzapam, Ativan, Lorapam, Lorazapam

look it straight in the eye and instead tried every available form of numbing intoxication. My only motivation was to feel nothing. In this way I tried to keep my head above water.

When I finally went under, admission to a psychiatric hospital seemed the only way out. Whether it really was I don't know. But I do know that in my case it helped me in curing my dependence. During my stay, which lasted two and a half years, I stopped the medication step-by-step. When I arrived at the hospital I had to hand over all my pills to the medical team who then took responsibility for them. This step was not easy for me because it was the tablets which gave me the feeling of having some form of control. When I handed them over I handed over everything, including myself.

The first thing that my carers did was to regulate my medication consumption. I was no longer able to swallow pills whenever I needed them. I was now given them at set times, about five times a day. They prescribed me a much larger amount of another tranquilizing agent which was much less addictive. At first it was like the blow of a hammer, I slept almost all day. The dose was then reduced little by little. They began with the time of day when I felt least bad (early morning), the amounts at the other times remained unchanged at first. When that went well the other doses were reduced. I remained at this level until all withdrawal symptoms were gone. As soon as I was more or less stable the dose was again reduced and again during early morning when I felt best. So I reduced until the point came when I was taking the pills only four times a day instead of five times a day. Then I succeeded in getting from four times to three times and so on until I was finally free of them. All in all this process lasted about six months. That is not really very long when one remembers that my addiction had lasted for about three years.

Withdrawal did not go smoothly. At each step my body reacted with withdrawal symptoms: shaking, dizziness, severe agitation. Everything I heard had an echo and there were waves in everything I saw. The most difficult moment was the hour before my next "shot" because I felt I would be overwhelmed from emotions in a deep slumber in myself—the monsters from the past–and finally go totally mad. On a few occasions the withdrawal went wrong and I lost my head. There was no boundary between me and my surroundings. I was swallowed up by the images and sounds around me and disappeared into them. Fortunately there was always someone around at these moments to bring me back. Someone held me, someone spoke to me. And then slowly, everything returned to recognizable proportions.

I also got free of my alcohol addiction during my hospitalization. It was not possible to drink secretly in the hospital and I had to stop drinking the large amounts I was used to. At the beginning I was occasionally allowed a small glass in a pub near the hospital but when I had to stop the pills this was over too. For many years after I did not touch a drop out of fear of becoming addicted again. Neither did I use soft drugs during those years. I didn't want the intoxication any more. I didn't want to risk slipping off the rails again. I wanted to keep both feet on the ground and not loose control over my life again. But I am not a teetotaler. As I gradually found solid ground under my feet, the threat of renewed dependency disappeared. Over the years I learned the difference between "to enjoy a drink" and "to drown the misery." I now know exactly when it is dangerous to drink and when it is not.

The process of freeing myself from dependency went hand-in-hand with getting a handle on my life. This is a two-way process. I had my life better under control because I wasn't taking drugs anymore. But I was able to reduce my consumption of drugs and psychiatric medication because I had gained control over my life. This process of reconstruction was possible because I dared to look back at my life and face what had happened to me. During the years I developed the courage to face what I tried to cover with all my dependencies. I fought the monsters of my past, and to be able to do this, first I had to admit them and look into their eyes.

In the meantime I have become the mistress of my own life. Among other things this means that I no longer need to be afraid. No rampaging monsters or debilitating dependencies. Since my period of withdrawal over more than ten years ago I have taken hardly any psychiatric drugs. This has not always been easy. There were times when I wanted to be anesthetized, to not feel anything for a while. At such moments I made clear to myself that swallowing drugs meant having to stop them again. Psychiatric drugs solve nothing; they only allow you to close your eyes for a while so that you don't have to face reality.

Translation from the German by Mary Murphy

Katherine Zurcher

Second Fear

Neuroleptics / Antidepressants / Tranquilizers

I was dependent on benzodiazepines for two decades. During those twenty years of dependency, I not only ignored and repressed who I really was, I was blind to how much misery the tranquilizers caused in my life. I believed I needed them. I was certain I would go crazy if I stopped them. And I *did* go crazy. During the stages of withdrawal, I knew I had never known such anguish and despair before, except, perhaps, during my first experiences with psychiatry as an adolescent.

In 1970, when I was seventeen years old, I began to suffer from feelings of depression, anxiety and inferiority. I was an American living in Switzerland, which meant that I had no family or trusted adults to turn to with my problems other than my parents, and they had their own problems.

My parents had begun therapy with a psychiatrist, and one day I asked them if I could see the psychiatrist myself. They agreed. I had no way of knowing that I was making a disastrous mistake.

The psychiatrist prescribed antidepressants for me at first. The more I went to see him however, the worse I felt. Soon, I was afraid to see my friends at all and at one point I no longer wanted to leave my bedroom. This was when the psychiatrist took me to the psychiatric hospital. I thought the hospital would help me feel better. That's what I had learned hospitals were for.

It didn't take long at the hospital for them to label me schizophrenic and treat me with neuroleptics and insulin treatment. I became more and more frightened because the treatment with neuroleptics cut me off from my own feelings and motivations. I knew less and less about who I was, what value I had, what possibilities were open to me. The psychiatric drugs created a burning anxiety in the center of my being, an anguish I had never known before. I attributed this to my "mental illness" as the doctors had convinced me to do.

The effects of the psychiatric medicine were frightening and confounding. One day I found that I could no longer walk. I kept falling down, unable to stand up again. At unexpected times my tongue stuck out of my mouth in a painful spasm. It was impossible to put it back into my mouth. These so-called side-effects terrified me. They would begin abruptly without warning and just as quickly disappear. Once I found myself crawling on my hands and knees to my room, desperate to get to my bed and hide. With my tongue sticking out of my mouth, I knew, I looked the part of the crazy person I supposedly was.

Another time, I started to notice a white liquid coming from my breasts. I didn't know what was happening to me. For days I tried to catch the doctor as he hurried down the hallway, to tell him about this "white stuff" coming from my breasts. He finally ordered a nurse to have me taken to a gynecologist. The gynecologist was rude and hurried as she examined my body. She had the cold speculum inside me before I could explain that I had come to inquire about the white liquid running from my breasts. When I was finally able to tell her about it, she said it was milk and dismissed it as a side-effect of the psychiatric drugs. The psychiatrist had put me through this humiliating and frightening examination when he could have told me the same thing himself. I felt betrayed and angry.

I decided not to take the psychiatric drugs if they caused such bizarre things to happen. Every day I was given several pills. I didn't know what they were, and I wasn't sure which one caused the side-effects, but I suspected a large orange pill and began throwing it away every day. I finally told the doctor that I threw it away. He didn't know which pill I was referring to, so he took me into the pharmacy, unlocked a large cabinet, and took out a dozen or so vials of pills and showed them to me, asking me which ones gave me the terrible. He didn't show me the orange one, but mysteriously it disappeared from my daily pills after that.

One day I was told that I was to talk to a professor. This was a big deal according to the nurses. I was to be on display in front of 10 or 15 resident psychiatrists while the professor asked me questions. I took special care with my clothing and make-up that day. But as the "important professor" asked questions and the others listened, I began to understand that it didn't matter how well I was dressed or how clean my hair was. They all saw me as a mental case and whatever I said would be interpreted in that light.

When asked what I thought was wrong with me, I told the professor about my family life and my father's alcohol problem. As I told this part of my story to the professor, and as the others looked on, I began to cry uncontrollably. But instead of taking into account that this was a family problem: alcohol, denial of problems and no permission to express feelings or talk about what might be wrong, the professor recommended insulin therapy for me.

Why did I and my parents accept? Because we truly believed that psychiatry could help. Because believing in psychiatric labels and its chemical therapies is so much easier than getting down to feelings and truth, easier than examining our family problems, easier than finding compassion and acceptance. And yet if my family and the mental health professionals had tried these things, they might have helped me find a sense of my own worth.

The insulin therapy consisted of shots in my thighs every morning which left them covered with bruises. After about forty-five minutes during which I would read or try to write in bed, I would begin to tremble uncontrollably. When I was trembling so violently that I could no longer see the page I was reading, a nurse would come in with a tray of very sugary food. After eating this food, I would fall into a deep sleep for hours on end. That meant that at night I would often have trouble sleeping and sometimes when this happened, the night nurse would give me more sugary food. I got fatter and fatter. Even I could see that this therapy tended to make me act strangely. I laughed a lot over very silly things. I enjoyed playing practical jokes. A psychiatrist came in every morning and asked me questions. I laughed and cried and made no sense at all. Once he accidentally broke the back of his chair and this sent me into such fits of laughter that he finally got up and left.

For the next four years I was in and out of the hospital, still taking brain-damaging psychiatric drugs. Neuroleptics, benzodiazepines and antidepressants. I was still dependent on, and living with my parents. My personality changed even more. I tried to cut my veins several times, I had outbursts of anger. I now know that the psychiatric medication, the very thing that was supposed to be helping me, was causing me to act this way.

I badly needed affection and a sense of my own existence. The only way to get this was to go to bed with just about any man who picked me up for sex. I always drank alcohol to do this because I was too shy otherwise. It showed much self-hatred, I realize now, to allow myself to be used by men in this way and some of them were quite cruel and could have been dangerous. I continued this behavior compulsively however, even though I had little or no sexual pleasure. I suppose I was hoping to find someone who would love me. I was extremely lucky at that time to meet a man who cared and wanted a long-lasting relationship with me. (I am still married to him.) I left the hospital and went to live with him. He kept pleading with me to stop my psychiatric drugs and finally I did. I was still very anxious and troubled but I was feeling a lot happier. Then several months later I got intolerably anxious and the psychiatrist gave me benzodiazepines. From that time on, I took them every day for years and years.

In spite of this, my situation improved. I managed to get a job, to live like everyone else, although I still had inferiority feelings and anxiety and stress which I handled with tranquilizers. After ten years of this dependency I managed to stop taking tranquilizers. It was when my husband and I went to live in California for a year. The atmosphere was so much more relaxed there and I think that helped a lot. I also did yoga exercises every day in order to relieve the physical tension I felt during withdrawal. I experienced some irrational anger and anxiety but after a few months I felt much better.

When my husband and I came back to Switzerland a year later however, I began to have intense anxiety and dizzy spells. I was once again incapable of relaxing. I had never truly learned to relax because the tranquilizers had always done it for me and so I had a tendency (often found in people with low self-esteem) to push myself too far, trying to be the perfect housewife, the perfect employee. Unable to live with the dizziness and anxiety, I went to see a doctor who prescribed benzodiazepines again. I was defeated by this. It made me feel I would never be able to live like a normal person and would always need tranquilizers. And so, I took them for ten more years during which I suffered more and more from dizziness, agoraphobia, anxiety, nightmares, tension, fatigue... I didn't know at the time that the tranquilizers were causing what I now know to be called "rebound anxiety." In past years I have often read accounts of people on tranquilizers suffering from these symptoms. Interestingly, agoraphobia, the fear of leaving home, or being out in public, is very common in people who take benzodiazepines. I suppose that is logical, given that these tranquilizers cause symptoms which can be very frightening in public places. Psychiatrists tend to look for obscure psychological reasons for agoraphobia. I know that it is caused by the very normal reaction of the brain to what it has perceived in the past to be a dangerous situation. I believe the same to be true of panic attacks.

I refused to increase my dose when the doctor told me it could help, but I now know that my addiction to tranquilizers was in fact demanding that I increase my dose. My brain, my body, had been trying to make up for the tranquilization by becoming hypersensitive and so I suffered more and more. I often felt as if I were on a boat that was rocking, or I felt myself sinking into the floor and sometimes as if I were floating several feet above the floor. Every movement of my head or movement of objects around me created an intense dizzy spell. Often, I saw immobile objects moving. Needless to say this greatly drained my confidence, made me constantly tense and over-vigilant. It tired me so much that I spent a lot of time resting, and I worried endlessly about what could be causing it. I went to dozens of doctors looking for help. I had dozens of tests done. The doctors never once suggested that what I was experiencing could be caused by the drug I was taking.

At times I felt I could stand it no longer and must give up. All I wanted was to lie down and die, just stop everything. But some self-preserving part of me told me to avoid this at all costs. I knew that if I gave up, psychiatrists would probably take charge and I could end up in the hospital again. And so I worked all day even though I was dizzy, even though I was tense and felt inferior to everyone, even though I was often afraid to leave my office simply to walk down the hallway to the toilet, or terrified to go to the supermarket. I just kept forcing myself. I took tranquilizers to get me through many situations. I planned every frightening task (and there were so many that frightened me) around the brief moments when the tranquilizers would have a calming effect. I was also very ashamed that I took tranquilizers and I hid myself to take them. I felt like a shameful drug addict. Which I was.

In my late 30s, at long last I began to cut down my dose of benzodiazepines. I found a therapist who was not a medical doctor or psychiatrist. He used sophrology[1], relaxation, visualization, neurolinguistic programming and other methods. It was his compassion and respect however, that helped me the most. He told me something very simple which no one had ever thought to tell me before: my feelings, my opinions, my values are the most important, the most valid and the only truth *for me*. There was no "crazy" or "normal" or "inferior" or "superior," there was just me. But my therapy with this man caused a lot of old fears, anger and resentment to come up and a terrible struggle in my unconscious made itself manifest. At the same time, I was cutting down drastically on tranquilizers. I was suffering withdrawal, which caused my symptoms to worsen and caused new and frightening sensations of unreality which seemed like true madness.

The worst part was doubting my own mind, because when you lose trust in your own thoughts, you feel as if you have lost all of yourself. I was constantly questioning my sanity. A general practitioner that I consulted, wanted me to take antidepressants. He said I was in the middle of a nervous breakdown. I refused. Perversely, I went to see a psychiatrist and neurologist. It was as if I were, in a way, "turning myself in" to psychiatry. When I told the neurologist that I had dizziness and a rocking sensation practically all of the time, when I told him of my anxiety and of feeling myself floating above my bed at night and hearing strange noises in my ears, he did not attribute this to withdrawal from tranquilizers, but said that these were psychotic traits and that neuroleptics could help me. I was very frightened to take neuroleptics again. I still remembered the adverse effects they had caused in my youth. But he told me that they would help me to stop benzodiazepines and there was nothing I wanted more than that, so I agreed to try the neuroleptics for two weeks.

Although he prescribed a very low dose of neuroleptics, they brought on an even worse feeling of anxiety. It was as if I knew reality had once existed

---

1 Type of therapy and/or personal discipline involving deep relaxation and positive suggestion

for me but was incapable of experiencing it. This was the most frightening sensation I had ever known and I was sure I was truly mad this time. I was terribly frightened that the neurologist and the psychiatrists had always been right. I was a psychotic, a schizophrenic, a defective human being incapable of sanity, a machine whose wires were crossed. There was no hope and there was no way to feel better.

My compassionate therapist however, was able to calm me. He was, I think, somewhat disappointed that I had resorted to going to a psychiatrist and neurologist, but he helped me understand that I had returned to these professionals because I had something to learn from the experience. I had old wounds that I needed to heal and long repressed anger to express. He helped me understand something important: the damage that belief in psychiatric labels such as "schizophrenia" had done to me. And suddenly, I was certain of one vital fact: It didn't matter what psychiatrists called my problems, it didn't matter what they thought they should do about my problems, the fact was, they were incapable of helping me and they had greatly damaged me. It was this realization that finally liberated me from taking psychiatrists' or doctors' advice and helped me through the final terrible withdrawal stage.

Withdrawal

I was aware, of course, that I had many emotional problems from my past to work on, but for now, I had to concentrate on getting through each day without letting tension build up to an unbearable degree. I went through a period that I now think of as my "So what?"-stage. If anything, anyone or any thought began to make me feel bad or unworthy I simply said "So what?" If things got hectic or stressful in my life, I told myself simply, "I refuse to get upset about this." I did my utmost to relax and accept everything that came my way. I was going off tranquilizers. That was my highest priority. I would not let anything distress me. I couldn't *afford* to.

My withdrawal symptoms were quite simply the same symptoms I had always had while taking tranquilizers but were even more exaggerated.

I got a lot of help from a book I had in my possession that I had bought years before in the United States. It was called "Peace from Nervous Suffering," written by an Australian woman, Doctor Claire Weekes. I had read it before this, but I had continued to depend on tranquilizers while trying to follow its advice. This time I was determined to succeed on my own.

Dr. Weekes had so many patients with symptoms similar to my own that it made me wonder how it could be possible that all of the doctors I had consulted in my life had seemed to be so unfamiliar with them. All of my symptoms were described here in this book. With relief, I read of the "sensation of lurching, swaying, or of being pulled to one side while walking." (Weekes 1972, p. 2) I read the accounts of people who felt the pavement heaving as they walked, and of patients becoming so worried about what was happening to them that they feared a brain tumor, a fatal disease or madness. The book described the increased anxiety and increased intensity of symptoms upon waking that I had often experienced. What a relief it was to read about other people having experienced the same odd, frightening sensations I had, and to read that these feelings were perfectly normal reactions to stress and anxiety. According to Dr. Weekes, there were millions of people who suffered like this from "nervous illness" as she called it. Why had I never met a doctor who could tell me at least that much? It could have helped me feel less lonely and crazy.

Dr. Weekes explained the origins of all nervous symptoms; from weakness in the legs to difficulty swallowing, to agoraphobia. She even explained the causes of obsession, personality disintegration, loss of confidence, agitation, feelings of unreality, grotesque thoughts, depression, all in a way that was so utterly logical, understandable and reassuring. According to her, the main cause of all of this suffering was very simple: "sensitization."

Dr. Weekes' definition of sensitization was: "a state in which nerves are conditioned to react to stress in an exaggerated way." (ibid.) She told of her many patients whose nerves played various tricks on them. Their nerves, she explained, were so "well-oiled" and "trigger-happy" that they were always ready to respond to the slightest stimulus with alarming rapidity. Her patients had become not only upset by the actual stress in their lives, but perhaps even more upset by the *symptoms* of that stress. What is more, they worried that these symptoms could worsen. They had added fear upon fear, stress upon stress. They had become *nervously ill*. This was all immensely reassuring to me. I already knew that taking tranquilizers and neuroleptics caused a person to become hypersensitive, because the brain creates new receptors to make up for the ones blocked by the drug. Now I realized that I had been exacerbating the problem with my own fear of what was happening to me.

The solution was acceptance as Dr. Weekes explained:

> "It is strange how we keep a grip on ourselves by being prepared to release it. We cannot keep the right kind of grip by tensely holding on, as so many suppose. By abandoning ourselves to whatever our body may care to do, we release the tension that fatigues the nerves controlling muscles and blood vessels, so that they recover their ability to function normally, and strength gradually returns." (ibid., p. 39)

In just about every situation now, I realized, I was withdrawing in fear from the physical sensations I was experiencing, adding what Claire Weekes called "second fear," becoming bewildered, afraid of the reactions of my own body to stress, and those reactions were easily brought on because my senses were so finely tuned to them. When I had even a slight dizzy spell, the disappointment and dread it brought could overwhelm me. This had been going on for so long that it had become a reflex. No wonder I was in such miserable condition, I thought, I was adding stress upon stress upon stress, fear upon fear, to a point where even relaxation had become frightening to me, and so difficult to achieve.

Dr. Weekes' precious advice continued:

> "You must be prepared to accept the ultimate. Practice acceptance of all of your symptoms until even panic holds no threat to you. Be prepared to go through the absolute worst with acceptance." (ibid., p. 148)

She compared this acceptance to the hardest lesson an airplane pilot has to learn. When the plane goes into a fall, he must resist the temptation to tip the wings in the opposite direction. "To draw away like that is fatal. To go with the fall is to flatten out and recover balance." (ibid., p. 65) And applying this to my dizziness was one of the hardest things I have ever done. I had to learn to let the dizziness come, "fall into" it and pass through it. For me, this was as frightening as falling in an airplane.

Dr. Weekes also warned about letting setback throw you into complete despair, and I realized I had done this many times. Setbacks, she explained, are unavoidable and should be accepted and passed through as calmly as possible.

> "They gradually fade from the scene when you no longer fear them. They lose their meaning and are no longer truly setbacks, but reminders of how you once suffered and how much you have progressed." (ibid., p. 182)

I realized that as far as dizziness was concerned I was going to have to accept it more fully than I had before. I was going to have to be willing during my dizzy spells, to fall down on the ground if necessary. It had become a deeply ingrained habit to go tensely through life trying to keep my grip, rushing to get the worst over with as quickly as possible. It was inevitable that I would fall back into that sort of tense reaction many times before I truly mastered acceptance. But I kept at it. I had to learn to accept failure too, and not to be devastated if the dizziness came back in spite of my perseverance.

When I woke up in the morning and felt the rocking motion start up, I did my best not to be affected by it. When I got out of bed and felt myself fall to the right as usual, I accepted it totally, leaned into it, took a deep breath and let myself feel dizzy. Every step I took, I relaxed my muscles, I accepted the heaving ground, I accepted the ringing in my ears, the palpitations, or whatever symptom my adrenaline-filled body was capable of. When I had a recurring strange or ugly thought, I accepted that too instead of being bewildered by its return. I eventually realized that many thoughts returned at the same stimulus, it was only a memory, a habit that my tired, frightened mind could not let go of.

When I went out on the street, to my job, or to the supermarket, I stopped trying to control my fear, I accepted the fact that it would come, I even welcomed it, because it meant that I had a chance to practice floating through it.

I regularly did relaxation exercises and made a habit of breathing deeply and calmly in all situations.

Surprisingly soon, my dizziness decreased in intensity and in only a few weeks, I had no more fear of going to the supermarket, or anywhere else. I no longer had that fear at the top of the stairs before going out, no longer had to plan meals days in advance, because I felt free to go down to the store at any time. I actually looked forward to going there!

In a matter of weeks also, I no longer felt the chair I was sitting on going up and down, I rarely felt the pavement heaving, and if I did, it was a warning to me that I was getting too tense, and I immediately let go of my tension. As time passed, the only rocking motion I felt was when I was particularly anxious or when I was lying down. I found though, that if I refused to worry about the rocking motion, and concentrated on my breathing and on relaxing my muscles, it usually left me in peace after a while.

The above account of how I managed to pass through withdrawal may make it sound fairly easy to do. It wasn't. If the physical symptoms were harrowing, the psychological symptoms were even worse. I felt very crazy, very unsure of myself and felt much self-hatred and shame. I was unable for several weeks to sleep for more than four hours a night. But I learned a valuable lesson from that. I learned that even without much sleep one can still function and sometimes it even helps to be tired because one just doesn't have the energy to be anxious during the day. To help me get to sleep, I used a meditation technique consisting of "filing" my thoughts away into three categories: past, present and future. It helps enormously to empty one's mind in this way. I also used deep breathing and concentrated on relaxing each muscle in my body.

But, when I had been off tranquilizers for one month, I was elated. I wasn't taking tranquilizers and I had no more agoraphobia and practically no more dizziness. What would the doctors have to say about this? I felt that I had won. I also knew that I had been to hell and back.

I was amazed at how much better I felt. I had more energy and enthusiasm. Physically I felt much younger. But the most amazing thing to me was that *I still had all of my symptoms*. But now they were normal, or near-normal, in intensity. Just as Claire Weekes' book had reassured me, they had all been normal reactions and emotions, exaggerated by sensitization.

No more doctors

In all, I took benzodiazepines for twenty years. During that time, I had seen many doctors. Some doctors had scorned me for being dependent on tranquilizers, others had liberally prescribed them, still others had given them to me in such small quantities that I was forced to visit their offices several times a month. This was humiliating and frightening because I needed tranquilizers so badly and worried that the doctor would suddenly decide to cut off my supply. Once, a gynecologist told me that I didn't deserve to have children because I was dependent on tranquilizers. As it turned out, I was never able to have children. But I didn't really want children. To me life was just too much suffering. Why would I want to bring a person I would love dearly into a life like this? None of the medical professionals I sought help from ever admitted that members of their own profession had gotten me into this addiction. I was only able to stop tranquilizers altogether when I got so angry with all the psychiatrists and doctors I had ever known, that I vowed never to be dependent on them again. I preferred to die rather than see a doctor, and for two or three years after that I didn't see a doctor for any reason whatsoever.

But I was never ill! I felt better and better. I no longer had anxiety as soon as I woke up in the morning. I was free of "rebound anxiety." I was finally able to gain the confidence that I had never learned to have. I learned to relax and overcome the dizziness and self-consciousness. I learned to accept myself, go out and meet people without covering up or acting from a false self. I learned to stop caring what others thought I should be and do. I even managed to lose 17 kilos! At long last, I was becoming myself again.

It seems incredible to me now when I remember my first hospitalization, that a young girl with an alcoholic father should be diagnosed schizophrenic without considering the problem within her family. My father was showing me that alcohol was the way to overcome problems and the psychiatrists were showing me the same thing. They just replaced alcohol with tranquilizers. Often, I used both, even though I was aware of the dangers involved in mixing alcohol and psychiatric drugs. The insulin treatment made me very fat as did the neuroleptics which also gave me pimples. An adolescent girl needs to feel good about herself. It was almost as if they were *trying* to give me a bad self-image. None of them ever thought to help me gain self-esteem, or to develop my talents. On the contrary, they made me feel even more inferior and defective. They helped me lose twenty years of my life feeling like an inferior mental case, incapable of living without psychiatric drugs and incapable of making any valuable contribution to society.

Nowadays when I tell this story, even mental health professionals are surprised that I was ever considered schizophrenic. As a teenager I was just very sad and frightened and shy. Not long ago, the psychiatrist that knew me as an adolescent said that he had been mistaken in diagnosing me schizophrenic at age 17. As far as I could tell, the sole basis of his judgment that I had never been schizophrenic was that I had managed to hold a job and to stay married for so long. He seemed to think that the mistaken diagnosis was not a serious error on his part. He didn't even realize that I lived for twenty years in almost incapacitating shame, secrecy, and loneliness, with extreme doubt about the integrity of my own mind and with a dependency that drained my self-esteem every single day.

Even though I have overcome many of my problems, I will probably never entirely eradicate the doubt that something is wrong with my brain (there very well could be now because of all the drugs that I have taken). I still have difficulty with my memory and concentration, which I have read is one of the things long-term benzodiazepine use can cause. This inhibits me in many areas of my life. I still experience hypersensitivity, tension and dizziness from time to time, although I have learned to relax and live with these less fearfully. Sometimes I worry that there is permanent brain damage due to the drugs. Also, I will never feel entirely comfortable with, or close to other people who have not experienced psychiatric treatment, because they could never understand that suffering. And because there is still a lot of prejudice attached to having been "mentally ill," I often keep my story a secret.

Michael Chmela

Escaped

Neuroleptics: Cisordinol, Dapotum, Haldol, Leponex, Melleril

In 1983 at the age of 25 I had a difficult time in my life. Suddenly I became ill with a "psychosis." My condition was classified as delusional, and I was admitted to the Graz psychiatric hospital (Feldhof), where I was quieted down with drugs. Ten days later I was discharged with Melleril. After my father, who had just traveled 700 km, had seen 30 to 40 people in hospital attire standing in line waiting for their psychiatric drugs and had seen me locked into a bed that was more a cage than a cot, with steel sides to lock me in. He suffered a heart attack on the following night; he died five years later as a result.

In 1983 I broke off my medical studies which I had commenced seven years previously. Shortly after I was again admitted to the hospital, this time near Constance in Germany. From 1983 to 1991 I was locked up more than 20 times in various psychiatric units, each time for an average of about three weeks.

I was given Melleril and Haldol which caused me great suffering. This was not only because of the physical side-effects, but also because of the loss of drive combined with an inner restlessness. The neuroleptics cut me off from (social) life in an indescribable manner, even from life within me. I was desperately aware of this but incapable of doing anything about it.

So I stopped taking the psychiatric drugs and the torturous state disappeared. But the next "episode" came three months later. Now I was in a vicious circle. The crises became more excessive, like happenings, although I never became violent.

Yet again I had to interrupt my studies (social science) for more psychiatric treatment, more neuroleptics, this time Dapotum *(neuroleptic, active ingredient fluphenazine)* and Cisordinol[1]—the worst of the lot, and not just according to me; almost everyone who has ever taken it agrees. Again I suffered seriously under the treatment, but no one could imagine or understand the mental pain and despair caused by the psychiatric drugs. When I described this state it was interpreted as resistance or as a symptom of my illness. They destroyed my quality of life, and my zest for life sank to zero.

But I knew that if I stopped taking the neuroleptics, the pharmacological depression would go away. Years later (1990/91), when I found another neuroleptic and insisted on trying it, I had no "resistance," since it did not have the effect of wiping me out mentally. This drug was Leponex *(neuroleptic, active*

---

1 Neuroleptic, active ingredient zuclopentixol, marketed as Clopixol

ingredient clozapine). I took Leponex continuously from the end of 1991 until about the end of 1994. Since then my quality of life has improved. If I were still on Haldol, Cisordinol or Dapotum I would still be stuck in the revolving door of psychiatry or by now I would have been physically and/or psychologically at rock bottom. Leponex was a step towards freedom. The minimal dosage, approximately 2 to 3 mg once a day (evenings), did not impair my quality of life. Of course I noticed it, but it was not particularly unpleasant. In fact, I would have been quite happy to continue to live with this dose.

Since 1992 I have had no psychotic crises and I have worked continuously since then. In our psychiatric units daily Leponex-doses of several hundred milligrams are usual—600 mg are by no means unusual—but I only "prescribed" myself one evening dose (= daily dose) of 2 to 3 mg for two years, and it was effective. But it was a long time before I got that far.

From 1984 to 1986 I lived through my worst period of crises. In 1990/91 my "Iraq crisis" followed and in the summer of 1991 I had a "trip on the wild side" to Milan, Italy; this was my last psychotic episode. The worst thing in all these years was the insoluble dilemma: if I take the neuroleptics I will be falling apart inside and painfully chained and miserably depressed (the same symptoms as a cerebrally localized psychotic syndrome, i.e., a negative personality change as a result of organic cerebral disease). I will actually be paralyzed and cut off from the simplest things of life; despair and pain will grow to unbearable proportions. On the other hand I know that if I stop taking the neuroleptics I will be thrown back into the psychiatric mill.

Caught up in the wheels. Classified, stamped and labeled, with negative prophecies for the future, accusations and contempt. But what to do? Personally, I couldn't find a way out. Approximately 30 acquaintances, including male and female friends, have committed suicide in situations exactly like this: they hanged themselves, knelt down in front of a train, died from an overdose or cut their wrists. Such deaths cannot, however, be called voluntary.

With well over 100 people among my acquaintances and friends still taking neuroleptics I am connected to intensive encounters, experiences, and friendships (from shared apartments, self-help groups, shared psychiatric admissions etc.). There is in fact nobody in this circle who was able to withdraw from the neuroleptics permanently. Some of us were healthy in the sense that we were able to carry out satisfying work or start families.

After my third admission I received the diagnosis "schizoid psychosis." Today this would be called "manic depressive."

How did I manage to get off Leponex? By achieving a continuous state of stabilization and building up a robust and positive personality. Then I decided that I was no longer going to damage anyone, including myself, with further exaltations. Finally, I was prepared to present myself voluntarily for treatment when the whole attempt became too much for me and the forces and energies became uncontrollable. Even the preparedness to take intolerable medication grew. It was on the whole a kind of surrender, in other words, I accepted my powerlessness in many areas, whether health or social. I accepted a power that was stronger than me, in fact, a supernatural one, and became (and still am) convinced that this power is a loving one. It is probably not possible to understand this but only to experience it.

My 15-month stay in a therapeutic community (Haus Weizenkorn, Allgäu, southern Germany), where I also learned to do practical work, helped. Since 1992 I have lived in my own apartments and have had jobs I enjoy and which are interesting (in a library, an archive, gardens, a book-bindery, the post office etc.). Work is a valuable factor for health and consequently for withdrawing from psychiatric drugs because one's surroundings must be right!

Withdrawing from Leponex caused no problems because I took 50 and then 25 mg for a few weeks and then reduced to 1 to 3 mg (!), in fact just a crumb. Even so there was a short but intensive rebound but without serious consequences.

I had gained the ability to get through the rebound experience during the previous ten years. Like a Jack-in-box, I never gave up on therapy and self-help groups but kept working on myself. I drew strength from my belief in a loving God. I was fortunate, because although the rebound might have been short and intensive, my fate was hanging in the balance. Withdrawing is a holistic undertaking; it doesn't just depend on the weeks before and the weeks after, and the withdrawal process is not only a chemical process. It depends on many factors: my surroundings, my psychological state, my personality, my attitude and behavior, my values and my strengths. And it depends on my motivation, and on whether the world appears to be worth living in or not, whether I can envision a satisfactory life outside psychiatry, whether I can accept my limitations (my own and those imposed on me) or not.

During the rebound it was fortunate that I was strong enough to consciously chose "my route into the psychosis." (In the spring of 1992 when I went through my last episode of psychosis, I consciously decided to be psychotic, and went to Milan, intensively but dangerously.) In the winter of 1993/94, when I stopped taking Leponex, I consciously decided against a psychotic relapse. When I became aware of the changing mood (that "taking off," which is both manic and conscious), in other words, the breakthrough to another world, I thought about what I might gain from it. At the same time I remembered the tasks I was committed to in the near future, but which I would not be able to complete if the psychosis broke through. I thought about the repressive power in the psychiatric units and the general lack of understanding for me and my situation that I encountered. A major reason for my decision not to allow myself to be driven into psychosis lay in the fact that I did not want to cause any more pain to those I love and who love me, which my "taking off" and the ensuing drama of being admitted to a psychiatric unit would entail. And I had a lot to lose: an occupation and many wonderful experiences and things in this "normal" world. I weighed up and it helped.

It was absolutely essential for me to leave a damaged and damaging family. I have drunk no alcohol for ten years and do not take drugs. The alcohol abstinence is very important, since alcohol can push you from instability into catastrophe. In addition, the conscious abstinence gave me strength. Now I barely notice that I have further developed in a (in the widest sense) drug-free culture. Getting to know EA-groups and the twelve-step program was also important. I still observe it today and it allows me to grow more strongly in a basic positive mental attitude which I then find reflected back at me.

Put simply, as I grew older I became calmer. Not necessarily more tired, but more aware and more mature. The way forward is more inwards and upwards without giving up one's convictions and efforts. One becomes more modest and wiser by seeing that we cannot change everything and by taking pleasure in the developments that have occurred. Having lived through almost a quarter of a century politically aware allows me an overview. In the Taoist sense I have been set more free.

Translation from the German by Mary Murphy

Bert Gölden

With Patience

Neuroleptics: Melleril, Truxal / Antidepressants: Anafranil, Equilibrin, Ludiomil, Saroten, Sinquan, Tagonis, Tofranil / Tranquilizers: Tavor

Since my childhood—I was born in 1955—I have suffered from obsessional behavior and thoughts. The most prominent manifestation is an obsessional compulsion to wash. The condition was first diagnosed when I was 18. At that time the issue of "obsession" was relatively unknown and unresearched in professional circles—and I was confronted with a great degree of uncertainty regarding the diagnosis among specialists. Therefore, psychiatric drugs were the only treatment used. I took the following psychiatric drugs for more than twenty-one years: Tavor *(tranquilizer, active ingredient lorazepam)*, Tofranil[1] and Saroten *(antidepressant, active ingredient amitriptyline)*. Many other drugs were prescribed experimentally but the unpleasant side-effects were severe. I remember what the prescribing doctor said: "The prescribed drugs do not cause any damaging side-effects and can be taken on a long-term basis without any risk." I was young at the time and trusted the specialist blindly, which later turned out to be a great mistake. The use of Tavor led to the known and to-be-expected "dependency and addiction," which must be taken seriously. Years of use finally led to a gradual impairment in personality. Since then, I like to call benzodiazepines the opiate of the people. Use of these "happy

---

1 Antidepressant, active ingredient imipramine, marketed as Imipramine, Melipramine

pills" only succeeded in creating an artificial harmony. The cause of my problems remained hidden and was never treated. In the end, I went down a long solitary route to break my dependency on tranquilizers. The doctors were only prepared to deal with the withdrawal on an inpatient basis in order to prevent symptoms of withdrawal, especially shock. Since I have stopped taking the psychiatric drugs, which are useless for me, I have made a more self-confident impression on other people.

But before I go into the details of my successful withdrawal from psychiatric drugs I would like to deal with my condition which is known as an obsessional state. There are various forms of the condition. As I mentioned above, I was suffering from a chronic obsession with washing associated with a control obsession and obsessional thoughts. An obsessional state is characterized by constantly recurring, intrusive and unwanted thoughts. Or irrational, ritualized and repetitive actions are carried out, which cannot be stopped despite an inner resistance. The recognition on the part of the patient of the pointlessness of the thoughts and actions is also characteristic of the diagnosis. Obsessions are very time-consuming conditions which can also lead to symptoms of anxiety and depression. The washing obsession is triggered through fear of contact and comes to the fore in association with certain objects or situations. Instead of fear, feelings of disgust are often at the forefront, perhaps when touching door handles when there is a fear that they might be dirty. In such situations I regularly experience the desire to wash my hands again and again. Sometimes it's necessary to soap and rinse them two or three times. Doorknobs or similar objects must be regularly cleaned with a wet cloth. These difficult moments are often accompanied by control and thought obsessions. After every completed task I have to check and think through every possible detail. I run the just-completed task across my mind like a dream. Only then can I consider the job completed and begin something new. This severely impairs my daily routine; the condition also has a negative effect on my dealings with other people, my leisure time and my job.

The "chemical straitjackets," better known as psychiatric drugs, are prescribed far too readily by many of our classical medical practitioners. They regularly cause serious, often permanent organic damage. I also suffer from depression and existential anxiety. Tavor was prescribed to establish inner calm and to deal with my various fears. Tranquilizers relieve anxiety and are calming, but they do not affect the depression. Anxiety and agitation were made bearable by the drugs and were thus indirectly reinforced, but through all the years the cause remained hidden. Today, now that I no longer take any psychiatric drugs my existence is accompanied by anxiety. In other words, I sacrificed twenty-one valuable years of my life hoping pointlessly for an improvement or a cure. I find myself at the beginning again and have to find a new treatment with the difference that I now refuse psychiatric drugs and will only work with a specific therapy that is suitable for me. Psychiatric drugs have caused me a great deal of mental pain and pushed me into isolation. The reward was social chaos and an inability to work, which I shall have to deal with on my own now because I am not prepared to accept this situation.

Because of my use of psychiatric drugs, my life has been characterized by a permanent sense of absence and an inner coldness. "Normal behavior" often appears quite different. Feelings, the expression in one's eyes, the general impression made and external appearance are all impaired to a shocking degree. Throughout all the years I could never develop warm-hearted feelings. I had no self-love and, of course, no love for others. I managed the first changes in this situation by founding a self-help group for people suffering from obsessions. This was the first step in a new stage of my life; but the way is still stony and long. The best medicine for the soul and the psyche of a person in my opinion is a balanced life full of love, harmony, security and recognition. The use of psychiatric drugs leads to exactly the opposite, i.e., loneliness, isolation, rejection. Those years confirmed my self-image as a loser and a failure.

What happened at the time: systematic destruction

Severe blows of fate in 1990/91/92 were the trigger for my withdrawal. After years of unemployment, my wife sued for divorce. Then began a fight to retain the home I loved. During this very difficult period I was committed to the Rheinische Kliniken (*Rhineland Clinics*), in the region where I live in Germany, at the behest of my neurologist at the time and the relevant authorities—and all without my ever indicating that I was thinking of suicide. In addition, this was undertaken using an ambulance, the police and handcuffs.

The destruction of my existence through this inconsiderate intervention took its inevitable course—systematic destruction and all perfectly legal. An experienced neurologist would not have allowed such a professional error to occur. Someone suffering from a washing obsession should under no circumstance be committed to a locked psychiatric ward, because the generally unhygienic and catastrophic state they find there can only lead to a serious worsening of their condition. Thus, for example, there is the situation of having to use the toilet and finding excrement beside the toilet bowl. There was only one toilet and therefore no way of avoiding it. Another situation was having to use—under the threat of "there'll be blows if you tell tales"—a washbasin after someone had used it to pee into. A further stressful situation was the fact that as a non-smoker and suffering from allergies, I could not get away from the smoke. In my case smoke represents another dirt factor. That the situation described here is also detrimental to other people with other diagnoses who have been forcibly committed should also be noted.

Just fourteen days on this admissions ward were enough to reduce me to a state of paralysis. The forced administration of various psychiatric drugs finished me off. My last reserves of energy were used up. It says in my discharge report: "The state of the patient has improved, in particular with respect to the washing obsession; the patient no longer appears compelled to wash his hands repetitively." This statement illustrates the ignorance of many psychiatrists: why should I wash my hands or care for my body at all when I was exposed to filth and dirt day and night. There wasn't one square foot in the whole ward that I could describe as clean. As a result, obsessive washing made no sense—the doctor simply did not listen to me and did not think of me as someone capable of thinking.

The washing obsession was only worsened by my premature psychiatric commitment and I suffered even more. During therapy the therapist gently introduces exercises which are gradually increased in difficulty but do not use force. No psychological problem was ever cured by force.

After my discharge, I was a mental wreck. It took me three years to gradually deal with the psychological chaos I found myself in. The fight with the powerful creditor mafia was too much for me after this experience, and I could not prevent the loss of my house; I simply didn't have the strength because the psychiatric drugs sapped my energy and prevented me from making decisions. The drugs were stronger than me.

Recognition and understanding

Worlds have to come crashing down before one is able to recognize one's own suffering. The specialists had failed me and I no longer trusted them. My head said: recognize your suffering and be your own therapist—help yourself, because no-one else will. So I recognized that specialists such as psychotherapists and doctors could only be my guides and teachers but could not on their own be my healer. Neither do psychiatric drugs represent a cure for me; at the most are aids to be used for a short time. The work of the doctors and the possibilities of the profession are not often understood by patients. I am my own healer, and on my road to improvement or health I can only be helped by an expert as long as I believe I need this help. The guiding help can only be a stimulant to mobilize the self-healing force in my body. This recognition is important in order to dissolve blocks to healing. From this point on I collected information on my illness and on the psychiatric drugs I had been prescribed. I looked for contact with others who had suffered as I had, and I read reports in books and journals, thus gaining in experience and knowledge and becoming my own expert in the area of obessional conditions. My decision had been made: I had to ban psychiatric drugs from my life.

Over a period of twenty-one years I had taken Saroten retard 25 mg capsules as well as Tofranil 25 mg coated tablet and Tavor 2.5 mg and Tavor 2 mg tablets. I had also been given as an experiment: Melleril, Truxal *(neuroleptic, active ingredient chlorprothixene)*, Ludiomil, Sinquan, Anafranil[1], Equilibrin[2] and Tagonis[3]. But none of these drugs changed anything. Either they had no affect at all or caused

1 Antidepressant, active ingredient clomipramine, marketed also as Clobram, Clomipramine, Clopress, Placil

2 Antidepressant, active ingredient amitriptylinoxide, apparently not currently marketed in AU, CA, GB, NZ and US

3 Antidepressant, active ingredient paroxetine, marketed also as Aropax, Aroxat, Oxetine, Paroxetine, Paxil, Paxtine, Seroxat

strong side-effects. Therefore, I was prescribed the standard psychiatric drugs until 1992.

My route to freedom

So I reduced the psychiatric drugs: withdrawal from Saroten retard capsules went easily within four weeks. The usual dose was 3 x 1 capsules per day (morning/midday/evening). Withdrawal dosage:

Week 1 and 2	2 capsules per day (morning/evening)
Week 3 and 4	1 capsule per day (morning)

I did not notice any unpleasant psychological or physical withdrawal symptoms.

The Tofranil coated tablets were withdrawn over a period of eight weeks. In this case the dose was reduced gradually to a dose of ¼ coated tablet. It was relatively simple to cut the coated tablets into halves and quarters. I placed the coated tablet on a chopping board and using a paring knife took the blade and the coated tablet between two fingers and pressed gently; it was easy. The standard dose was 3 x 1 coated tablets per day (morning/midday/evening). Withdrawal dosage:

Week 1 and 2	2 x 1 coated tablet daily (morning and evening)
Week 3 and 4	2 x ½ coated tablet daily (morning and evening)
Week 5 and 6	2 x ¼ coated tablet daily (morning and evening)
Week 7 and 8	1 x ¼ coated tablet daily (morning)

In this case too I suffered no unpleasant psychological or physical withdrawal symptoms.

Care was advisable in the case of Tavor due to the expected withdrawal symptoms. At a time when I was less experienced I tried to withdraw in a few days. The result was terrible: withdrawal symptoms occurred in the form of trembling hands and a twitch at the corners of the mouth. The latter was so severe that I had to bring spoons with liquid as well as glasses and cups to my mouth with both hands. In addition, the following occurred to an almost unbearable extent: anxiety states, inner restlessness, lack of confidence in social contacts, outbreaks of sweating, apathy, erratic blood pressure, disturbances of vision, etc.

After that I intended to carry out a very gradual withdrawal over a period of one and a half years. The usual dose was 3 x 1 tablet per day or 3 x 1 tabs (morning/midday/evening). The then new type of tablets, Tavor Tabs, made withdrawal easier because they had an notch scored in them.

The switch from the daily dose of 3 x 2.5 mg normal tablet form to 3 x 2 mg Tabs was thus the first step and was maintained for two months. Further withdrawal doses:

Month 3 and 4	4.5 mg per day	(3 x ¾ Tab morning/midday/evening)
Month 5 and 6	3 mg per day	(3 x ½ Tab morning/midday/evening)
Month 7 and 8	1.5 mg per day	(3 x ¼ Tab morning/midday/evening)
Month 9 and 10	1 mg per day	(2 x ¼ Tab morning/evening)
Month 11 and 12	0.75 mg per day	(1 x ¼ Tab morning + 1 x ⅛ Tab evening)
Month 13 and 14	0.5 mg per day	(2 x ⅛ Tab morning/evening)
Month 15 and 16	0.25 mg per day	(1 x ⅛ Tab morning)

I began with the withdrawal of Tofranil and Tavor simultaneously. No symptoms occurred at all because of the gradual withdrawal. There were no psychological or physical symptoms at all. What are sixteen months gradual withdrawal in comparison with twenty-one years of psychiatric drugs. I accepted these sixteen months willingly, and it was worth it in the end.

Nothing is impossible

I have been free of psychiatric drugs since 1994 and intend to stay so. My zest for life and the quality of my life have increased. I see many things from a different perspective, I can implement ideas, and decisions are easier. The obsession is still there but I have learned that psychiatric drugs cannot provide sufficient help. Early psychotherapy is much more promising and is not accompanied by side-effects. In contrast to many experts, a good psychotherapist always focuses on the individual case when selecting the method of treatment. And of course nothing must be done without the agreement of the patient.

In the self-help group I founded I gained further positive knowledge. The chemical substances in the psychiatric drugs cause personality changes which I discussed earlier. I can, therefore, only offer the following advice:

- collect information on psychiatric drugs and their mode of action
- collect information on the condition involved and on the possible causes of the problems
- then consider whether the time has come to start reducing the psychopharmacological treatment.

It is only then that one will start to feel emotions again and life will start to take another course—in other words "object-oriented" thinking and acting.

As a final word, two quotes from Albert Einstein: "In the middle of difficulty lies the possibility."—"In order to be a blameless member of a flock of sheep, over and above everything one must be a sheep."

It was important for me to get out of the flock. To this day I do not regret the step.

Translation from the German by Mary Murphy

Counterweights

Una M. Parker

Talking, Crying, Laughing

Neuroleptics: Haloperidol, Modecate, Stelazine / Antidepressants: Protiaden

In 1972, at the age of 37, I was taken to a mental hospital as I was behaving in ways my family found difficult to tolerate or understand, and which puzzled my GP.

I had returned from a five-day course on group dynamics, believing that I was dying, and had kept my husband awake by talking all night. The doctor came, at my insistence, very early in the morning (I was wanting to ensure that if I died, my family would not have any regrets about not having done all they could). During the rest of the weekend I felt supercharged with energy at times and felt an urge to run up and down the stairs, and did so many times. I was writing about this in a journal during the rest of the weekend, and about what had happened in the days on the course, where I had been painfully excluded from a group. In what I wrote I referred several times to schizophrenia as I tried to understand what was happening to me. I did lie down and try to rest, but did not sleep.

At the hospital on the Monday morning was seen with my husband for ten minutes (during which I lay on the floor with my feet against the wall as I was feeling very tired). Then he was seen alone and told that I was schizophrenic and they needed his agreement to treat me with ECT if I did not respond to drug treatment. I was treated with haloperidol and had seven ECT treatments. I left hospital after about a month, feeling like an empty shell and went on a short holiday with the family, but became deeply depressed and returned to hospital within a month. I was again treated with ECT (eight treatments) despite having said when I was readmitted that I did not wish to have ECT again, my resistance worn down by the psychiatrist when he found me crying three weeks after admission. (To me crying was a relief—I was feeling again after being numbed; the psychiatrist interpreted the crying as a symptom indicating a need for ECT.) I was discharged three weeks later, in October 1972, with a prescription for Stelazine[1] and Protiaden[2].

Soon I started to ask my GP when I could stop taking the drugs, but was told "We do not know what might happen if you stop taking them." This made me more cautious about it but I continued to ask on my regular visits, and dropped the Protiaden first, when my GP agreed. I had not been told of any possible adverse effects from the drugs, but did not want to be taking drugs for any longer than I had to. The hospital psychiatrist had told me that I had a biochemical imbalance, but I thought that I had a good idea of what had caused my disturbance, and that such a thing was unlikely to happen again; and I was sure that an emotional upset might well cause some "biochemical imbalance." About six months after my discharge from hospital I learned what the diagnosis had been, and soon after that my doctor agreed to try reducing the dose of Stelazine. I was taking 3 mg a day, so I reduced it by 1 mg at a time over a year to nil by mid 1974. I do not recall any withdrawal effects, but I think I felt more alive. By then I had read various books by Ronald D. Laing, Mary Barnes' story (Barnes / Berke 2002), and "I never promised you a rose garden" by Hannah Green, which had all helped in my wish to get off drugs.

Other support we had from October 1973 came from a Christian psychiatrist called Frank Lake, who used bio-energetics and Gestalt in counseling me; and when in January 1974 my husband learned about the peer counseling

---

1 Neuroleptic, active ingredient trifluoperazine, marketed also as Suprazine, Trifluoper, Trifluoperazine

2 Antidepressant, active ingredient dothiepin, marketed as Dopress, Dosulepin/Dothiepin, Dothapax, Dothep, Prothiaden

method (Re-evaluation Counseling)[1] the psychiatrist encouraged us to get into classes. He also gave us work to do together between our monthly visits to him. We saw him about four times, perhaps six.

S taught me co-counseling as he started going to classes in March 1974, and I spent many hours talking about my experiences in the hospital (especially ECT) and listening to him in return. I went away myself to a basic course in October 1974, and have been a co-counselor ever since. It has made a very great difference to me, and I think that the support I have had from regular co-counseling sessions not only kept me out of the psychiatric system but also helped me be much more effective in my life. In August 1974 we met Jerome Liss who had worked with Ronald Laing, and did psychodrama[2] with him about my experiences in hospital.

In January 1975 I had another experience at a group relations course which triggered a further episode in which I had strange beliefs, and all kinds of adventures in a waking dream that would have got the label "psychosis." This lasted a total of ten days. Stelazine and Modecate were prescribed by Frank Lake when we went to see him on the fourth day. I took one tablet of Stelazine and refused to take more. The next day I was taken to stay with K, a co-counselor, and his family for three nights to give S, my husband, a rest, and our daughters had already gone to stay with friends. K and others did what they could to get my attention out of the waking dream nightmare. I had slept only a little, but when S came with a friend to take me home, I fell asleep on the two hour drive home, and went to bed and slept when we got back, so that the doctor who called decided not to give the Modecate injection. The next day S contacted a meditator we had met the previous August; the meditator spoke to me on the phone, and recommended that I find a large stone

---

1 Re-evaluation Counseling is a way that people can learn to exchange effective help with one another, agreeing to take turns to listen to one another and to allow and encourage the natural ways of healing past hurts, by talking, crying, laughing, angry storming, trembling, and yawning. The relationship is of equals and is empowering because of that, and also because the process enables people to think more clearly. (U.P.)

2 Psychodrama allows the focus person in a group to examine some past event or aspect of her/his life by enacting it in a drama with other participants, and experiencing different roles. A director is required for this group process. (U.P.)

or a ball and rub my insteps on it. He also meditated with me in mind. Two days later I was free of delusions. I do not know whether the meditation was directly helpful; it is impossible to know, but I was aware that someone was caring about me, and I think that was important.

Five weeks later, in March 1975, I got a 20 hours a week job in a local school (not having taught since the birth of my first child in 1961). Soon I was working full time when other teachers were absent.

In August 1978 my mother died whilst I was away at a co-counseling workshop, and I went into a state again where I was not fully in touch with the reality that others were experiencing, though I had my father and brother over for a meal, and went the next day to help my father make funeral arrangements and also went with my brother to see my mother's body. That night my husband came home to be with us for the funeral, and recognizing that I was not fully present with him, spoke sharply to me, so that I burst into tears and came out of the waking dream state. No doctor had been called, and I slept that night and next day went to the funeral.

This happened during the school holidays. I returned to work in September and continued to teach full time in the same school until I took early retirement in 1991.

Now I lead workshops on mental health, and speak about the effects of ECT because I find people think that it is no longer used. It can still be given compulsorily to people who are not voluntary patients, is still given to children and young people under 18, and there are difficulties about what is "informed consent" for voluntary patients. Some people do apparently find ECT helpful, but these are probably about one third of those treated, and another one third feel it was no help, and one third consider that it has damaged them in some way. People have memory loss most commonly (even those who think it was helpful experience memory loss, but discount it), sometimes losing several years of memory, others losing weeks. Many continue to have difficulty with memory, particularly for new learning. Others lose particular abilities, such as knowledge of the alphabet and use of dictionaries, indexes, and telephone directories. Some people lose their ability to find their way about the place they live (a taxi driver was unable to carry on working because of this). Others suffer a change of personality, distressing to themselves and their families. Another very important effect is that for many there is a disastrous loss of confidence following the experience.

Occasionally I am asked to lead a training session for social workers, and work voluntarily for Mind, the forward-looking mental health organization in England and Wales. It is clear, I hope, from what I have written that I have not taken any psychiatric drugs since 1974, except for the one single Stelazine in 1975.

Nada Rath

To the Convent Instead of the Clinic

Neuroleptics: Impromen, Sigaperidol, Taxilan / Antidepressants: Saroten / Lithium / Carbamazepine: Tegretol

My own experience with psychiatry began 1990 when my son was just doing better after his experiences with psychiatry. After years of struggling with the institution of psychiatry and with mobbing at my work place, I suffered from a "paranoid response," as the psychiatrist called it. Looking back, I would now describe my condition as "powerlessness plus fear and horror in the face of an overpowering public service system and the threat of unemployment." I was fifty years old and not as productive as I had been. I was all alone as I had to cope with the stress of illness and death in the family. (My husband had an operation for a bladder tumor, and my mother and sister died during the time when M. was being pushed from one place to another in the psychiatric system.) At work no one was interested in what I had to cope with privately. The pressure increased as I became less productive.

The doctor prescribed Impromen[1] and then I was able to work another six months. A deep depression landed me in the closed psychiatric ward and I

---

1 Neuroleptic, active ingredient bromperidol, apparently not currently marketed in AU, CA, GB, NZ and US

was prescribed Saroten *(antidepressant, active ingredient amitriptyline)*. After fours weeks I entered a new day clinic where I was able to try out several kinds of psychiatric drugs. Tegretal *(mood stabilizer, active ingredient carbamazepine)* gave me a skin allergy, Taxilan *(neuroleptic, active ingredient perazine)* made me tired and sleepy, Sigaperidol *(neuroleptic, activ ingredient haloperidol)* caused restlessness and states of fear. In the end lithium was prescribed and I was able to work another year.

The feeling of being packed in a wad of cotton and of being a stranger to myself became less and less bearable. Suddenly from one day to the next I quit all drugs (lithium, the hormone L-thyroxin and the hormone compound oestrofeminal). The decisive factor that led to this was that I did not feel well at all during the period when I had been taking the medication. I lived like a robot, as if programmed to carry out certain tasks. Besides my daily tasks I had no desire nor need to undertake anything else. I slept away most of my free time. A final push to change my situation came with the recognition that I had become a machine that was used up more and more each day and thus was becoming obsolete. Rather than being afraid, I felt freed and relieved. My whole life long I had never liked taking medication. I slipped into an elevated religious frame of mind and felt as if I were guided and protected by God's hand. These high spirits were interrupted periodically by states of fear, but I was able to overcome the fear with meditation and prayer. The experiences with my son as well as the insights about my psychosis gained from my psychotherapist served me well. I accepted my condition as an alternative state of consciousness. It hardly bothered me that the doctor whom I sought out to testify to my illness diagnosed my condition as a "schizoaffective psychosis" and wrote me a referral for a psychiatric hospital. I rejected the idea and entered a convent at the recommendation of another doctor whom I trusted. She said her colleague was wrong and that I didn't belong in a psychiatric ward; she gave me Bach flower drops. I lost my job, but I had gained a new feeling of freedom and independence.

While I was in psychiatric treatment—twice in closed or half-closed wards in regular hospitals and twice in outpatient clinics—I felt that my feelings and thoughts were determined by those who were treating me because their behavior had a constant effect on me. But in the convent, something unique happened. It was during a prayer weekend during which everyone was silent; it was a special kind of silence. We took our meals together, which were ac companied with meditation music. I was a guest there. I didn't take part in the program, so I was free to occupy myself solely with my own inner being. I once heard the large group praying together outside my window; they were standing in a circle around a glowing candle. I experienced this as a prayer personally devoted to me, and I, too, began to pray. The next day I went to the library and discovered Hildegard von Bingen as my healer. From now on I was no longer alone, and I began to recognize the thoughts and feelings that came from inside me—as opposed to those originating outside of me, as I had experienced in the past. I wrote a letter to a nun, in which I described my transformation. She spoke with me and let me know that my need to inter-vene against the war then raging in my home country, Yugoslavia, was a very real need. She encouraged my to find a way to satisfy this need. From then on I directed all my thoughts toward the heavens and ask God to show me the way and to be my guide.

Hildegard von Bingen was now a sister to me, guiding me where ever I went. I felt that she touched me and healed me. It was two years before I was able to distinguish inner reality from an outer reality. Today, I no longer con-fuse my inner world with the outer world. Prayer and meditation have be-come an important part of my life. I now have a more distanced view of the war of my new home against my old home, the home that I experienced as a vision in my soul in 1990. The sight no longer makes me ill. I am now in a po-sition to be of help wherever my help is needed; I no longer take off or go searching for the "secret service" in order to intervene. Instead, I am actively engaged with different peace organizations. I keep in touch with both Ger-man and Serbian communities, and I am thus better able to unite these two different sides of myself. Instead of waiting for world peace, I am able to find my own inner peace with God. I believe in His truth and justice, and only thus am I able to bear the world that has been created by the people—or, more exactly, the politicians. They, if anyone, belong in the closed wards, rather than those people who have almost been broken by their bungled poli-tics. The church and the convent were always a refuge; today they should be more than ever for those whose souls have suffered. Since the world has been threatened by the megalomania of politicians, I have come to see psychiatry as a very good place to treat their illness—even for those politicians who have been elected according to democratic rules. But how would it be possible to have them committed involuntarily, given that they are the ones who determine the laws regarding psychiatric committal?

With this kind of an attitude, I made myself ineligible for my job with a public agency. But I gained a new feeling of freedom and independence. I sought help in individual consultations with people who were engaged with spiritual subjects, including clergy, doctors and social workers. Most important were the conversations with (ex-)users and survivors of psychiatry who had comparable experiences and a similar attitude towards the world. This helped me to overcome my feelings of loneliness. I also learned the wonderful effects of meditation, prayer and dialogs with myself. Writing became the best medicine for me. My voluntary work in the (ex-)users and survivors of psychiatry movement and later in a humanitarian aid organization for victims of war in my home country made psychiatry and its incapacitating medication obsolete for me. A network of (ex-)users and survivors of psychiatry became my social net and I feel comfortable there.

I don't miss contact with my former colleagues and friends; it was the best thing for me to integrate the recent changes into my life. After I was allowed to experience being a child and a youth again through my psychosis, I am now more mature and more composed. Since 1995 I have no longer had any psychoses; my life has become meaningful and fulfilled. The meaningless work I used to do has also brought something good with it: I now have a secure pension and can devote myself to tasks that are important to me. Above all, I am able to organize my life as I want to, without institutions or psychiatric drugs to determine the structure of my time.

Translation from the German by Mary Murphy

Katalin Gombos

From Electroshock to the Voice of the Soul

Neuroleptics: Fluanxol, Haloperidol, Imap, Piportil

My "paranoid schizophrenia" began in 1984. I had already driven myself too hard for half a year, by days I learned, by nights I worked, I had no sufficient time to sleep. Several times I collapsed, the ambulance took me to the hospital. There they did not find proper meaning in my exhausted speech and began a course of ECT. I got three shocks weekly for two and a half months. Then I was discharged with a maintenance treatment with neuroleptic drugs. I took haloperidol in various doses.

For three or four months I felt very tired, all the daytime I was sleeping. Beside that I could do some shopping and nothing else. But the real problems began when I started to work again. After being diagnosed with schizophrenia, feeling enormously tired, I did not dare to continue my job as a computer operator, and my bosses did not dare it either. "Forgetting" about my qualification, they employed me in an auxiliary position, I had to run through the town with various official papers. Then, months after my first hospitalisation and massive treatment, in 1985 I had my very first brief "paranoid" experience. Being shocked from it I went to the hospital because there was no other help available. I spent half a day there, then they sent me to the outpatient unit.

These professionals' response to my distress was a chemoshock, a combination of various neuroleptics including haloperidol in huge doses and Fluanxol[1] depot injection. Immediately I began to suffer from Parkinson symptoms. After several months my menstruation became irregular. Then, with the aid from a doctor, I withdrew haloperidol, but still received Fluanxol de-

---

1 Neuroleptic, active ingredient flupent(h)ixol, marketed also as Depixol

pot injection every three weeks. Nevertheless, I felt much better than during the haloperidol treatment 1984.

I began to study again, I was rather successful, but the effects of the psychiatric drugs made it difficult to learn. Then I was treated with Imap *(neuroleptic, active ingredient fluspirilene)* depot injection (since the imported Fluanxol was replaced with this Hungarian product, due to financial reasons) every second week. I tried to stop taking psychiatric drugs in order to improve my learning skills. A couple of months after the withdrawal I experienced frightening symptoms, I could not sleep, I could not concentrate on my diploma work and I had endless chains of symbolic ideas I could not control. I tried to write down these associations. For days I was wandering around the town, full of paranoid fears. I was hospitalized again, got a chemoshock again. I experienced failure in my life again, I felt that in spite of my good marks, I would never finish my studies as an applied mathematician. At the time I did not know about withdrawal symptoms and about rebound, I began to believe that I was really ill. After my discharge my doctor withdrew the pills and introduced Piportil[1] depot injection (25 mg). I received one 25 mg injection every six week.

My second trial to withdraw neuroleptics was in 1995, after 11 years of almost permanent treatment with neuroleptics, most of the time with depot injections. I met my future husband and he supported my trial. Our main motivation was that we wanted children and did not want to risk their future health. For half a year everything went wonderfully. I moved in with him, and in the beginning of our common life I faced new difficulties in my life. Then my sleeplessness occurred again. After a few weeks of insufficient sleep I had uncontrollable laughs. Still we did not know about rebound or delayed withdrawal symptoms and were frightened. Instead of our scheduled wedding, I went to the psychiatric hospital and postponed our marriage.

During my time in hospital my husband spent his time studying biochemistry of neuroleptics (at the university he had already studied biochemistry for two years) and we learned about the rebound effect.

---

1 Neuroleptic, active ingredient pipotiazine

After being discharged I stopped taking psychiatric drugs. By this time we learned a lot how to relate to my "paranoid" experience and uncontrolled laugh. I became his wife and more busy in an association of people with mental problems and their families. Users/survivors were a minority there and we had serious conflicts with the majority (family members and professionals). Due to an acute crisis in the board my husband became very depressed, my sleeplessness came again. Unfortunately, we could not help it and after two weeks of lack of sleep I got so tired that I began to collapse, my paranoid experiences came back. I went to another hospital, where I hoped that I found he serious mistake! Their response was another chemoshock with two months stay in the hospital. Finally I was discharged on my own responsibility. This was an important step, since then I lost my remaining illusions about the psychiatric help they could provide.

Then came important months in my life. I became more involved in self-help and together with my husband established Voice of Soul, a user/survivor only self-help association. A consciousness-raising process took place in our life. Surviving several emotional and spiritual crises together we got very close to each other. We invented various techniques to handle "paranoia." We met a herbalist who helps sleep difficulties with herbs. We made several friends whose support is invaluable to survive difficult periods of a potential rebound. Now I am much more conscious and aware of the difficulties. This is important, because one can organize the needed support only if he/she knows of the difficulties. And I hope that now this will be a long-term success.

Iris Marmotte

The "Blue Caravan," on the Road…

Neuroleptics: Haldol / Antidepressants: Aponal

When I became ill in the spring of 1991, a girlfriend, with the advice of a doctor, brought me to a hospital. I knew "something was wrong" and my outlook was pretty dismal. I can still vividly picture that day when we went to the bus together, and I thought to myself: your mother, one of your friends, and the object of your unrequited first love are sick, and now you are too. It seems important for me to make it clear that in contrast to other people whom I have met with mental illnesses, I admitted from the beginning I was ill. When I described my symptoms to the emergency room doctor in very clear, professional terminology and he replied, "schizophrenia," it was just as I had anticipated. I had feared this diagnosis for years as I felt I was becoming ill. Initially, nothing pointed to a particular problem. I was simply quite interested in various types of illnesses and was attracted to people who were not quite normal. Thus, I ended up working in the area of child and youth psychiatry. At the age of 23 I already had a great deal of responsibility for psychiatric patients and children and youths with behavioral problems, some of whom were not much younger than myself. I had to manage difficult late shifts on my own and in this way got to know the symptoms first-hand rather than only from text books. I was eventually able to recognize the symptoms in myself. Although I knew—and this knowledge was fed by the German Democratic Republic's (GDR) one-sided biologistic view of humankind—the prognosis for psychiatric patients is rather bleak, I somehow also felt certain that for me, it would not last as long as for some of the long-time patients I had known; I would get better soon!

From the beginning, I wanted to reunify my body, which had been visibly torn apart. To the pleasure of the nurses and doctors, I went jogging everyday across the Finnbahn, I did brush massages, kept myself physically fit and thus tried to stay mentally fit. I took all my medication on time, prayed, and was concerned particularly at the beginning to accomplish not only the prescribed occupational therapy but also to practice a strong work ethic as therapy. The other workers didn't notice because I had made this my own personal task. Back then I thought that if I just disciplined myself and humbly do menial labor I would become healthy again. So there I sat, sorting screws, dusted and repacked silverware or fumbled around to put something together. I felt so miserable and performed my work slower and slower. The breaks for bad coffee and a smoke were too short. The same old babble among fellow patients was unbearable and the pay was lousy. Everything reminded me of my time in prison which I had left behind me a few years ago when I was freed from the most infamous women's prison in the GDR after serving one and a half years. Yet, things seemed even more hopeless now, since there seemed to be little possibility of a change and ultimately things could only get worse. I asked myself, did you come all this way for this, risking danger and strange places, losing friends and acquaintances, only to land in prison again—this time in a psycho-prison? Inside of me things looked darker and darker and I saw no future anymore, no hope, no meaning. Within two years I had mutated into a patient who was constantly spinning through the revolving doors of the hospital. The nurses were disdainful because I neglected myself and didn't get up out of bed anymore, not for breakfast, for our morning walk, or for any kind of therapy. It got so bad that my hair became matted from too much lying around and it had to be cut; after that they got a nurse to wash me. During the course of my wash-down my question was always the same: "Will things ever get better for me?" The nurse, who was younger than me, laughed optimistically: "But of course, Mrs. Marmotte." I wanted to believe her but couldn't. As a nurse, I knew this was the only possible response she could give to such a question.

When I got out again, I sat in my kitchen in front of the water-faucet, thirsty yet unable to pour myself a glass of water. I could not bite into the bread that had become stale and hard. The supermarket was not far away, but I couldn't manage to go. I wished I were simply dead so I would have some peace at last. I was broken by my illness. I saw it as a punishment for two dark points in my life. Worst of all was the vicious circle of endlessly recurring psychotic patterns of thought. I tried again and again to think of something else even for just a moment—but it didn't work. My thoughts always revolved in the same circles, a hundred times a day, sometimes at a time-loop tempo in slow motion, other times constantly accelerating until my brain was spinning. That was hell for me, the devil's game. I felt damned and abandoned by God with no hope of salvation. I could do nothing but suffer through this film, my life, lying down. I knew that I had to learn to have faith again, but I couldn't, and so I tried to end my life.

When I was brought to the hospital again, my friend couldn't visit me anymore. We didn't have anything to say to each other as I angrily thought to myself: Not even she can remain faithful to me. This idiotic psychosis was able to do what the Stasi *(secret police)* couldn't accomplish with their long interrogations: to alienate us and play us out against each other. *Why? And how?* I could make no sense of it. I ran around the ward in circles, always in the same pattern, very tense, always with the same questions in my head: *What if… and if you only had…*Especially at night, I marched around, but also afternoons while the others sat in front of the television or slept, engaged in their senseless discussions about relationships, or blamed this "shitty society" or more often their "shitty parents" for their illness. I saw it all differently. I thought about various points, but came to the conclusion that if society was responsible, I would have gone crazy before while in prison or in the GDR. And the misery of my family situation? What can you expect and who can you blame if your was ill herself and nonetheless had to work so hard? If anything, bad genes were to blame, and I didn't want to pass them on to another generation. I also noted that so many people had a false image of themselves. They felt as if they were unrecognized geniuses who should have earned Nobel prizes, but ultimately they had nothing better in mind than to satisfy their urges as fast as possible with the least amount of effort and, of course, cheaply! And all the while they had no idea where they were headed each time. They celebrated themselves as true human beings with ideals and souls who were better than those who were consumption-oriented; they quarreled and tricked each other, scrounged through, and thought themselves smart—yet they were not able to keep even the smallest goal in sight long enough to reach it.

I didn't want to grow old with them! Of course, there were exceptions; I am only describing that which helped me to recognize what I wanted even if I felt at the time that I didn't know anything anymore. In the meantime I had gained weight quickly due to the medication, weighed double my original weight, couldn't get up the stairs anymore or think a sentence through to its end, couldn't occupy myself with anything except my own misery. And so I was brought to a ward for chronic patients where they teach you the basics again—things like tying a shoe and getting dressed. Imagine that, after having studied and even having worked as a tutor! Then I knew for sure: "This is it for the rest of your life. It's a long one—the statistics say another 40 years

—that's a life sentence!" My girlfriend didn't want me to go, she asked lots of questions, asked me if I really wanted to go there. I said it's really all the same where I lie around. She asked me once again later: "Do you really want to stay here, running around looking so ruined? Is this what we survived the prison for? Is this what we envisioned for us when we were young?" I gave a stubborn answer: "Yes, leave me here. What should I do out there? Out there you're the lowest of the low, here you fit in and are taken care of, I get my meals, and I don't have to worry about the rent and the authorities. This is the only form of freedom I have left." We didn't see each other any more after she left with the words: "Good, then I won't come for awhile." She had to look out for herself for a time because she was taking exams, she was pregnant, had a job, and her mother was terminally ill.

Life went on in all respects, but I was caught in a vacuum. When some caregivers showed up to ask if I would be interested in a sheltered community where I would receive care, I thought this was a fine idea. Much later, I found out that my girlfriend had arranged for them to try to convince me to leave the chronic ward; she just couldn't accept that I was living there—for her it was the "end of the road." She had enough professional experience in psychiatry to know there was little hope of a recovery in the chronic ward, a place of bottled up misery and "cases" that had been given up on. In order to live in the community, I first had to take a kind of test to be accepted there. I found it grotesque that even here there were tests one had to pass. Later, I learned that they had accepted a punk with a rat before me, but because she only stayed for one night, I had been accepted as their second choice.

At first I kept a certain distance to the others living there. They didn't read, they were trivial, uneducated and dependent upon alcohol, cigarettes, and coffee—primitive. One could see right away they were losers and they always had been. And me? No one liked me anymore either, no one could see my joy in life and my competence; I had never wanted to turn out like *this*. I slept a lot, and the caregivers had to come get me for the daily meetings. It was torture getting through them, and I had to vomit regularly, because of the pills and because my life disgusted me. I constantly struggled with heartburn, salivation, stomach aches, difficulty swallowing, and restlessness—it was not really what I would call living. Early in '93, I had to go to the clinic again but did not stay as long as before.

In May of '94 I tried to stop taking my medication from one day to the next, despite the warnings of the caregivers. I wanted to get better *right away*, to mobilize all my energy—and the pills only paralyzed me. My old fighting spirit had been reawakened. I thought it would be easy, I was optimistic, and I was happier.

My doctor always told me there must be a counterweight in my daily life in order to be able to withdraw gradually from the pills. What kind of daily activities did I have? Not many. Sure, I had appointments, but they were only appointments. My contention that I couldn't be active as long as the pills kept slowing me down didn't convince the doctor.

I finally was experiencing a good phase, and I wanted to make use of it. It was May, a time to awaken and begin anew, and I had been living in the community for some time now.

I left my bed to do the shopping, fed myself on cans of beer and broiled chicken from the grill around the corner—I was hungry for them every day. I heard my friend had just given birth and I even made it to the hospital with a bouquet of roses for her. I was able to think coherently again across larger spans of time and space. But, I became nervous again and smelt bad. When my girlfriend celebrated her birthday, a few days after giving birth, exhausted from the birth and with a sleeping baby next to her, I went to celebrate, but ended up spoiling her party. I had to leave again after the cake, because, I had fits of crying and couldn't control myself. Seeing her moved me so much, I had not experienced such an emotional reaction in the past years since my body had become a lifeless robot. The problems had come again four or five weeks after I stopped taking the pills. I thought I had my life under control—I was somewhat manic, having arranged one appointment after the other with psychologists and therapists listed in the telephone book or by recommendation from acquaintances; and then the endless phone calls with my insurance to find out which therapies and therapists they would pay.

In short, I had done everything possible to get my body fit again, to feel something down there because this seemed to be missing thus far in my recovery. But then, the moment I wanted to proudly show off my cleaned and straightened room to one of the caregivers, I suddenly couldn't remember any more what it was that I had so desperately wanted to show her.

It was immediately apparent that my withdrawal from the pills had not worked and the caregivers were right about a grace period of four to six weeks until the problems would come again.

My condition: short of breath, fearful of suffocating, panting, restlessness, inability to sit still, autistic movements, disjointed thoughts, lack of orientation, jumps in thought, a racing heart, laughing and crying simultaneously, pressure in my chest and heart, nausea and vomiting, sores caused by stress, eating problems, lack of appetite, fear of falling or fear that the earth would drop away or open up when I walked—all of this was back again. In addition, I had difficulties concentrating and remembering things. I didn't understand what the caregivers had just said to me and had to ask them to repeat it again and again. My surroundings disappeared in milky or dark shadows, but mostly, they were flooded in light until they came into focus again. I was taken to the doctor immediately and given a high dosage depot shot. I raced the whole way there with my caregiver, holding tight to my bicycle, all the while crying and swearing at the fact that you can't get around being insane, not by praying nor by working nor with clear goals and desires, and suicide is not an option for ending the nightmare. It was a torment.

But, I still knew who I was. We had had positive experiences together as a community, always pulled together, cooked often. And independently of the caregivers, we supported each other and dealt with our own problems like everyone else does. Back then I tried to create the sense that we unfortunates could also have a normal life, for example, by having a "Sunday roast," "Birthday parties," an "Easter/Christmas dinner." I cooked more and more often, mostly casseroles or meat balls, which everyone loved including the guests who sometimes showed up for dinner. I also let a fellow soul share my small room with me for a few months—without the knowledge of the caregivers, but with the blessing of the other community members.

Later, I cared for the garden: hoeing, planting, watering and digging. That was satisfying. I had the most fun with my favorite community member, an original character who was a big kid at heart and a former sailor. He understood me and could make me laugh with his tall tales, his weird philosophical thoughts that always ended with little aphorisms. I liked to read to him and cook for him when he asked me to. I could make his big eyes twinkle, and when his stomach was full he would say, "And now we'll pump the globe 'til it's empty!" I knew he had never had a home nor a real childhood. I was increasingly annoyed with the caregivers and their language and gestures; they never saw the source of our problems but rather "addressed" problems we didn't have. We had many arguments with them.

Around that time, I began taking the train, then the bus to visit my girlfriend who now lived in the countryside—a trip that was exhausting for me, but also good training. She had moved because her room had been too small for her and the child, she was overburdened, the father wasn't helping out, and also because she felt cut off from cultural life. I said to myself: Ok, if you can't help yourself anymore, if there's no real life out there for you, then you can at least devote your life to being of service to your girlfriend and her child. Even if I couldn't do a lot, at least I could push the baby stroller around the countryside so she could have some rest and time for herself.

During my last stay in the hospital I had met a new friend with a fate similar to my own. She had spent much time visiting me in the community. We would lie in bed or sleep arm in arm, talk about earlier times and about our professors, what kind of women we had been then and how we had looked. We showed each other the clothes we had outgrown and old photos, and we talked about everything including heavy philosophical topics that were inherent to our depression.

We ate and drank together, she was my soul-mate in suffering with whom I shared everything. I went to the movies for the first time again with her, and she let me talk her into going shopping for shoes with me, because, I knew she needed some in order to take her first new steps. Later, we would go to our favorite bar where we would spend the entire night, because, we couldn't sleep anyway. They served warm meals at any time of day. It was a bar for gay men, and that was good for us. She had more problems with men than I did, but there, we felt they accepted us and didn't bother us. We had our best conversations there, exchanging information about our earlier studies and experiences or about the books we were currently reading. I told her about my weekend with my other friend and her family, about the music I listened to, and about what I thought of the caregivers and the community. We were often very distanced from things or laughed a lot and were quite cynical. I think we developed some kind of an identity for ourselves. We may have looked like slobs, wearing the same t-shirt and not washing for weeks. This didn't bother us, we were free of superficialities. We knew no one else would like us this way and we would never live as a normal man and wife couple with children and money. For us there were other standards, we lived as if in a carnival and devoted ourselves to whatever seemed important at the moment.

In addition, we also talked about death—we had even wanted to commit suicide together at one point earlier. When I visited her at the intensive care unit and they noticed that I was psychotic too, one of the nurses—a father-like figure—pulled me aside to speak with me. He asked me what we were hoping to accomplish with this. I said: "We want to get out of this living hell and be with God." He answered that he had seen so many lives end here and God was not over there, but right here. A Bible passage occurred to me as he said this: "You should search for Me not among the dead but among the living." I had heard this many times in church, but this time it struck me. From then on we decided we should accept life because it is probably much harder to die, than to accept the life one has. We didn't try any more experiments. Our lives consisted of eating and drinking beer at the "Beehive" and talking about the past and present. At least then we were no longer lying in bed. The taxi driver who took his breaks at 4 a.m. at the bar would drive us home.

That would kill another evening. We would then sleep until the caregivers came to get us up, we went shopping and then read whatever we felt like reading. Thus the weekdays passed.

The weekends were like another world for me—more like a normal life. My girlfriend cooked good food—she didn't use any canned food—and thus my thoughts also had better "nourishment." I wandered about the countryside with her child Diogenes, regardless of snow or rain or shine. I felt responsible and needed. And, if I couldn't keep walking, I parked the stroller somewhere and waited until the agreed upon time to return, so that my friend still had the time off. I even developed a certain ambition about staying outside as long as possible. Ambition?! Now, that was something I hadn't experienced in a long time.

I watched Diogenes growing up, I experienced nature again and the change of seasons. I didn't feel like an evil alien who was locked out of nature's cycle. There was a purpose for venturing out that was bound to something beyond my self. A living being connected me to a life with tasks and a structure, making me tired and satisfied at the end of the day. I didn't worry so much about my own fate anymore, because this created meaning for me beyond painting yet another silk scarf or weaving another basket that no one needed anyway.

This was how I spent the first half of 1994. Then in the summer I heard my psychiatrist was planning a three-week trip through the former GDR with patients and professionals who were interested in the subject "Border Crossings." The tour was to be on a "Wüstennarrenschiff" *("desert ship of fools")* called The Blue Caravan that would travel along the Elbe River, the Middle Land Canal, and the Weser River. Without hesitation, I decided to go. The Blue Caravan (like the blue of the Romantics)—it sounded like a fantastic fairy-tale; I imagined the ship to be a blue camel that could float on water. It was to sail through my former home, where I was previously not wanted nor allowed to reenter even before my illness began. For me this was indeed a "border crossing" in various ways. It harbored the possibility of something wonderful and interesting, but also had a purpose, namely to support others, gather new perspectives from people who are different, create something new together, and direct the public's attention toward "an ever-growing minority" (Dr. Pramann)—a minority of the sick, handicapped, unemployed, foreigners, welfare recipients, all those searching for something, i.e. those people who have been designated "crazy" due to their skewed position in relation to social norms, lifestyle norms and the work ethic. The "crazy" are the ones who don't fit in with these norms and who haven't found a place in the market economy, those who live in poverty despite a supposed high standard of living, those who are hated by the majority of society: social parasites, the asocial, cripples, idiots, foreigners. Here's where I felt I fit in. A Christian-humanist project—after all, I, too, belonged among the "lepers." The past few years I had not known any normal people anymore; everyone I knew had somehow been burned.

Despite all my enthusiasm, I was still afraid I might not be able to handle the trip. Too many people, too many different places to stay overnight, the timing of the trip would not suit my problems. Just to get myself to move my fat body around, to hold out, and at the same time to take my pills regularly (for the past 6 months my dosages had diminished to 10–0–25 mg Aponal *(antidepressant, active ingredient doxepin)* and evenings 1 mg Haldol). I wanted to keep this dosage at all costs to avoid a repeat of my condition in June. For the first time in years I was going on an adventurous trip. The backpack I had carried throughout Europe during my travels was no longer going to hang idle in the hospital; instead it would be honored again. It was now bursting at the seams. I was very excited. This trip would suit my identity as a "wanderer" who knew the streets and the nights and nature.

I never thought I would be allowed something like this again. I sat happily in the bus that took us to Leipzig. One of the social workers told me she had taken her final exams with one of my favorite professors and she had liked him very much. For years as I lay in bed, I still remembered his beautiful, interesting lectures, his charm and his talent for speaking with all manner of people. I imagined he would be very sad to hear what had become of me. I would have given anything to be able to sit in one of his lectures again, happy amd healthy. Everything this social worker had before her in life I, unfortunately, already had behind me. But I had glimpsed a sign of life from my professor again, and this cheered me the rest of the bus trip. Much of what I had learned from him went through my mind again later on the ship—including his lectures on the "Narrenschiff" *("The Ship of Fools,"* original 1494) by Sebastian Brant that was full of fools from "Foolsland." I was very aware that we, too, were on a ship of fools and that back then it hadn't gone so well for them. And I knew this was not just literature, it was also a metaphor and a premonition of the later journeys to concentration camps, to ill-reputed clinics, to death.

I couldn't stand people who desired to live a ready-made, normalized, and therefore rubricated, administered life. I was more interested in exotic people; normal, average people were dull. Maybe I didn't even understand what that is—normal—and thus only saw the terrifying aspect of it. One of the artists whose photo I had seen in the conference program in Leipzig interested me enormously. In the photo he had long, stringy hair, bad teeth, big, wide-open eyes—and a curriculum vitae to match. I wanted to know if he had arrived yet, so I asked one of the organizers how I could recognize him in the crowd. She laughed and said, "You'll recognize him right away—he's impossible to miss!" I spoke with the others in Leipzig about him and noticed they all liked him, too and even worried about his alcohol consumption. My interest was peaking. I went to the Leipzig stadium to get some water for our tent and asked a long, thin man with a watch-cap who was coming out of the restroom if it were free. He didn't understand my question, even though I repeated it several times. As he walked away irritated, I got a glimpse of his teeth and knew it was him.

I lost him in the crowd, but I knew we would see each other again. I walked around the stadium but none of the events really interested me until I wandered into a tent. This is what I saw: a tall, thin man who looked like a thief; a half-grown woman with a tambourine, violin, flute and drum; a strong, fat woman with a shaved head in a dark, flowing gown with a big drum; a cute black woman in a wheelchair whose leg had been amputated and who was playing the flute; and a banjo player. The tent had been made into a den-of-thieves and they were all thieves. They sang about anarchy, for example, "The thieves from the Bohemian Forest" about a journeyman tailor who had tricked the devil. I was fascinated. The audience wanted an encore. I could have watched forever. And when he put his long arms around his people to say farewell to the audience, you knew this was not a pose, but a true gesture that went beyond the average musician's etiquette. This image of a "family" so impressed me that tears ran down my face. I was spellbound as I watched them packing their things together and wasn't able to leave, because I wanted to stay and meet the "Leipzig Riff Raff." My soul already belonged to them. Was there ever a family to which I felt I belonged during all those years in the East, in the West, among the psychotics? No, I had siblings who were eleven years younger, but they had other worries and desires I did not share. Living in a family was something that had been difficult for me, even before my illness, though I had tried again and again and was always disappointed. Did I ever have a mother? No, mine was far away and had no idea how fat and sick I had become, or how I thought about things. It wouldn't have helped anyway. I hadn't seen or spoken to her in five years, not even a phone call.

Did I have a father? A spiritual father in the East and one in the West, but I had no regular contact with them. I couldn't simply show up, I'd have to plan a train ride and arrive for office hours with an academic question in mind. In short, I found my family to be the "Leipzig Riff Raff." There, I had siblings of different skin colors, a mother who worked as an artist, but also had children, kept up with a household, and cared for other children as well. I had a father whom I was able to tell everything and whom I could trust. And, there was even another father: the first husband of my mother who was lying in bed paralyzed, but able to paint beautiful pictures and who called himself the "father" of several children from other fathers, and who even tolerated, in addition to a dog, my mother's alcoholic live-in lover whom she also took care of. But nonetheless, there were financial problems. Enough money could hardly be raised by playing music in the streets, an occasional concert, show, poetry reading or theater project in order to pay for the doctor's appointments, operations and other medical expenses for a daughter who had cancer. Money was also short for cigarettes, alcohol, Rebecca's saxophone lessons, or just for basic living expenses. I knew about financial problems from the time of my childhood as well as from the time of my illness. I also had a mother who played the violin and a little nephew who was mulatto.

Perhaps this family was exactly what I had been missing and searching for without even being aware of it. It suited me. That's why I was even more excited when Jens-Paul and a musician from the Caravan accompanied us to the markets and helped us attract attention for our camel Wüna. At first, I was embarrassed that Jens-Paul was always listening nearby during the interviews about my illness, because at that point, we had not yet had closer contact. When one of the caregivers asked me at the bar one night what I liked best about the project, I answered: "Jens-Paul."

He asked, "Does Jens-Paul know that?" and I replied, "No, I don't have the nerve to say it; we don't know each other that well." Then he said to Jens-Paul as they were drinking beer, "There's a handicapped woman who would like to meet you." I overheard this and got so angry that he called me handicapped I got into a quarrel with him near the restrooms. He said he didn't understand what I was talking about, that's not what he really said, etc. I was so hurt, above all because, he couldn't understand how it made me feel.

I suggested, for example, what if he were in the same situation as me and I told the woman he was interested in that he's handicapped—that would destroy all chances of being treated fairly by her. He didn't seem to understand my analogy. I was so angered and hurt that I wanted to show him and everyone that I intended to become healthy, attractive, and competent right then during the Caravan project.

My problems began with my forgetting my pills, but got worse when there was no quiet place for me to sort my daily dosages into the small boxes to be taken at different times of the day. In addition, I didn't want to get ill. I wanted to stay strong and fit in order to show the caregivers who I really was. The idea of having to prepare my pills like a sick woman—let alone having them prepared by that particular caregiver—was not acceptable. I wanted to live, to be healthy, to amuse myself and to be interesting and worthy of love. It was possible for me without having to make a big fuss. I was able to gather the TV crews around me and make them see in me a figure among the Blue Caravan with whom everyone could sympathize. I convinced people at the markets that one is not necessarily dumb, because one is mentally ill. I drank all night long with Jens-Paul, I even out-drank him. I then sat down along the Weser River with only the moon staring at me, and I finally felt happy again.

Often the Caravan would only stay in one place for two hours before moving on. I met so many different kinds of people with whom I had discussions or danced with, like I hadn't done for years. I defended to the teeth the lifestyle of Jens-Paul in a discussion with a sheltered, bourgeois student from Ottersberg, and I never asked for help from one of the caregivers. Caregivers were a fact of life I knew all too well from the past. Instead, I made an arrangement with another woman whom I had met during the Caravan that we would take care of each other in the case that either of us had a psychotic episode during the trip. We promised each other we would leave the ship and find a quiet place under a tree and there decide what needed to be done—without the help of a caregiver. Having found a partner who was on the same wavelength, gave me a feeling of security during the trip. I also met and spent time with a bubbly journalist, whom I later introduced to my community in Bremen. I enjoyed her childlike expressions as we listened to the tales along the way and thus, understood the motto of the Caravan literally: "Everyone may join in." No one knew how many people had joined the project, not even those who managed the youth hostels along the way. I loved the chaos and the funny situations that grew out of it. I was of course there for every show my "father" performed in.

After the trip, there were only a few remaining hours with the project members and Jens-Paul and his family in Bremen. I was becoming more and more sad, because I realized how much I loved them, and also that I may never see them again. I didn't want to say anything because I thought it might hurt or possibly annoy someone. I cried as I lay on the riverbank, but I wanted to take action instead because one thing was clear: How will the others ever know how much they are loved if they are not told in this lifetime? The tip that led me to finally say this came from the girlfriend with whom I had spent so much time in the "Beehive" bar last year and who now seemed much healthier than back then. It was something I had to do on my own, however, and only after a lot of grumbling was I able to get myself to do it. It was the most difficult thing I did during the Caravan project.

Jens-Paul and his girlfriend understood my gesture. To thank me, he took me in his arms and invited me to visit them in Leipzig. He wrote "It doesn't have to end!" on the CD he gave me and then his address. That was the most beautiful reward for this difficult task I had accomplished, and now I knew where I could find my "family" and I was invited to visit them.

Now it was up to me to have enough trust to take up the offer. After the Caravan, I was able to keep up the wonderful feeling of joy. At the monthly meeting with my psychiatrist, he was not at all happy I had once again simply stopped taking my pills without gradually tapering them off. He had learned from experience that during a vacation things first seem to go well and some people decide they won't take their pills, only to find they will need a double ration later. I was not afraid, however, and became so active I was able to make true what I had told a journalist before we parted. He had asked me, "And what will happen next for you?" I said, "I think something new will begin." One month later I was elected to the board of the newly formed project "Nachtschwärmer" *("Night-Revelers")*. I was responsible for correspondence with prospective members, sending invitations, putting up posters, calling the authorities, preparing for the bi-monthly meetings, group discussions, and PR in schools, hospitals, health centers and associations for relatives of the mentally ill.

Life seemed to call out to me from everywhere. I traveled a lot—to see, for example, the "Leipzig Riff Raff"—and consequently, I started losing weight and was invited to many different places. Others in my community also started withdrawing spontaneously from their medication, which meant the caregivers saw me as the ring-leader. I replied, "I've heard that before." I was now well again, there was no task for them anymore. I had held a mirror up to them in which they became more aware of the true nature of their work in the community. The next argument we had confirmed this, as we couldn't agree upon the simplest facts. I wanted to know what kind of an understanding of human beings these caregivers had such that they are incapable of negotiating in situations in which most people with a healthy attitude toward others know that negotiation is necessary. They seemed, in contrast, to "make an issue" of everything that is otherwise self-evident. I never got an answer on this, because, in a one-on-one conversation I was asked to move out; the reason for this they gave was they were of the opinion I was healthy.

I was healthy after six months of having quit my medication—healthy and full of contagious vitality. Yet, I was still not sure if I could make it in an apartment on my own. I received help from my new friend from the Caravan who had decided shortly after the trip to move to Bremen and was now looking for a better apartment. We already spent a lot of time together, so we started looking for a place together and found one in a familiar neighborhood. We looked out for each other because our promise from the Caravan journey still held. We kept an eye on her hair loss and my bad skin, as well as her extended hours at the typewriter during which I had to remind her to eat by calling her for a warm meal. She noticed when I had stress sores or when I got hyperactive, and I massaged her feet for hours. Sometimes we would prepare a bath with lemon balm in order to calm down or to "bathe the soul," or we drank tea together or maybe a bottle of beer or wine.

I learned from her to look after my own health and take seriously any signs of stress (herpes, cold sores, hair loss, skin problems, never-ending colds). We realized at some point that the many purported friends going in and out of our apartment were not really friends nor available to us and that it was time to clean out our "nest." This meant we no longer offered free, warm meals to these people, and those who exploited our home as a cheap place to get warm were also no longer welcome to come. I didn't miss them, because they only stole time from us. We used the time more constructively for meeting with our "Die Therapie-Resistenten" *("Therapy Resistant")* group, which was a music group made up of various personalities, all of whom had experience with psychiatry. They simply liked to make music and have fun together, as well as to engage in projects without therapists for guidance. Of course, people still came and went within the group. After all, if a group could not establish a good working relationship, then small or big events were impossible to plan. I enjoyed the process very much. I was finally able to do the kinds of things I had wanted to do when I was younger, but was prevented from doing by circumstances in my life. Today we are a group of five people who meet regularly for rehearsals and we are lucky enough to have a space and drinks provided for free. Sometimes we invite guests to our group as well.

It is amazing to see the many different situations and contexts we have invented for our rehearsals, for example, imagining that we are doing a live show in a studio, etc., and how we have learned to improvise, especially when someone is sick. We try to involve people who fear they will never get a job, or who have lived on welfare or social security for years, but nonetheless, are talented musicians or otherwise active in private circles. I am proud we have held together for three years now. I love to research the older texts we use, combining them with new texts or making something new out of them through music, song and a kind of acting up in response to them. I was fortunate to be able to attend a QiGong course at the AOK *(general public heath insurer)* taught by an excellent teacher, where I learned a means of confronting psychosis with the body. Shortly after leaving my community, I also returned to an activity I had participated in during my studies, namely, working at the Red Cross. I applied to volunteer at the AWO *(Arbeiterwohlfahrt, a charity organization)* in my neighborhood. For me this work was very satisfying because I was able to do something concrete. For so many old people who didn't have anyone any more, my visits were so important and made them happy. This work also gave me a glimpse of many different ways of living and interacting with others, and it distracted me from my own problems. Sometimes it was physically and mentally exhausting, but most of the time I enjoyed it. I got to travel all over the city in all different seasons regardless of the weather; I was even invited to some of the grannies' birthday parties. In addition, at the urging of my friend from the "Beehive" days I decided to fulfill my dream of going back to college. With the help of medication, she had even been able to finish her masters degree—and this inspired me. Since leaving the community I had been able to support myself without welfare, and thus I was able to enroll again at the university with full student status. I finally saw my old professor again. He said to me, "You haven't changed a bit—it's just like old times." Of course, when I came to his office to discuss the topics for my exams, he asked me why I hadn't been back for so long. He had heard from a friend of mine that I was very ill and he wanted to know what illness I had had. I was not ashamed as I handed him the letter I had written to Peter Lehmann Publishing describing what had happened to me in the past five years.

As the semester took its course, my professor was at first very distanced. But gradually, we restored our familiar old working relationship. After a successful semester, I had the courage to sign up for my exams. The only problem I had was that I was often very tired and fell asleep over my books. Today, I work as a substitute nursing assistant in a hospital. In addition, I do work in the area of pedagogy in a residence for the mentally ill, and I still take care of a few grannies, though not as much as previously. I convinced my father from the East to move to Bremen, and he now lives in my neighborhood. I live together with my brother, slovenly but harmoniously. I can withstand living with pressure and stress, and I have few problems. I have not needed to go to my psychiatrist since 1995, but I still see him at the lobbying lunch every Friday in the Café "Blau." The rifts in my body have closed up and my sexuality has returned. My exams will soon be completed. The medication I still kept for emergencies—10–10–25 mg Aponal and 5–5–5 Haldol—expired in 1997. I never needed to take them. I didn't realize it, but what I needed was perhaps a family instead. In Bremen I have established that and now I feel at home here. I find it most difficult to part with egocentrism because it is inherent to the illness.

I was lucky to have had a true identity before the psychosis set in, which I was able to hang onto. Also important, was that I had a girlfriend who loved me, who was honest with me and who didn't desert me even when I almost made her sick, too. I was also lucky to have lived in the community with a roof over my head and less to deal with alone. I was fortunate enough to have no real problems with addiction, and I had a revelation leading to a concrete and realistic goal during the Caravan. I had the luck of finding Dr. Pramann, a doctor who does not just prescribe pills but who is a well-meaning skeptic, who takes up the challenge with his patients. I thank him for this, as well as my "family" and friends. It is my wish that you may read this report and find hope for yourself and/or for your family.

Translation from the German by Christina White

Harald Müller

Twenty Years Later

Antidepressants / Lithium / Tranquilizers: Valium

Today is January 2, 1998, one of the most important days in my life and one that I celebrate like a kind of birthday. Tomorrow the friends who have accompanied me through the past twenty years will visit me. Twenty years ago today I stopped taking psychiatric drugs and have never taken a single medication since then that has an effect or a side-effect that alters consciousness or mood. Before that, I had a thirty year "career" of medication use (or to be exact: abuse) that can best be described as iatrogenic, that is, an addiction that was brought on by a doctor's prescription.

It began with medication for migraines and pain killers. My night-time panic attacks caused severe insomnia such that I also "had to" take large quantities of sleeping pills every night for fifteen years. In addition, there was the then-new Valium and later the whole spectrum of benzodiazepines as well as antidepressants including lithium. I always had doctors who were well informed and who provided me with the necessities and the latest drugs. All my attempts to quit during those years ended in failure. Over time I needed more and more and "stronger" pills.

By the end, the fatty degeneration of my liver was like that of an alcoholic, and I had kidney problems and problems with absorbance. There was no iron left in my sternum, and my intestinal tract was becoming unable to absorb the medication so by the end I had to take shots. I was unable to work by the time I was forty years old due to migraines, depression and insomnia (which was ultimately caused by the medication misuse). Then I reached a point where I had to make a decision: either I would die from the medication, or I would dare to attempt withdrawal—against the advice of all my doctors, who warned me of a massive danger of suicide should I withdraw.

Shortly after Christmas in 1977 I entered a hospital run by the German federal employee insurance company which was recommended to me as "progressive." The head physician advised me to quit my medications on January 1. When I went by the nurses' station on my ward, I saw that my old dose had been put into the pill container for my room. When I reminded the nurse that I had stopped taking medication, she excused herself for having made a mistake. A few days later, I went by the medication dispensary again and saw my pill container was full again. I got angry and complained about the "sloppiness." Later I found out that this was done with all patients in rehabilitation: they could interrupt their withdrawal at any time without a word being said about it. The logic behind this was that anyone who was unable to voluntarily quit in the supportive atmosphere of the hospital would be certain to slip up once they were at home. In that case, it would be better to never begin a withdrawal in the first place.

In the first four weeks I slept two hours a night at the most, and during the day I was also unable to sleep. At night I ran through the stairwells on all seven floors of the hospital because I couldn't stand it in my room. During the day I walked around or went swimming a lot in the hopes of making myself physically tired.

In this hospital I became aware that the withdrawal was only the beginning. From then on the psychological problems that had led to my symptoms—migraines, insomnia and depression—became more visible again. While still at this hospital I applied for a place at a renowned hospital for psychosomatic medicine, knowing they had a long waiting list. I was accepted very quickly and entered therapy there for ten months. Success was, however, very limited.

In those thirty years of medication abuse, I had not developed at all. I needed at least ten years of intensive confrontation with myself to make up for those years. In particular, I had to find out the causes of my symptoms and then get rid of them.

When I look back today at the last twenty years, the first thing I feel is thankful. The richness and value of my life without psychiatric drugs is so great it cannot be measured. My depression has been gone completely for the past eight years. I have migraines perhaps three times a year for which there are clear, massive reasons. The periods free of fear and thus with normal patterns of sleep are getting longer and longer.

But, the price of all this was high! On several occasions I was within a hair's breadth of suicide. In the first years after withdrawal my life was a torturous hell without any glimmer of light. If I had known what was coming I may not have even tried to withdraw. For this reason, I could never make an unqualified plea to someone else to quit their medication. You've got to have a lot of courage, endurance, toughness and persistence. Most of those I've known in the past twenty years who were dependent upon medication did not succeed with withdrawal because they were "compelled" by their old symptoms. I unfortunately had no role models from whom I could have learned or who could have given me courage to continue along my way.

Self-help groups were very important to me. Emotions Anonymous (EA), however, was not very helpful. About half the members there have been prescribed psychiatric drugs by their doctors. They therefore reacted very negatively—from a lack of understanding to outright aggression—to my chosen route of abstinence. NA (Narcotics Anonymous) was somewhat helpful, but there were rarely others there who were dependent upon medication. I learned a lot at AA; I experienced sobriety and recovery there. The spiritual twelve-step program of AA was (and still is) one of the most reliable foundations for my recovery. This had to do with my recognizing a power greater than myself (a higher power, God) and anticipating help from it for my recovery.

The details of my route out of addiction to medication are beyond the boundaries of this contribution; I would have to write an entire book to tell that story. Helpful for me was the indescribable pressure of my suffering at the end of my long career of medication that ultimately pushed me to attempt withdrawal. In the first years of my being clean it was important for me to guide others through their withdrawal in hospitals; under no circumstances did I want to have to repeat that process myself again!

In this way, the memory of my own withdrawal was preserved. The fifty years of my experiences with and without psychiatric drugs can be summed up in one sentence: There is a way!

Translation from the German by Christina White

Gerda Wozart
Adversities

Tranquilizer: Tranxilium

For many years I was chasing after an image of myself created by the environment around me. I complied, I was very active, never tired and with arms wide-open I flew towards other people, took them up, took them in with a glow, carried their burdens and cooked for them.

The autumn began to creep into my bones, a little more every year, and with it darkness, mourning, homesickness for a place inside of me, a fear of death, a death wish-life and air were seeping out of me. The nights sat like great burdens on my chest, fantasies of having a heart attack made me shudder, and I feared a self-fulfilling prophecy. It became difficult to make it through the day with ease. My large family (and in addition my husband's office in our home) should not be punished for my weaknesses, I thought to myself. My guilty conscience began a hopeless spiral out of which I thought I would never be able to escape.

A latecomer was on the way. I showed the whole world with my pregnancy, my swelling belly, my (thereby proven) youth, my light-footedness (despite my heavy body). I embodied the complete opposite of other pregnant women's whining and tales of suffering—it was me against the rest of the world! This, too, was the living out of a self-fulfilling prophecy, but in a positive form. Living like day and night.

Small annoyances had crept up again and again in the past years that I had not taken very seriously: intestinal cramps, stomach problems, infections of the esophagus, etc. When I informed my doctors, they responded by prescribing me sedatives. I was actually happy about this because I had the feeling I was being supported by the medications. I was no longer alone with my struggles, and finally this business about getting to sleep at night was no longer an issue. For many years I lived with various drugs and varying degrees of success.

My little child was born and developed splendidly. I exerted unending energy fighting off the know-it-alls and those trying to give me advice; I exuded a proficiency that was meant to silence everyone and everything else. Thankful for the nightly "disruptions," I smothered my baby with closeness and care, while trying too hard to not make my older kids jealous.

Of course I felt guilty on all sides and thus increased my efforts to make my family happy by cooking and organizing family events. My husband was a "traveling man." Before the birth we had developed a wonderful clarity about how we would organize our lives as parents: a true partnership, no fixed roles, modern, etc. We had always been such good theorists! Stupidly, my husband's career developed away from home and the earlier good times were overshadowed now by his constant absences. I intensified my efforts to make up for the lack; my husband withdrew even more, feeling as if he had been booted out; frustration set in. It was a familiar frustration, but with a new manifestation; with our older kids (two families thrown together!) there had been similar scenes of daily life.

My husband ended up in a hospital for psychosomatic medicince for three months. This had been long in coming. There were the usual grim doubts, outbursts of emotion and rage, etc. These were hellish, dark months that had been building up for some time. I became co-depressive. My "strength" was only an affront to him, there was no other way than to go through this with him quiet and busy and keep the whole "show" running at home. My husband was prescribed Saroten *(antidepressant, active ingredient amitriptyline)* and has been taking it in large doses for years.

My heart troubles got worse again, mainly at night. One EKG after the next was done; some results were good, some just okay. I readily believed the poor results; the fear of every night was a horror, and Tranxilium[1] was a true companion. The quiet nights were initially comforting so that I did not mind the increasing dosage. I had become very "sure" of myself; I had pills in every pocket, and sometimes all I had to do was hold them in my hand and I was calmer already. If I had forgotten them on a trip (even just to go shopping), I turned around in panic and picked up my source of life and my savior. For a long time I was certain I could not live without them. I was able to manage my life, I could withstand all the commotion. I tried to be a loving mother who could—and had to—raise her children to be free of fear (!). I was fine with the image I had of myself, I had gotten used to it.

My "own" work, creating texts, remained an embarrassing secret that I didn't want to let out. I struggled to find a few hours in which I could disappear to my hidden writing nook in our big house. A difficult undertaking. My whole life this craving had been with me, but I never wanted to admit that pen and paper are the source of true meaning in my life. As a smoker (addicted), a wine-lover (addicted), user of tranquilizers (addicted), a writer (addicted), a fighter against authoritarian structures (addicted), and individualist (addicted), I came to see myself as a burden for those around me; my nightly encumbrances grew until I could hardly breath anymore. EKGs every week, prescriptions for Tranxilium every month. Swinging between highs and lows, light and darkness—was this to be for the rest of my days?

18 months ago I got a hold of the book "Schöne neue Psychiatrie" *("Brave New Psychiatry")*. A copy of it was lying around at my brother's, who is best friends with the author. "Peter Lehmann," that interested me.

---

1 Tranquilizer, active ingredient clorazepate dipotassium, marketed as Clorazepate Dipotassium, Gen-Xene, Tranxene, Tranxilene

I read it in one night. I was trembling and shaking, and a realization struck me like nothing ever had. *You are addicted. You are addicted.*

That hurt, it revolted me, it was an attack on me.

The recognition that I was tied up in addictions needed a catalyst to become conscious and for me to admit it. It became clear to me I was poisoning myself, the chemicals were changing my body, my soul, all my expressions of life. Only then was I able to initiate a change. I put away the Tranxilium and never touched it again. Though one shouldn't abruptly withdraw from benzodiazepines, I did so in a second. I never had any problems associated with withdrawal.

My addictions are not gone, but they are different now. I can observe them with calmness, and that in itself helps me to control them. With a certain euphoria and pride in my own strong will, I was able to navigate through the first weeks of being free of Tranxilium. But the old fears and the familiar nights soon had me by the collar again, though not as severely. Autogenic training, reflection, publications and natural remedies helped me through the difficult times. I have harvested quite a bit of St. John's wort by now. My fears, my loneliness and some discontentment are still there, but I know now that hard times and easy times, pain and pleasure all belong together and are all a part of my existence. And the deep abysses? Of course I could name them: relationships, marriage, they could also be called "a lack of roots," "homesickness," "speechlessness," "dissatisfaction." But why ask the same old questions again? We are on our own, called upon to live in a responsible way. We are not only sentenced by others, muzzled by others. We always have more forces (and self-helping forces, too) available than we might have thought in dark days. We only have one life, and death is a part of it. I now say "yes" to myself, to my own determination. The autumn has forfeited its darkness. I write and publish, keep my head up and my feet on the ground. I dream, work, *live.*

Each and every problem is still there, but they don't have a hold on me anymore. I can look at them straight: *I live.*

Translation from the German by Christina White

Ulrich Lindner

I Ran for my Life
How I Healed my Depression

*Neuroleptics: Taxilan, Truxal / Antidepressants: Anafranil, Saroten /
Antidepressant-Tranquilizer Combination: Limbatril / Lithium /
Tranquilizer: Valium*

The decisive question on my four-year road to health was whether I could live without psychiatric drugs. It was this chemical staff which comprised the bars of the prison cell in which I had been buried for 33 years. I could only find my route to freedom after I had sawed through them.

My problems started at my conception. My mother already had her hands full with four boys and then I came along as number five. If only I had been a girl! All the more astounding that she accepted and brought me up so loving-ly. For my older brothers I was the fifth wheel on the wagon, completely su-perfluous. When I was an adult my mother said once that she had wanted two or three children at the most. Through the whole of my childhood she sat at my bedside every night and prayed and read me bible stories. My favorite was the volume entitled "Vom lieben Heiland" *("Of the Loving Savior")*.

My father was proud of his sons. Of course he expected them to be as capable as he was, the academic whiz kid in his family. As a successful general practitioner and obstetrician as well as a committed Christian, he wanted three lives: the first one for his family, the second for his profession and the third for his church. During the Third Reich he exercised passive resistance. He refused the Hitler salute and instead only said "Heil!" The explanation in his family was that: "Heil comes from our Heiland *(Savior)*."

As with my brothers, my father practiced the latest "scientific" know-ledge on me. Thus, my mother was not allowed to breastfeed me since practical baby food had been invented. I spent most of my time in my carriage on the balcony screaming myself into despair. Irritated neighbors were told this was necessary to strengthen my lungs. My father dealt with my continuing bedwetting by spraying my genitals with ether and calling out "cold, cold."

I was five years old when my father killed himself. After several weeks his body was found in a small channel in Hamburg. I can still see my mother banging her head on the bedroom wall and crying: "How could he do this to us!" A year later my hometown disappeared in ash and rubble in an RAF air raid.

I had crises to deal with in the postwar years too. Among other things I entered a marriage which made neither me nor my wife happy.

How to turn an acute crisis into a chronic one

I owed my mental and religious development to my generous, pious parents, but also to my church. My baptismal motto included God's words: "And I love you." My confirmation motto was the triple love motto from Mathew 22, 37– 39: "Love thy God, thy Lord with all thy heart, and with all thy soul, and with all thy mind" (in the original Greek literally: "with your whole understanding"). This is the most important and biggest commandment. The other one is very similar: "Love thy neighbor as thyself."

I was thus given the key to my life. It was to be my undoing that I understood it as a double command to love. I had to be there for God and for my neighbors. That I can only love both if I accept myself with love was something I only learned on my route to health. Before that, I did not know what to do with myself and most importantly I didn't know that I had to fight for my own vital interests. Self-discovery and self-development were foreign words to me which I could not harmonize with my Christian existence. Thus, in my Christian life, along with the helpful things, I came to know much that caused illness.

From autumn 1959 I suffered horribly time and again from depression. When I was a student in despair, I turned for a long time to four helpful professors of theology. The best known was Helmut Thielicke. His several-volume work on ethics and religion is impressive. I got to know him in the first place as a great preacher and pastor. How often I listened to his sermons in the packed St. Michaelis church! I based my second thesis on his sermons on the Lord's Prayer. His practice-related basic rule was: "you have to start with people where they are at." He gave me a great deal of time. If I was overcome by tiredness at lunchtime, he allowed me to sleep on a camp bed in his room during the theological seminar.

Prof. Thielicke visited me at the beginning of my stay in the first clinic and took me for a long walk. When my university teachers heard of my family stress, in their misplaced belief in science they all advised me: "They have discovered such good drugs. Go to a psychiatrist! They'll fix everything in the psychiatric hospital." When I told Prof. Thielicke about my thoughts of suicide, he comforted me with the lot of Saul: "Remember too the disciples Paul, Martin Luther, Kierkegaard and Jochen Klepper! You are in good company!"

I was a student assistant to Prof. Leonhard Goppelt. It seemed that one could not understand Jesus without understanding his miracles or his healing of the sick. This fascinated me. Could those miracles come true for me? Far from the truth! Because, as the great New Testament scholar taught: "Jesus" miracles are limited to his earthly life and early apostolic life." I asked my superior what he thought about the pastor Johann Christoph Bumhardt (1805–1880) and his healing works in Möttlingen and Bad Boll. That was quite different, he explained to me. So I told myself then that I could not hope for a miracle.

Up to that point I was fine, and I really had everything I needed. But during the winter semester 1959/60 everything became so difficult. Everything took much longer. My energy was gone. My drive grew weaker and weaker, paucity of thought and lack of concentration took over. I only managed the written version of my paper with difficulty and my exam sermon was not ready on time. Bible reading and prayer left me empty. I had lost my belief.

A third professor of theology advised me:

> "Alsterdorf is a Protestant hospital, and the medical director of Ochsenzoll is a Protestant whose own wife suffers from depression. You'll be in the best hands there."

Yes, those friendly hands kept writing me new prescriptions for neuroleptics, antidepressants, tranquilizers and sleeping pills. What a miracle that I did not become addicted to Valium, Limbatril[1], Anafranil, Saroten *(antidepressant, active ingredient amitriptyline)*, Taxilan *(neuroleptic, active ingredient perazine)*, Truxal *(neuroleptic, active ingredient chlorprothixene)*—none of them helped and only made me tired and unimaginative. None of the doctors told me anything about the damaging consequences. It was difficult to understand what was written on the package insert and it did not interest me anyway.

Because I had taken the psychiatric drugs I could explain everything: I was without doubt mentally ill! "Thank God," I said. Now I no longer need to have a bad conscience. "It's not your fault that you are ill; you cannot do anything about it. You just have to take your medication regularly," explained the doctors. For two "episodes" I was given leave for three semesters from Hamburg University.

When I then wrote a good thesis for my first major exam, I heard the diagnosis for the first time: I was now "manic." This way I fitted easily into the pigeonhole into which they had already wanted to put me. Initially the talk was of "vegetative dystonia." Then my case notes in the hospital contained the term "MDI," and I learned that it stood for "manic-depressive illness." Why should I be manic or mad? I was told by the ward doctor that it was the standard term.

In fact, the periodic course of my condition was impressive. For more than a year I remained symptom-free. I did not expect to be ill again—a typical symptom of my new diagnosis, I was told, a mere lack of understanding of my condition during the manic phase. Weren't the traditional psychiatrists right after all? In summer 1963, when I was to begin my curacy, I could not work because of a renewed severe depression. What else could I do other than throw myself once again into the psychiatric mill? My church superiors continued to show understanding.

We had managed it: the theologians, the psychiatrists and the unstable young adult. The chronically ill psychiatric patient was born, but unfortunately I had not yet discovered myself.

---

1 Combination of the antidepressant amitriptyline and the tranquilizer chlordiazepoxide

Paths to healing

Two psychoanalysts brought me a great deal. However, I had broken off both therapies with suicide attempts when my respective therapists were on holiday in 1965 and 1969. On both occasions I almost did not survive the intoxication with strong sleeping pills. Following my suicide attempts I had to go through hell with appalling hallucinations and physical pain. I could hardly believe that on both occasions I had not been allowed to die…

From 1969 to 1989 a lithium medication more or less "stabilized" me. During this time I developed terrible headaches and a backache. They were fought with pain killers. In the end I developed urological complaints when passing water. For this too I was prescribed a drug. There were also drugs for the beginnings of a goiter.

Today I know that at that time I had not yet discovered myself. My pious excuse: "with God's help things will work out," proved to be unsustainable. Even then I could not live beyond my limits. Without knowing it, I was fleeing from myself. But I could not achieve this insight from my Christian faith. In fact, both the church and theology had done a great deal to contribute to my helplessness. Luther's "alone" had become a trap for me: "alone out of mercy, alone through belief, the Holy Scripture alone, in all: Jesus Christ alone." That meant: you, Ulrich, are nothing and can do nothing in the end. The Luther text "Es ist doch unser Tun umsonst, auch in dem besten Leben" *("All our actions are for nothing, even in the best of lives")* had a catastrophic effect on me.

When I told my wife in 1990 that I was on the way to a cure and was about to stop taking the psychiatric drugs, it was the end for her. She created a huge scene so that I could not think of anything else to do other than to move out of our apartment and leave her and our son. What should I have done? There was nothing left for me other than to become healthy. I had told myself for long enough that my illness was incurable.

My spiritual healing

Up to that time I had received pastoral support from two capable people. But these withdrew their support when I stopped taking the psychiatric drugs and decided to convert to Catholicism. "Think of your family and start taking the medication again," wrote my confessor before he broke off contact with me. Right from my first visit in 1986 to the Protestant monastery, Bergkirchen, I sensed that from this point on my life would change and I would be healed. And this route to healing began in earnest through meditation.

It was Thursday, January 19, 1989 when I began nightprayers in the chapel of the monastery and remained alone on my meditation bench. Time and place sank away. All at once the face of Christ lit up the dark in golden contours. HE appeared to me in unspeakable love. I watched HIM, fascinated. I watched and watched and lay then with my face on the ground, transformed. Now I was rock solid in my conviction that I was on the right road. I began to become a new person.

On that day I experienced several wonderful forms of guidance. I was taking part in a meditation course given by the Benedictine priest Anton von Mühlhausen. He invited me immediately to his monastery. In time, I entrusted him with my experiences on the road to healing. On the one hand he gave me courage in his role of confessor, and on the other hand he was cold and rejecting. Finally, I decided to take part in a meditation course given by Father Anton. Prior to that, I had a decisive mystic experience in Bergkirchen. I would just like to refer to the audition *(inner hearing)*, which particularly strengthened my certainty. During a meditation I heard Jesus saying to me: "I will heal you." Again and again I asked: "How will you do it?"

I still felt helpless in the face of my depressions. Psychologically I had recognized that I had created a demon through my depressive, self-destructive behavior which now ruled me. Feeling down, I started on my journey. As soon as I set foot in the monastery I was able to breathe. The prayer said at the canonical hours impressed me more and more. The abbey church began to fascinate me. The meditation exercises gave me unbelievable peace. Only the depressive dullness still got me down. How was I going to get rid of this "fiend?" I reproached Jesus for his promise. "You have promised me, 'I will heal you.' But how?" For a long time the Communion service had been of special importance for me because I experienced the nearness and love of my savior intensely. But I still felt so unworthy. With every fiber of my being I wanted to give myself to HIM. But I told myself that HE could not possibly accept me with my self-destructive behavior.

Father Anton had planned a Mass in the meditation room for Saturday. The Protestant course participants were also invited. While preparing the offerings I experienced my healing vision which was totally unimaginable for me as a pacifist. Suddenly the "fiend" stood before me in a very threatening form. I had a dagger in my hand and killed him with three stabs. He collapsed and disappeared. So I had killed him! An incredible feeling of happiness, an ecstasy came over me such as I had never experienced before. The summit was reached when I received the "Body" and "Blood" of the Lord and became one with Jesus Christ.

Thus on the evening of June 10, 1989, I experienced the key mystery of my life in unique intensity: mystic oneness, the *unio mystica*. I only realized bit by bit that what had happened to me is described in the New Testament as a "rebirth." For days, all physical and mental pain disappeared. As had happened with my first vision of January 19, 1989, wonderful acts of providence and guidance occurred. I experienced all senses far more intensely and in a deeply satisfying way. In the end I understood that I was completely loved and reconciled with everything: with God, with the world and with me. I was a new person, so it seemed to me.

In fact, the basis for my new life was not yet strong enough to bear a new life. To my horror, in my new home I experienced two serious bouts of depression lasting several months: in September 1990 and in May 1992. The people who had supported me did not know what to do. I felt deserted by everyone. Even the telephone help-line could not help me. A life-saving welfare and social organization was at least somewhere I could go. Once again I visited a psychiatrist and had psychiatric drugs prescribed again. They didn't do any good at all, just like all the other devilish stuff that I had had prescribed for me over thirty-three long years. I did not doubt the deep faith experiences, but they did not help any more. Prayer and medation now brought me to hopeless despair. I would have tried to take my life for a third time had not something unexpected happened.

The new horizon: self-help and an integrated approach

On a November night in 1990 I had made all the preparations to kill myself. Suddenly, the doorbell rang. My brother Thomas with whom I had had no contact for some time was standing at the door: "You are in a bad way. I'll have to take you to stay with me for a few days." "But Thomas, you can't possibly know that." He had obviously experienced it telepathically.

Thomas is ten years older than me and had gotten out of psychiatric treatment ten years before me. He lived 30 kilometers away. He came to my aid on two more such occasions. His advice seemed to me to be cruel and absurd, but opened up a new horizon: "Nobody can help you, including me. You have to pull yourself out of the swamp of your self-destruction by the hair of your head—just like Munchhausen." And: "Anyway, I can only tell you that the mentally ill person has to use all means at his disposal if it helps him get better."

From my faith I received a similar answer. I asked Christ repeatedly why he deserted me. The reply I received was: "What you can do yourself I can not do for you." I understood that my piety had often been an escape from independence. And, furthermore, I gradually understood that religion is not everything in life. I remembered my Confirmation motto. The triple commandment to love is aimed at wholeness. By the time everyone had proven to be helpless in the face of my mental suffering, I understood that I had to help myself. The concept of wholeness is closely associated with self-help. It was difficult for me to recognize this horizon and even more so to bring it to life.

My physical healing

I am not by nature a very sporty type. Nonetheless, even at school I had forced myself to perform physical exercise and had, for example, started jogging years before. I started jogging again in Obertalheim in 1990. In view of my depressive apathy, this was especially difficult for me. The encouragement I had from my brother Thomas helped me. Still, I had to practically beat myself out of bed every morning. I told myself that it only depended on the next small step. From the start, I prescribed myself a daily run in the woods in all weather. Again and again muscle cramps and tears stopped me. I began to suffer from a backache. The doctor and the masseur both said that what I was doing was mad.

Over the years I experienced an increase in my physical fitness. My performance increased quite rapidly. As if made for me, the route of my slow, hour-long run that I have been taking right up to the present begins directly outside my front door.

In any case, my self-esteem has been increased massively through my physical healing. Without doubt, it is the experience of happiness which is triggered by the expression of the endorphin hormones. I had experienced this before. But the euphoria was considered to be unhealthy. I had heard this from the psychiatrists, from my former wife and occasionally from pious people. But, in fact, the literature leaves no doubt that jogging is the best anti-depressant.

At the beginning, I was afraid to be seen in a track suit. What on earth will they think of me? For a long time I hated running in the early morning in the pitch-black woods. What if I have an accident? Now in the winter I take a powerful torch with me.

It helped me a great deal that I came up with the solution: "I'm running for my life." I don't care what the others think. They don't help me out of my misery. In fact, they hinder me. They are probably indifferent to me.

After four years I finally did it!

Complete healing includes the mental-psychological, emotional-cognitive, artistic-creative, social-human and religious-spiritual. At last I understood the meaning and task of my life. I could only find this healing route for myself. And, something especially true of (ex-)users and survivors of psychiatry, I can now encourage other people with mental crises and illness to find their own way out of the hopelessness. My encounter with literature, with music, in particular with singing and painting also opened up sources of healing to me. As well as these relaxation exercises, which I performed daily and passed on in self-help groups, I began breathing and muscle relaxation. I found the basis for my self-help program later in the books of two professors from whom I learned much for my work: Reinhard Tausch, "Hilfen bei Streß und

Belastung" *("Help with Stress and Pressure,"* 1996), and Michael Dieterich, "Wir brauchen Entspannung" *("We Need Relaxation,"* 1997).

After four years, my psychiatrist said when I visited him at the beginning of 1993 for the last time: "I can imagine that you will never need psychiatric care again." That was many years ago. The last prognosis that a psychiatrist ever made for me has been completely fulfilled so far.

My way out of psychiatry and my "coming off psychiatric drugs" has finally succeeded. Thanks be to God! I now say that I am healthy and happy, healed and whole. Yet, I must add: the status quo only pertains because I implement my self-help program each day anew. I have learned to accept myself with my limitations and deficits. There are times I do not feel capable of writing a paper or a sermon—a similar situation as back in 1959 when I had no choice but to give in to my depression and take a medical leave. Now I simply put off such tasks or drop them altogether. Fortunately I do not need to earn money. In any case, it is clear that our society with its relentless demands drives people to crisis and illness. This is especially true when they can not relinquish their perfectionism.

In my extensive self-help work, the question often arises of how to avoid becoming victims of stress and pressure. Life will always be associated with difficulties. In my volunteer work I often receive thanks but also encounter failure and rejection. I try to accept it calmly and do not allow myself to take offense or to be made ill. I agree with the words of the German poet Hermann Hesse (1877–1962) who freed himself from severe mental suffering:

"Des Lebens Ruf an uns wird niemals enden...
Wohlan denn, Herz, nimm Abschied und gesunde!"
("Our life's calling will never end... Come then, heart, say farewell and recover!")

Translation from the German by Mary Murphy

To Withdraw with Professional Help

Eiko Nagano

Nishi Therapy—A Japanese Way

Neuroleptics: Perphenazine, Chlorpromazine, Methotrimeprazine, Promethazine / Antidepressants: Amitriptyline / Tranquilizers: Flunitrazepam / Hypnotics: Phenobarbital

I was born in 1953. When I grew up, there were seven people in the family —my parents, my older sister, one of my grandmothers and two of my aunts. When my parents got married, my father moved into my mother's house, where she lived with her whole family. That is, by the way, an exception in Japan. The common practice is that the wife moves into the husband's family, except when the wife has no brothers.

Growing up in a family of aliens

Both of my aunts did not work and they were at home all the time. Supposedly they were too weak to go to work. They were not married either. If they would go to a psychiatrist now, there would be diagnoses for them as patients.

My sister is five years older than me and ever since I was a small child, both my aunts were bored all the time and my sister always made fun of me. During the meal they would say something like: "Look at her, the way she eats! She thinks that it's cute to move her mouth like that." This is just one example. They made such comments to almost every move I made. That was the kind of atmosphere in which I grew up. So I was always nervous about the way I did things and I was afraid of making the smallest mistake. I knew that they were waiting for the chance to mock me.

When I was a child, I used to believe that these people came from a different planet and kidnapped me. And I remember well that I thought about committing suicide when I was five years old.

I was also very much pushed by the family to achieve things. They expected me to be successful at school. I had to have good notes. I went to a private junior high school for girls and when I was in the ninth grade I was too exhausted and could not go to school any more. I did not want to go there, was always very tired, felt sick and could almost not move any more. But everybody just told me to go to school and they forced me to go so I thought I would rather die. This was my symptom.

The internist I had to visit did not find anything so I became a psychiatric case. I was sixteen then, in 1969, and it was the beginning of my long relationship with psychiatry.

Starting a psychiatric career in childhood

As far as my body was concerned I was healthy. So I was brought to a child psychiatrist. And what he said was that I was too childish, that I had to become mentally independent of my mother and that I was spoiled because my mother did too much for me. And he said also that I should not behave like a spoiled child, that I must go to school and do a lot of sport. These words of this psychiatrist have followed me like a nightmare all my life, and I almost think that the cause of my depressive insanity might be the result of this child psychiatrist's mistake. If you are sick and go to a doctor, an internist for instance, he or she would not say such things to you. But as soon as you go to see a doctor because you feel mentally sick, you get accused of your mental attitude and your personality.

I thought myself that I was mentally ill, and I believed at that time that psychiatrists were there to help somebody like me. But the reality was different. What the psychiatrists did was just to blame and to accuse me of being the way I was. Under their influence the sense of self-denial became stronger and stronger and the guilty conscience became deeper and deeper.

I was seventeen when I stayed in a mental hospital for the first time. Between nineteen and twenty-six I received neither psychiatric treatment nor took any drugs. But then I had a relapse into depression and since that time I had taken all kinds of psychiatric drugs for about twenty years. I was really a junkie, but a legal one. In these years, as I got older, my condition kept becoming worse and worse. But all my psychiatrists could do was just to increase the doses of the drugs which I was supposed to take. By 1999 I had to take in the morning perphenazine[1] 2 mg, chlorpromazine[2] 25 mg, promethazine 25 mg, and in the evening perphenazine 4 mg, amitriptyline 25 mg, levomepromazine *(another term for methotrimeprazine)* 5 mg, chlorpromazine 25 mg, flunitrazepam 1 mg, and a combined drug with the ingredients chlorpromazine 12.5 mg + promethazine 12.5 mg + phenobarbital 1 mg.

At that time I believed everything that psychiatrists said. So I thought, even if I feel myself that I am not sleeping, if you look at it objectively from the scientific point of view, then I am actually sleeping. If that is true then it means that my senses are affected by the mental illness. It means that my emotions and my thoughts are also affected. As a result I started to think that I had to check whether everything that I thought or felt was right. So I began to ask my nurse before I did something. For example, when I felt cold, I asked at first if it was really cold and if I should put something on. This behavior was, of course, recorded as a symptom. At home I was tired of hiding myself and my feelings and acting in the way how they wanted me to be. And the psychiatry contributed in this way to extinguish my ability to show feelings completely. No wonder I got more and more depressed.

For example, I tell you one story which happened in the mental hospital one day. A nurse came in the evening to give me a sleeping pill. I told her that I did not need it because I could sleep without it. She accepted this and said: "Okay, if you can sleep without it, then you don't need to take it." The doctor who was in charge, however, said to me: "You think that you can sleep, but you are actually not sleeping at all." So I had to take the pill.

---

1 Neuroleptic, marketed also as Fentazin, Trilafon; component of Etrafon, Triavil

2 Neuroleptic, marketed as Chloractil, Chlorpromazine, Largactil, Thorazine

I want to die! That is always the first thought when I wake up in the morning. The hell starts all over again today… Since I was fourteen it has been like this every morning for about thirty years. I used to have a comic or an easy book to read near my pillow, so that I could reach them right away after waking up, hoping that I did not have to think about dying. I could not begin a day without this ritual. "Depressive illness"—that was the name of my disease. The psychiatric treatment of the last thirty years could not heal this pain of mine.

On the long way to liberation

Since my late twenties, I have been a member of a national organization of psychiatric patients called Zenkoku Seishinbyosha Shudan. When I got to know this group of psychiatric patients, I saw one day that somebody in the group was angry, and I was very surprised. Until that time I had always thought that psychiatric patients should not get angry. I was convinced that to become angry is a symptom. For me, it was very liberating.

Through the activities of the patient's group, I finally managed to regain the self-dignity which psychiatry had taken away from me. Moreover, I was able to find the simple truth, that I am the main person in my life. It may be that I would not have been so damaged by psychiatry if I had had more experience in society and had been older and able to look at psychiatry in a relative way. But the prize of having become a psychiatric case in my teens is this big. I really hope that the young people do not get this damage that I got, and this hope becomes stronger and stronger every year. I am also hopeful about Nishi therapy, which I am now testing under the instruction of Miss. T, one of the first members of Zenkoku Seishinbyosha Shudan where I got to know about Nishi therapy.

What is Nishi therapy?

Before the World War II Katsuzo Nishi, who was not a medical doctor, introduced his special therapy. He was a doctor of engineering who designed the underground train system. Ever since he was a child he had never been healthy. So he used to read all kinds of medical books about Western and

Oriental medicine and studied different ways of treatments. As a result of his research he introduced his special therapy. Its theory is quite complicated. My understanding is based on the instruction of my friends and on books about Nishi therapy.

Human civilization began when Homo sapiens stood up on two legs and, because of that, the function of the spine was forced to change. As long as human beings were going on all fours, the spine had the function of a beam but now it had to take on the task of a pole. Through this development human beings started to have such problems as the distortion and the dislocation of the spine. In addition, the internal organs dropped, twisting the intestines and wrinkling the intestinal walls. This creates blockages in the intestine causing an accumulation of wastes while also overheating the food. As a result, the human body started to have a lack of vitamin C, which the human body is not able to produce on its own, and it became necessary for human beings to eat more in order to take enough nourishment in. This burdens the internal organs and quickens the aging process. We started to wear clothes which led to the inability of the human skin to function satisfactorily. This decline in the ability of the skin to breathe causes a lack of oxygen and an increase in carbon monoxide in the body which can in the end cause cancer. The development of human civilization, away from the primitive way of life on all fours, made human beings become vessels of diseases. Like a lot of doctors in the middle ages, Nishi says that the causes of all diseases originate in the excrements which are accumulated inside the intestines, and also the lack of oxygen in the body, the distortion of the spine and the lack of vitamin C in the body.

In comparison with modern medicine, Nishi therapy looks at the body as a whole unity and tries to get rid of the cause of the illness instead of looking at each internal organ separately to cure the disease. In addition, it says that the symptoms are the most important steps to the recovery, so that the treatment is rather to support the natural course of the illness. It also says that all the bad things must come out completely before the illness can take the course of the recovery. So far, it is not that unconventional. In Western medicine, Florence Nightingale also said that the symptoms are the process of recovery and that the symptoms must not be mixed up with the illness itself. If the patients are suffering then they are not getting the right care. What is interesting about Nishi therapy is that it not only theorizes the principle of the natural recovery but also explains exactly what you should do to have the best result.

Under the instruction of Nishi therapy there are several different ways to deal with these problems. To deal with the distortion of the spine, you have to sleep on a hard board bed, use a hard pillow and do several exercises. To enhance the function of the skin, you have to do the "naked therapy" and use the hot-cold-bathing method. In order to avoid the accumulation of the excrements inside you, you must always eat a small portion, you have to fast, take some magnesium hydroxide (the only drug you have to take in Nishi therapy), eat fresh vegetables and drink fresh water.

In March 1999 I fasted with Miss T. for one week, following the teachings of Nishi. I was not allowed to take any of the psychiatric drugs which I had been taking. Ever since, I have not yet taken any medicine again, and the hell, which I felt every morning, has not come back yet. What was the treatment of the last thirty years? I want to shout: Give me my youth back! So far I am happy with the result of Nishi therapy.

Nishi therapy in practice

It is not easy to follow the rules of Nishi. I would like to introduce the daily plan, which my Nishi therapy specialist gave me to follow when I visited him in October 2000.

You have to sleep on a board and use a pillow like a short wooden pole. For some people it takes some time to get used to it but I actually liked it and, since sleeping with the hard pillow, I do not have stiff shoulders any more. Next you have to do the so-called naked therapy, which Mr. Robery, a Frenchmen, has designed. In the morning you first have to open the window and undress yourself naked. Following the instruction tape, you have to put the blanket or the bedclothes on and off yourself repeatedly. When you do not have the blanket on you, you do your exercise, and when you have the blanket on you, you stay quiet. The exercises you have to do are the special Nishi therapy exercises like the gold-fish-exercise (lie on one's back and move head and legs left and right like a swimming fish), capillary-exercise and prayer-footsole-exercise (lie on your back and join your palms and soles of your feet together and move your arms over your head along the floor and move your legs along the floor). You are supposed to do this "naked therapy" for thirty minutes and after that you have to do the so-called back-and-stomach-exercise for five minutes. You are to take the magnesium hydroxide to smooth the movement of the bowels. Breakfast is supposed to be not good for you, so you should skip it. In the evening, you are to repeat the "naked therapy" again and take a hot bath and a cold bath alternately. As far as the meal is concerned, you should always eat a small amount, and avoid oily food and meat as much as possible. You should eat mainly unpolished rice or dark wheat bread. You are to take 250 gram to 300 gram of fresh vegetable every day, and you should allocate them to two meals. You have to take the leaf portion and the root portion of five different kinds of fresh vegetables in equal amount and mix them in the mixer. And you are to drink one liter of fresh water and one liter of persimmon tea every day.

I think you can see that you need to have real determination and the discipline to be able to follow this schedule every day strictly. But when you do it incorrectly and come out of the rhythm, because you had a long business trip or you ate too much of your favorite things, then your body shows you immediately. You will become sick again.

My doctor tells me that I have to do the "naked therapy" and all those exercises three times a day, but I hardly manage it. It is also difficult for me to drink one liter of water every day. I manage to mix my vegetables in the mixer for the evening meal, but for lunch I just chop them up and eat them without mixing them in the mixer.

When you read the books about Nishi therapy written by the doctors who practice it, you find all kinds of incredible reports in which they tell you that the most difficult diseases have been cured by Nishi therapy. These stories are so unbelievable that you might ask: Is it really true? As far as I am concerned, it was not that I found Nishi therapy when I was about to die, after all the doctors had given up on me. So, as to the other illnesses, I just cannot say anything. But what interested me, of course, was Nishi therapy's theory about mental disease. It says that such a thing as the human mind which has neither a form nor smell and of which existence is metaphysical cannot become ill.

"The mind cannot become ill"—is a very fascinating statement. But what's also wonderful about Nishi therapy is that it says that illness can be cured only by nature and never by a doctor or by medicine. And it is up to you how much effort you make to support the power and the process of the natural cure. You should neither just follow the things that your psychiatrists tell you to do nor should you rely on them. Your daily effort in a concrete form leads to recovery. Contrary to the pessimistic view of the psychiatric belief that I will have to take psychiatric drugs for the rest of my life, the optimistic principle of Nishi therapy, which shows me the exact way to the cure, gives me the energy. This is a therapy which can motivate those of us who have some kinds of mental diseases. When both modern psychiatric medicine and Nishi therapy are only hypotheses, then at least I would like to follow the instruction of the one that I am convinced of and where I make the effort myself. That is my basic attitude towards Nishi therapy and my condition has been dramatically improving.

Nishi therapy and the psychiatric patient's liberation movement

There are, however, subjects in Nishi therapy which are questionable. First of all, it requires for the patient a very strong will. The high cost of the therapy may be the second point and probably the biggest problem of Nishi therapy. In order to get a good result you need to stay in a hospital for about three weeks, and that is too expensive for most patients. In addition, you also have to pay for the magnesium hydroxide and the persimmon tea by yourself. As the third point you could mention the fact that—as a result of a homeopathy-like phenomenon of first worsening under Nishi therapy—your condition could become worse again at some point in course of making progress. In my case I do not know if it is the reaction of my body, which comes from the fact that I quit all the drugs, or if it is first worsening. Whichever the reason is, I have experienced the instability of my condition quite a lot in the first two years which is very hard to cope with. You can face some setbacks during the treatment so you would definitely need the guidance of a professional and experienced person. There are only a few specialists of Nishi therapy, and if you do not live near the places where these specialists are it is not easy to get hold of them.

I was first introduced to Nishi therapy quite some time ago. But the reason why I could not decide myself on it for a long time was my resistance, as an active participant in our liberation movement, against its pure biological theory which says that there is no such thing as a mental illness. I resisted against the way of thinking that the mental illness is a biological disease like any other illness. The biological attitude can be considered as the fourth critical point of Nishi therapy.

Like I mentioned already, I now think that my chronic depressive state of mind is the result of the psychiatric treatment. In addition, my condition at the time of the first psychiatric therapy was the result of the maltreatment at home. That's why I could never deny the importance of sociological and psychological factors when I talk about mental illness. It is essential to research the sociological and psychological problems in order to find out who you are and where your pain comes from, and this matter is also very important for our liberation movement. I had always denied the biological view of psychiatric medicine: to reduce everything to the physical constitution of each individual and just to say that it is a malfunction of the brain or the metabolism or the genes.

To try to mend the biological defect does not mean that you deny the psychosocial problems. For example, if you get an ulcer from too much stress and a chaotic situation at work, then the fact that you go to the doctor to get rid of the ulcer does not mean that you try to preserve the chaotic situation at work or don't do something to change the situation. In such cases, you just have to get healthy first before you can do anything else.

As to the effect of the therapy, I am also not sure if it would work for everybody. I am still testing it myself. I am convinced, however, that the improvement of the health care system so that anyone could try such an alternative therapy in the future is in the interest of the liberation movement of psychiatric patients.

Translation from the Japanese by Chie Ishii

Manuela Kälin

Home Visit by the Homeopath

Neuroleptics: Fluanxol / Antidepressants / Lithium / Tranquilizers:
Rohypnol, Valium

In 1981, after years of taking neuroleptics, antidepressants, tranquilizers and lithium with all their side-effects, I was extremely lucky to find a job which I really liked a lot. This then was the right time for me to stop taking the psychiatric drugs.

The fact that I was never really well and suffered side-effects, in the form of severe debilitating shaking, finally drove me to take action. I was quite shocked when my doctor declared that my treatment was long-term and had to be continued for at least another two years. He did not agree with me and did not offer me any help at all. His position was absolutely clear, and so I decided to bear the responsibility of taking action on my own.

A friend gave me the address of a good and experienced homeopath who agreed to treat me. At the time I was taking lithium, Fluanxol, Valium (as needed) and Rohypnol to sleep. Against the advice of the homeopath, who told me to withdraw gradually, I stopped taking everything from one day to the next; I had simply had enough of the medication.

At first I didn't notice much, but fairly soon after I became very restless and nervous and could no longer sleep. I developed very severe anxiety states which worsened with each passing day and developed into a psychosis. During a visit by the homeopath I was given an additional homeopathic treatment and because I was no longer capable of being on my own, I stayed with friends for the next while. Overall, the treatment was intensive and individually designed by an experienced homeopath to deal with my needs.

It was important for me to be able phone the homeopath at any time and to know where I could contact him. I frequently made use of this opportunity during the first week, including at night. As I was in a state of permanent crisis, this brought me back to earth each time. The homeopath became involved in a particularly humane way, and also encouraged me by having confidence in me and always being present when there was a problem. In particular, he didn't panic because of my state but neither did he act as if he were indifferent to my situation.

I couldn't sleep for a whole week. I had to stay awake continuously because I was convinced that I would die if I fell asleep. During the day I painted in a state of despair, I walked the dog and tried to deal with my restlessness. Although I was in a terrible state and on the point of hospitalizing myself, I always had the feeling that somehow I would make it. Apart from my dangerous inner state, I suddenly noticed that I was seeing the outside world differently. I saw the colors of fall, of the river and the heron, of the beautiful trees and the flowers and sometimes I felt really strong and happy. After a week I could no longer stay awake. There were flashes in my head and I had the feeling that the world was ending and I was going with it. But I woke up again and had one fear less to deal with. I was in almost daily contact with my homeopath and of course the support of my friends was extremely important. If I had been alone my anxieties would certainly have exploded.

After about two weeks I began to work for a few hours a day. At the beginning, even going to work was very difficult. I could barely concentrate, I was very slow and my body perception was partly disturbed. Everything had to settle down again: sleep, work, what I could do and what I couldn't do. Back in my own apartment, my therapy consisted of cooking and organizing my day in as stress-free a manner as possible.

The whole time—since 1981—I never had a relapse and no longer require psychiatric drugs. In fact I continued to become more and more healthy. This was also thanks to good psychotherapy, which of course has a much better chance of success if one is not pumped full of medication and can access ones emotions.

I would also like to emphasize the fact that when on psychiatric drugs, which cause dangerous side-effects, one never feels well. They are often used to calm the fears of doctors and nursing staff who no longer understand mental crises and emergency situations and so cannot deal with them. During therapy, I later learnt that one comes out of extremely dangerous states even without using medication. There are alternative treatments and it is very important to encourage these.

Translation from the German by Mary Murphy

David Webb
"Please Don't Die"

Neuroleptics: Zyprexa / Antidepressants: Aropax, Aurorix, Efexor /
Hypnotics: Heroin, Methadone

At the time of writing, in September 2001, I am 46 years old, living in Melbourne, Australia, and for nearly two years now have been back at work (part-time) as a university lecturer teaching computer programming. I am white, male and heterosexual and was brought up in an essentially comfortable, middle-class family with three elder sisters and a twin brother. Education was highly valued in my family and I went to what some regard as one of Australia's better schools (though personally I detested it). My personal history can be characterized as safe and abundant.

Background

In mid 1995 I "collapsed" into a despair, from which I did not recover until mid-1999. This was triggered by a relationship break-up, but also accentuated by being both unemployed and homeless at the time, though both of these were through personal choice. I was heartbroken by the failure of this relationship and unable to shrug off my sadness and pain and took refuge in heroin. I had used heroin on and off as a recreational drug for several years in my early twenties but had not used it for more than fifteen years when I turned to it for relief in 1995. The heroin did give me some relief from the immediate pain I was feeling at the time but, inevitably, it also led to more problems than it solved. I did not yet realize that I was suicidal. Again.

I had had a pervious suicidal "episode" back in 1979, again triggered by the break-up of a very precious relationship. I had again turned to heroin at that time but on this occasion it was almost immediately in order to use it to kill myself. My first attempt was a joke, giving me a nasty heroin hangover. My next attempt may have been successful except that I somehow set fire to the house, which alerted the neighbours. I woke up a couple of days later in hospital with extensive burns and the next year or so of my life revolved around recovery from these burns. I made one more attempt during this period, this time with all the medications that I had from the doctors, but this time was rescued by my mother who sensed I was not actually asleep and called the ambulance. After some more time in hospital, including a brief period locked up in a psychiatric ward, I more or less fell out of my hospital bed into the classroom at university to study computers. Somehow I graduated and started a moderately successful career in the computer software industry, returning to this same university to teach there in 1989. A pretty good life. Until 1995.

As I said, I did not initially realize that my suicidality had returned. But my pain and despair was only briefly relieved by the heroin and now I was having all the problems of heroin addiction and withdrawal. I became progressively more and more dysfunctional and eventually overwhelmed by the hopelessness and helplessness that so often leads to suicidal thoughts. I began planning my death. For some reason, perhaps I was a little more mature than I was in 1979, I decided to call for help and phoned my sister. This marked the beginning of what became a four-year struggle with my sadness.

Although at the outset I called my despair a spiritual crisis, the reaction to my cry for help was to be treated for drug addiction. This spiritual crisis had been a crisis with my deepest, most person and most intimate sense of who and what I am. It has been the question "What does it mean to me that I exist?" I had reached the point where these questions simply had to be answered in some meaningful and satisfactory way or I was going to die.

I went to various drug detox and rehab programs, attended Narcotics Anonymous (NA) meetings, went to live on a yoga ashram and, later, with some friends in the beautiful Australian countryside. While some of this helped enormously, there was no "cure" for my sadness. Whenever I came to the city I found myself using heroin again. A few times I thought I was over it only to fall over again. My despair was never far away.

Psychiatric drugs

I had briefly taken the antidepressant Aurorix[1] early in this four year journey but it had no apparent effect, either good or bad. Later, during the time I was living with friends in the country, I took Aropax for about twelve months. I was also having a weekly counseling session with a psychologist during most of this time. The most notable effect for me of this drug was how it disturbed my sexuality. Otherwise this was a fairly stable period for me and I was not using heroin or actively suicidal so most people, including myself, were content with this. I'm sure that the psychiatrist felt this was due to this drug but I felt it was more to do with healthy living, plus I was also training myself to just accept that life sucks. I decided to stop taking the Aropax at the same time that I decided to return to my hometown of Melbourne. I had lost all faith in the psychiatrist by this stage (his standard appointment was fifteen minutes and he was arrogant, sexist and inconsiderate) and so I didn't consult him about coming off the drug. I had been told again and again that these drugs were not addictive and I felt that they weren't doing any good, just deadening me sexually, and so I could just stop taking them. Immediately I relapsed into heroin, but actually I do not blame the withdrawal from Aropax for this relapse, it was just my suicidality resurfacing, though perhaps it was a factor.

After some time at another drug detox I agreed to try a new antidepressant, this time it was to be Efexor[2]. Given my history, I was started on what I believe was the normal full adult dose rather than the usual practice of trying the half-dose first. After a couple of weeks there were not noticeable effects—

---

1 Active ingredient moclobemide, marketed also as Arima, Clobemix, Manerix, Maosig, Moclobemide, Mohexal

2 Antidepressant, active ingredient venlafaxine, marketed also as Dobupal, Effexor

again, neither good nor bad—so my psychiatrist and I decided to double the dose to two 75 mg tablets twice a day. Within a short time I found myself unable to sleep. After about a week of virtually no sleep I insisted on seeing the psychiatrist about this. We considered switching to another antidepressant but as I was still very "depressed" (i.e. suicidal), this was considered somewhat risky as it would take a couple of weeks to detox from the Efexor and then another couple of weeks before the new drug (maybe) took effect. The psychiatrist recommended instead that we add another chemical to my drug diet. This drug was Zyprexa, one of the new "atypical" antipsychotics, primarily used in the treatment of "schizophrenia." My doctor said that this drug would "enhance" the effect of the antidepressant, plus it had some sedative effect that would help with the sleeping problems.

This all was a shocking lie. I now know that Zyprexa is a powerful and potent major tranquilizer (neuroleptic) that subdues brain activity with effects that are also not well understood. I also now know that it is in fact a common practice in psychiatry to simply increase the dose and/or the potency of these so-called treatments in order to subdue the symptoms. I also now know that all of these drugs only ever conceal, at best, symptoms and that none of them can truly treat the real causes of the suffering.

I now know that this was all a shocking lie. I now know that Zyprexa is a powerful and potent neuroleptic that subdues brain activity by chemical processes that are not well understood, usually with side-effects that are also not well understood. I also now know that it is in fact a common practice in psychiatry to simply increase the dose and/or the potency (i.e. stronger drugs) of these so-called treatments in order to subdue the unpleasant symptoms of despair. I also now know that this is all that these drugs ever do— that is, they can sometimes subdue the symptoms but without truly treating the causes, the real source, of the despair and suffering that I was experiencing.

The only so-called side-effect with Zyprexa that the psychiatrist mentioned was that I might "develop a bit of a sweet tooth." This proved to be an understatement. Over the next year while I was taking this drug I developed an addictive passion for Cadbury's Top-Deck ice-cream with vanilla custard and put on about twenty kilos. But the "real" effect of this drug, that is the effect that I now know is its designed purpose, was that I became a zombie, at home eating ice-cream and watching daytime television.

I'm not sure of the exact dates of all this but I think I had been on this drug cocktail for about a month or so when I finally burst and after three years of struggle made my first serious suicide attempt. I had made a few half-hearted and sometimes stupid attempts prior to this, but this one was "fair dinkum" (as we say here in Australia). I checked into a motel with a large stash of heroin and a bottle of whisky and, after drinking the whisky, gave myself what I was sure was a lethal shot. I woke up in hospital a day or so later—the motel staff had found me unconscious and called the ambulance. For a brief but horrible while my poor family did not know whether I was going to wake up. And I found out much later that the doctors were concerned about possible brain damage, not from the heroin but from all the medications that I had also taken, especially the Zyprexa.

It was at this time that I relented and went on the Methadone[1] program. It had been offered to me before but I had always refused, dreading its reputation as a more severe addiction than heroin as well as how it chains you to the daily visits to the chemist. I was now on a double-dose of Efexor, a sizable dose of Zyprexa and a "blockade" dose of Methadone. I was pretty addled by this daily load of potent brain chemicals and staggered around, dazed and confused and not really caring about anything.

It was my very good fortune at this time to find my living circumstances were comfortable and secure, sharing a house with a former lover. I settled into about eight months of daily Methadone, Efexor, Zyprexa, Cadbury's Top-Deck ice-cream (with vanilla custard) and the joys of daytime TV. I was sexually inert and severely constipated but otherwise "stable," not using heroin and not actively suicidal. Again it seemed that most people were happy to accept this as some sort of recovery although I knew that I was still deeply unhappy … but just didn't care. I was having occasional counseling sessions but not much as I was as disinterested in this as I was with everything else. I was zonked out, dull, lethargic and disinterested in anything, like

1   Hypnotic, active ingredient levomethadone

a zombie, and waiting for something but without thinking about what that might be or how it might come about.

What came next was that the owners of the house I had been living in returned from overseas after six months as planned. I had started having the occasional shot of heroin again in an aimless kind of way. It gave a little buzz to an otherwise dull and dead life. It was also very expensive (and probably quite dangerous) to get enough so that I could feel it through the fog of the Methadone. I was negotiating with family and friends about where I might go to live now, which confronted me again with the hopelessness of my situation. I tried to kill myself again, this time by taking an overdose of Methadone that I had been accumulating from the take-away doses over the preceding months. I had heard that a treble dose had killed so I figured that the twelve to fifteen times my normal dose that I took would be a certainty. Alas, no, this time I simply woke up in the motel room with the staff banging on my door.

I didn't know what to do. Waking up from a suicide attempt is a pretty peculiar feeling. I called my doctors who went in to damage control and insisted that I come and see them immediately. After checking that I was physically O.K., and to cut a long story short, before that day was over I was certified and taken under escort to a psychiatric hospital. This was a bit of a joke because after spending a weekend there, I was interviewed by the hospital psychiatrist who assessed my condition as an "existential depression" and therefore did not need to be there and arrangements were made for my immediate discharge.

Coming off

After a few days sleeping on the floors of friends and family, again my very good fortune took me to a rooming house (public housing for the disadvantaged), which is where I live today. I was a mess but very grateful for these few small square meters that I was able to call "home." Within a few weeks I decided that I was going to get off all these drugs. It's hard to say just where this decision came from. It was like I was stuffed without these drugs but I was actually more stuffed with them. I was going to stop taking all these poisons and if I died in the process then so be it, I didn't care. I called my doctors to go and see them and tell them of my decision.

Funnily enough, when I got there the head doctor (not the psychiatrist but the doctor who was supervising my Methadone and a wonderful person) told me that they had reviewed my file and decided that the current treatment plan was not working. I laughed as I told him that I had decided to get of all the medications. The truth was that I had been struggling with my suicidality for nearly four years and the two serious attempts that I had made were both made while I was taking this heavy load of psycho-medications. Despite this, and despite my hatred now for these despicable "medicines," I do not blame them for my suicide attempts. I was suicidal before them and it was exhaustion with my struggle more than anything else, I believe, that finally pushed me over the edge. So I do not blame these drugs for my suicidality, even though I have now learned that these drugs by themselves can trigger suicidal feelings. But it is clear that they did not help and that they in fact made the situation worse because while I was zombied out by these drugs there was no way that I was ever going to attend to the real issues behind my suicidality. As a dear friend from NA once said "if you can't feel it, you can't heal it."

I wanted to just stop taking everything immediately. The medical advice, however, was that this would be foolish and dangerous and that I had to withdraw from these drugs one by one and slowly and carefully. I had to agree that this made sense so we put in place a plan to first get off the Methadone, then the others. By this time it was the Zyprexa that I loathed the most and most wanted to stop taking but I was persuaded that I must get off the Methadone first.

Methadone is also very addictive. I had detoxed off heroin many times and yes, it is a very unpleasant experience. But it is nothing compared to detoxing off Methadone. I had been warned about this in advance, along with the other side-effects of the drug, and I have no bitterness at all to those who advised me to take the Methadone. I was well informed by them, including that it was an experiment that may not work for me, and I was in enough trouble with my heroin use that I took this chance. It didn't work but I do not blame the doctors for that.

The Methadone withdrawal plan was to taper off over three months. I later learned that this was actually a very rapid schedule—six months would be more typical for the dose that I was on (80 mg per day)—but I am actually grateful to my Methadone doctor for this rapid detox schedule. I had also heard at NA and elsewhere that no one gets off Methadone without using heroin again—that is, you use heroin to cushion yourself from the methadone withdrawals. I was no exception. I did well for the first couple of months. The chemist asked me from time to time whether I had "hit that wall" yet. I kept saying no, I was doing fine. Until my very last week of the detox. I was down to 2 mg per day and due to go to 1 mg then zero by the end of the week. I started to feel sick like I was getting a bad flu. Typical symptoms of opiate withdrawals. Normally when this occurs (and it almost always occurs at some time) they will re-stabilize you at this dose or slightly higher until you are ready to proceed. I was so close to finishing that I decided to go for it and just pretend that I was sick with a bad flu for a week or so or whatever it took. Although I am still happy with this decision, it was actually about six weeks before these withdrawal symptoms finally faded.

The symptoms of opiate withdrawal are well known. Aches in your joints, inability to sleep, diarrhoea, runny nose, hot and/or cold sweats, feeling like you are itchy on the inside of your skin etc. etc. I was familiar with these and just tried to put up with them as best I could. The difficult thing about Methadone was how long it took for these to pass. You would start to think that maybe the worst was over when suddenly you'd break out into a cold and very wet sweat. This was most awkward when it occurred out of the blue while you were sitting in crowded bus or whatever.

A slightly funny aside at this time is that, in my enthusiasm to throw off these drugs and to return to some semblance of "normality," I had applied for and been offered a vaguely high-powered job as a computer consultant at 400 Australian Dollar (in January 2003 approximately 200 Euro or 200 US-Dollar per day) a day. It seems laughable today that I actually turned it down because it was not enough money. It is doubly funny because if I had accepted it then it would have been a total disaster. The full impact of the Methadone withdrawals hit me about a week after the date I would have started the job if I had accepted it. Phew!!!

Meantime, I was still taking the Zyprexa and the Efexor. I found that I was starting to forget to take them, particularly the second dose of the Zyprexa. I recall a day when I realized that I had missed a couple of days and went to take a tablet of the Zyprexa and I broke it out of its wrapper and put it to my mouth. I just couldn't bring myself to swallow it. I haven't taken any since that day. I was still deep in the Methadone detox and I didn't tell my doctors that I had stopped taking these foul Zyprexas. I think I also stopped taking the Efexors too but I may have kept these up for a little while longer.

Whatever withdrawal-effects I may have had from coming off these drugs is probably lost in the nightmare of the Methadone detox. I stopped taking these psycho-meds before I should have, according to my medical advice, but I just could no longer keep taking them. This may have accentuated the withdrawals I was having from the Methadone and, as I said, I did take some heroin during this difficult period. My suicidality also returned, briefly I'm pleased to say, and my last intense suicidal moment was at this time on the Westgate Bridge urging myself to take the leap over the edge. It is impossible to tease out all the factors that led to this.

All this detox and withdrawal was supervised by another doctor who is a general practitioner and registered with the Methadone program. He was concerned about how rapid my Methadone detox schedule was and tried to extend it but I insisted we stick to it. Towards the end he urged me to get out of town for a while—he actually said that he knew of very few instances of people who have successfully detoxed from Methadone without getting away from their normal environment, away from easy access to heroin, for a while.

I had sleep problems during this time and he gave me some benzodiaze-pines to help with this, but this was the only other medication that I used during this difficult time. By the time the Methadone withdrawals had passed I had already stopped all the Zyprexa and Efexor and told the doctor at this time. He could only frown at me… and be grateful that it hadn't been a complete disaster.

I must add here that although today I am very critical of bad "medicine," especially that of the psychiatric profession, some wonderful doctors have helped me. This fellow is one of those. He was available (though never on time) and genuine and always honest with me. I remember him saying to me "please don't die," which is one of the most useful things any doctor has ever said to me. He did not pretend to have any miracle cures, but was prepared to assist with whatever skill he had. This sort of integrity was absolutely vital to someone like me.

Recovery

I feel that it is important in a story like this to tell you that today—since 1999 for more than two years now—I am no longer suicidal, am no longer "depressed" (a diagnostic label that I now find meaningless) and that I am no longer using heroin. I am not totally drug free. I remain a dedicated smoker, I love some wine with dinner (but do not like being drunk) and am seriously addicted to tea. After two years without psychiatric drugs in my system, I can say that I still have some problems with sexual function and occasionally with sleeping, which I never had before this horrible adventure. I am tempted sometimes to blame this on these drugs but again it is impossible to know. Some of these are probably just due to aging—indeed some call my crisis a male menopause, which I think is an argument with some merit. It may also be due to my heroin abuse.

I have now been able to return to part-time work for the last two years and am pursuing some research into the relationships between suicide and spirituality. I am also active in mental health consumer rights where I meet many lovely people with whom I find great comfort and support as well as sharing a concern for the abuses of psychiatry. But most of all, I am also now settling into a very special and lasting relationship with the wonderful Elaine. Life is good.

During my time of struggle, one of the most annoying things was all those people who believe that what had worked for them could also work for me. The path to peace and freedom is unique for each individual and very personal, I believe. Although I want to shout aloud to the world with the joy of my own liberation, I do not assume that my path is necessarily the path for any other person. I also now believe that the struggle for inner peace and personal freedom is intrinsic to a life well lived.

The issue is not how do we "cure" these "illnesses" of mental, emotional and spiritual distress, but how do we embrace them into our unique lives and how do we support each other in allowing us the full experience of whatever life brings us. I heard a story of a person who asked an Australian aboriginal elder what their culture did when someone was experiencing what our culture calls a "psychosis." The answer was so beautifully simple. He said "first, we allow them to have it (i.e. the psychosis) and we make sure that someone is always with them."

Hannelore Reetz

Addiction or Search for Self

Tranquilizer: Tranxilium

While searching for the causes of my addiction, I constantly come up against my childhood. I found the atmosphere in my home to be repressive and frightening. A great deal of emphasis was put on performance and cognitive thinking. Thus, at an early age I lost the access to my needs and emotions. I developed into an inhibited person who always put other people first. At sixteen I met my first boyfriend and we were married two years later. My first child was born when I was eighteen and I was pregnant with my second one three years later. My husband was unfaithful to me during this second pregnancy and left me and our two daughters for another woman. On top of the feelings of worthlessness came existential anxiety and the fear of failure which, even at night, never left me.

I had never learned to talk about my feelings and problems and I had no one I could trust. To be able to at least sleep at night I went to the pharmacy and asked for a sleeping pill. This was sold to me without any questions asked. It was a sleeping pill containing bromide sold at the time over the counter in Germany. At last I was able to sleep at nights and this gave me strength to keep going the following day.

After about four weeks I needed a higher dose to achieve the desired effect. I experienced severe feelings of guilt and was ashamed that I could no longer survive without sleeping pills. I went to all the pharmacies in my neighborhood. It would have been obvious if I gotten my supply from only one pharmacy.

As the date for my divorce drew nearer, I needed pills during the day also. That I might have become addicted to the pills and needed treatment never entered my head. On the day of my divorce I was pumped so full of pills that even my family noticed.

Under threat of having my children taken away from me I went to a psychiatric hospital for six weeks. It was 1967 and I was twenty-three years old.

At the hospital it was made clear to me that I was ruining my life and my health. I didn't know I was suffering from an illness and could only hope to be able to sleep naturally again. Unfortunately, even after six weeks my fears and anxieties had not disappeared and in fact were worse than ever. In addition to all this I was afraid that my children would be taken away from me if I talked about my problems. On the day of my discharge, when the children were asleep, I slipped out and went to the emergency pharmacy and got a supply of sleeping pills.

In 1976 tablets containing bromide were declared prescription-only drugs by the authorities. I went to a psychiatrist and deliberately hid my tablet career. He prescribed me Tranxilium *(tranquilizer, active ingredient clorazepate dipotassium)*, a benzodiazepine. At first the pills had no effect. I was calm, but I could not sleep at night. However, after about fourteen days my anxiety states had disappeared and I felt more free than ever before in my life. Gradually, I began to look down on people who had emotions and showed them. I didn't feel as if I belonged to the world but was somehow hovering above it. I functioned like a robot. I could work eight hours a day, run the house and look after my children. From now on I had no more problems. I even joined a fitness studio and performed superbly on the equipment. For the first time in my life I felt as if I was worth something. I was no longer anxious and could perform well! Very often I only needed to collect my prescription at the practice without seeing the doctor.

I became friends with a colleague and fell in love with him. We moved in together and married a few months later. I told him about my pill dependency in a matter-a-fact way, but he attached no importance to it. At the beginning of the marriage I was able to reduce my pill consumption, although in cases of conflict I needed a higher dose. Now and again my conscience got to me. Then I would simply reduce the dose and use alcohol instead. My husband was surprised that I could not hold any drink. This combination had a disastrous effect. Depending on my mood, the highs got higher and the lows lower. As I was approaching menopause this seemed to provide an explanation for the mood swings.

A feeling of absolute emptiness and pointlessness in my life began to grow. One day I lost control and swallowed a lot of tablets and washed them down with alcohol. I can no longer say whether I really intended to take my life at the time. It was my first despairing call for help. I was sent to the closed ward of a psychiatric hospital. I still could not find the courage to talk about my pill consumption. I was afraid of losing my husband and losing the pills.

The hospital stays became more frequent until I began to feel safe there. During my last stay in the Waldhaus clinic in Berlin, I hid my Tranxilium in the lining of my purse. When my supply was discovered I felt terribly ashamed. I was offered the opportunity of undertaking four months of therapy on the addiction ward. The idea made me feel miserable. For twenty-five years I had swallowed pills with only a few interruptions. I was forty-six years of age and could not imagine trying to live my life without their help.

The fact that I was going to become a grandmother was the key to my decision to undertake the therapy in 1990. I wanted to be clean for my first grandchild. Consumed by panic attacks, I started withdrawal.

The only thing I can remember from the beginning is the terrible pain in my neck. The fear was there. I felt scalped, with no protective skin. There were no more pain killers. I could not sleep at night. The only thing that kept me going was simply the desire to live.

There wasn't much time for brooding. The day began with morning exercise. Then there were lectures on the illness of medication dependency from a medical perspective. Walks, jogging in the woods and ergotherapy helped get me through the early phase. But the most important thing for me were the group discussions and the individual consultations with the therapist.

I lived very intimately with the others in the group. We were all under the pressure of addiction. It was very difficult to put up with both my own problems and the problems of the others. There was no opportunity to escape. One day I was close to breaking point. I wanted to go home immediately. I did something I had never done before: I talked openly in the group and made myself vulnerable. When the therapist accused me of wanting to start swallowing the pills again, I felt my anger growing. This was the first real emotion I had experienced. The ensuing sadness and the never ending self-pity opened my eyes to the fact that I was addicted and that I had to accept this.

I suffered from severe mood swings and had great difficulty in accepting my sensitivity. I had feelings of guilt and inferiority and could not bear criticism. It became clear to me that I was not only dependent on the pills but on the opinion and judgment of other. I so badly needed to be loved.

The clinic provided groups for relatives. My husband came regularly to these "parents' meetings" as I called them. From the beginning I talked to him about all my feelings and it was a great help to us. The time in the hospital went quickly. On my discharge I was already able to sleep four hours straight.

The therapist recommended that I return to work immediately. I was very agitated because I was so anxious at the prospect. With a beating heart I went to my boss and told her about my addiction. This helped reduce my fear of returning to work.

In the community I found a Kreuz-Bund *(caritative self-help organization for drug-dependents and their families)* group which I attended regularly. We talked a lot about feelings in the group. At the beginning I wasn't able to talk in front of the others. Listening was enough to start with. I was constantly being asked to talk about myself and after a while my heart stopped landing in my throat. I felt accepted as a member of the family in the group.

It was made clear to me that I would have to change my life. But I would have find out myself how I was going to change it. I didn't know my own needs. I had always functioned and lived according to what other people expected from me. My new life was accompanied by mainly negative feelings. Some days I was consumed by pressure in my head. I felt constricted and couldn't breath properly until I felt that 100,000 little demons were whimpering in the back of my head for the drugs. I had no choice other than to admit my addiction. I talked with these treacherous little demons and told them: "you're not getting anything, no matter how much you scream." This helped me through the most difficult pressure of the addiction.

I had discovered together with my husband that driving helped at such times. Because the Berlin Wall was now gone, we had the opportunity to get to know the surroundings of the city. Driving and then taking walks in the countryside calmed me.

I became a grandmother. I saw my grandchild once a week and really looked forward to these days. I took pleasure in the feelings of love I felt for this little being. How different it would have been if I had still been swallowing the pills.

Years of practice of suppressing my feelings meant that I now exploded for very small reasons in my day-to-day life. It took quite a long time for me to understand annoyance, anger, sadness or joy for what they were. I reacted irritably, often felt guilty, and was annoyed at myself for not being capable of distancing myself from seeming judgments.

I went to a weekend seminar offered by the Volkshochschule (*public adult education school*). It was called "dealing with inhibitions." I got a little closer to myself by recognizing that as a result of my upbringing I had become a perfectionist out of fear of punishment. In the long run it became strenuous not to admit to any mistakes. All of this knowledge did not make me particularly happy because I still couldn't do anything with it. I went to more courses, one called "learning to deal with conflict." I was at least proud of myself that I could attend without feeling guilty at leaving my husband alone some weekends. Water-color painting which I learned at the Volkshochschule brought me great joy.

After three years staying clean I still experienced the pressure of the addiction at regular intervals. When we moved apartments and I left my familiar surroundings, the "nasties" in my head tried very hard to pull me down. By a lucky chance I received the address of a group of clean, medication-dependent women and at the advice center "Schwindel-Frei" (*"Head-for-Heights"*) I met them for a preliminary meeting.

These women met once a week and during the first meeting I immediately felt that I would be better able to open up in this group. The group was run by a psychologist with experience in withdrawal from medication. I learned that after years of taking pills, withdrawal could take up to five years. On the one hand I felt relief at gaining this new knowledge, and on the other hand I looked excitedly towards the two years still to go.

I still experienced a longing for a life free of conflict. So many times I didn't want to see the path I had already put behind me; I wanted still more and I wanted it immediately. In this new group I learned to break down this "addictive frame of mind" in small steps. First I recognized my inability to keep my distance. I became unsure of myself when others wanted to unload their problems on me, and I only recognized later what was really part of me. I often became involved in other people's problems so as to avoid my dealing with my own.

The avoidance of conflicts, the compulsion to keep everyone happy and, if possible, never to lose my self-control always led to a build up of pressure in me. Sometimes I think I'm going to have to deal with this until the end of my days. A feeling, deeply anchored in me, of not having any right to exist is closely associated with this pressure. My fear of hurt and disappointment probably led to my tendency to self-destructive behavior.

At times I felt that all my cells were negatively programmed and I was astonished to realize that I couldn't deal with pleasant, happy emotions for long. The negative emotions were more familiar and I could deal with them.

Birthdays, Christmas, in fact celebrations of any kind, particularly family ones became a torture. I had always increased my abuse of alcohol and tablets at such times. These times represented a relapse risk for me. I had changed, but the others hadn't. I had learned to talk about my feelings with other members of the group, with my husband and with a few friends and found this stimulating and interesting. The "blabla" of normal society bored me. In such situations I often fell into my old role of playing the clown. I still kept my feelings from my family because I continued to see them as a weakness and did not want to keep digging around in them. For a long time I was the black sheep in my family, which no doubt suited them in view of their own inadequacies.

In the time after I had withdrawn I suffered badly from influenza-like infections. Many doctors I went to for help prescribed pain killers and antibiotics, although I always told them about my addiction. I refused the pills offered and took their lack of understanding in stride. I stopped going to doctors altogether and treated myself instead. Old traditional remedies such as inhaling, chest rubs or herbal teas are more time-consuming, and the colds lasted longer, but they came back less often.

I began to find my job more and more stressful. I had sat typing for years at the typewriter. I had constant neck and back pain, not just from anxiety but from wear and tear. The employment office offered me retraining as a bookkeeper. I attended school for a year and was proud of the good results I achieved. Unfortunately, without any professional experience and at my age I had no chance in the job market. In my disappointment I felt my stubbornness and defiance welling up in me. Thoughts such as "well, I could have kept on taking the pills" came to me and I thought them through to the end and I realized that despite all the difficulties, life without the pills was better than a creeping death. I applied to be officially classified as "severely handicapped" but was refused, the reason given being that since I had been clean for five years I was cured. I was given 20% recognition for the rest of my life for my bad back. Anger, bitterness and the feeling of being unfairly treated gave me no peace until I realized that I alone had to take responsibility for my illness which is not recognized by society. This recognition made me grateful for having achieved so much.

My route led to the twelve-step group of Alcoholic Anonymous. Here, at the beginning of 1996, I gradually found my way back to belief. "Worrying" caused me lots of trouble. It used to be the worry about getting the pills and more than anything keeping the pill swallowing secret. And now the compulsion of always trying to do right by everybody was still there. The belief in a higher power helped and the ability to entrust this power with my worries and problems. This step meant a kind of letting go. Many group members in Alcoholics Anonymous had been dry or clean for ten years or more and had a great deal of experience in the cunning of addiction and in gaining the skills to cheat it. I also found yoga and meditation helpful in finding my center. During meditation I learned to concentrate on my own thoughts and to switch off.

Looking back today, I realize that the path to sobriety and taking responsibility for oneself can only be managed with a good deal of courage, distancing and searching for one's own needs. For me personally, the most important thing was never to give up and to talk. The path is thorny but life is worth it.

Translation from the German by Mary Murphy

Better Sometimes than Forever

Mary Nettle
Having Control Again

Neuroleptics: Largactil, Modecate / Lithium: Pridal

I had my first contact with the psychiatric system in 1978 when I was twenty-five. I had a good job as a marketing executive involved with consumer market research for a large manufacturer of pet foods and breakfast cereals. I feel there were three trigger factors involved in my eventual admission to a psychiatric hospital. The emotional strain involved in getting married, I had a very difficult journey to work and, primarily, my workload had increased due to many of my colleagues having been made redundant.

I left hospital with a diagnosis of manic depression and a prescription for lithium. After several months I was very lucky to be given a job by the market research agency I used to work for. I was able to come off lithium as my psychiatrist at the time had the impression I was settled and may not have another episode. This was true for several years until I got another job, which stressed me out this time as a civil servant on an American air force base close to where I lived.

In 1982 I had another spell in hospital and my label was confirmed. This time I left hospital on lithium and a major tranquilizer depot injection Modecate. After a couple of years I stopped being given the depot injection but continued swallowing one thousand milligrams of Pridal *(mood stabilizer, active ingredient lithium)* daily. I had blood tests once every three months from my family doctor (GP).

I was told that as a diabetic needs insulin to live so a manic-depressive needs lithium to control their mood swings. I put on weight but was told this was because I was content now my moods were balanced, I was eating too much and should go to a diet club. This I did, without effect, as of course weight gain is a well-documented side-effect of lithium. The main side-effect was that I did not feel any emotions at all, I was unable to feel anything— happiness or sadness, anger or delight and I certainly was unable to laugh or cry. My marriage was a disaster as my husband developed into a chronic alcoholic. I took lithium for the ten years from 1982 until 1992 and put up with his quite unacceptable behavior because I was not able to express my emotions due to the medication.

About 1984 my GP told me that he did not believe in keeping people on medication indefinitely and did I want to try and come off it? I told him that I had been told that I needed lithium for the rest of my life and he should talk to my psychiatrist. He wrote to her and she replied that he had no right to interfere in my treatment and if I came off and needed admission to hospital she would have nothing to do with it and my GP would have to cope with the consequences. Needless to say I remained on the lithium.

Around 1988 I met up with some people who were members of Survivors Speak Out, a user group of people, who had experienced psychiatry and wanted to change the system. For the first time I talked to people who had challenged the system and survived, it changed my life! Due to the user movement I became empowered and tried to take control of my life.

My GP was amazed when I said I wanted to stop taking lithium. After he had recovered from the shock we discussed the pros and cons. He said that if I was an asthmatic and wanted to run a marathon and not take my inhaler, he would insist I did because if I had an asthma attack without an inhaler I could die. However the worst that could happen if I stopped taking lithium would be that I would have a spell in hospital. He felt I was in no danger of dying if I stopped taking lithium so he said "Go for it" and he would be there for me if I needed him.

So in 1992 after ten years of taking lithium I stopped. It took a while but I felt alive again and knew what it was like to "feel." I was in touch with my emotions again and it was wonderful! For my husband it was a disaster as I was no longer the passive wife who cleaned up after him without a word and did not mind having an emotional desert of a marriage. After two years off lithium I walked out of the house at 10.00 p.m. on Saturday 11th June 1994 to stay with my mother who lived 40 miles away. My mother and I both felt I could not cope anymore I had not been sleeping and had spent many hours on the phone to the Samaritans my GP had been as supportive as he could be and I had Valium and Mogadon to take if I needed. She was providing the safe haven that I needed.

After I stopped taking the lithium in 1992 my husband acknowledged that he was an alcoholic and in that year had two admissions to our local psychiatric hospital 25 miles from our home (a small village in the Cotswolds—a scenic part of the UK about 100 miles west of London). He undertook an alcohol detoxification (detox) programme and "dried out" each time in the same ward where I had my second and last (I hope!) inpatient admission for manic depression in 1982. This hospital was an enormous red brick Victorian lunatic asylum that took patients from many miles around and closed in 1995. The detox programme did not work and he continued to drink.

He was made redundant from his job and was unable to look for another one. He received incapacity benefit from the state because of his deteriorating physical and mental health resulting from the alcoholism. I survived the stress of this because at least he had admitted he was an alcoholic and I had the support of my fellow mental health system survivors and was developing my own self worth by being respected and valued within the growing user movement.

In January 1993 I celebrated my 40th birthday with a big party and was still hoping that my husband would accept help and support from his fellow alcoholics in their user movement. Then came a flood of unexpected stress triggers. In March my father died suddenly of a heart attack just after midnight whilst he and my mother were sitting watching television. When she rang with this dreadful news my husband was in his usual alcoholic stupor and unable to support me. In May of that year my mother developed serious heart problems, which totally disabled her, and in September she had a major operation to replace the mitral valve in her heart and was in hospital until Christmas time. In the October my husband was found by police in London slumped over the wheel of his car. He was taken to hospital where he had an epileptic type fit and lost his license to drive on medical grounds.

I believe it was not until June 1994 that I felt able to "breakdown." This was when I was sure my mother had made a very good recovery from her heart condition and was in a position to take care of me rather than the other way around. However by that time I had got so stressed that I had a major psychotic episode which meant though I was cared for at home because my mother knew that I did not want to go into hospital I agreed to accept psychiatric help and medication.

In 1996 I went to live in my own house in a small town eight miles from my mother's house. I have a different GP and psychiatrist both of whom want me to keep taking the lithium just in case I get another stress trigger. In the UK we have a system called the Care Programme Approach where if you are considered to be severely ill (i.e. a diagnosis of manic depression or schizophrenia) you are given a key worker to look after you and keep you in touch with the mental health services, currently my psychiatrist is my key worker. I have regular meetings with him and can contact him at any time (although I've not tried to do this.) However I am still empowered and in touch with the user movement and I have persuaded the doctors that I know myself. I am not taking lithium and do not intend to take it, the doctors respect my decision.

It was a struggle to convince the psychiatric system that it was safe for me to use the self management technique that is I dose myself with the horrible but effective major tranquilizer Largactil on the few occasions stress triggers lack of sleep. The way Largactil affects me is that it works by temporarily partially paralyzing my brain and limbs so that its really difficult to move even if you want to this is why it is called the "chemical cosh."

This is far better for me than having my emotions blocked all the time in case I meet a stress trigger. So far its working and, with the additional help of aroma therapy massage and co-counseling, long may this state of affairs continue and I will begin to love life and start to learn how to have fun!

Wolfgang Voelzke
Together with my Psychiatrist

Neuroleptics: Haldol, Melleril / Lithium

Since I became active in the self-help movement of (ex-)users and survivors of psychiatry in 1991, fundamental experiences have made it increasingly clear to me that it is normal to be different.

This is true also in dealing with psychiatric drugs. Before I describe my own journey in dealing with neuroleptics and lithium, I would first like to report on a few basic lessons gained through the experiences with psychiatric drugs among my circle of friends and the self-help groups. In the self-help group in Bielefeld, I got to know many who had experiences in psychiatry and who had often been patients in psychiatric hospitals in recent years. As soon as they were doing better again after being released from the psychiatric hospital, they had immediately withdrawn from psychiatric drugs, and a crisis—sometimes with a forced readmission—ensued after a certain period of time. Whether or not these were cases of classic relapse into the original complex of problems, or if they were directly caused by withdrawal was not examined. In any case, some people lost their apartments or their jobs. Today these people with experiences in psychiatry take very low doses of neuroleptics, they intensively confront their biographies and their life situations, and they try to deal consciously with their life, their limits and their possibilities. By doing so they have been spared further stays in psychiatry. Of course, it is difficult to determine if it was the neuroleptic dose that had led to positive developments, or if it was rather the fact that they had begun to live a more conscious life and had confronted their problems.

I myself was always able to withdraw from my neuroleptics for a mid-range term after each crisis and/or hospital stay. But this does not seem to be the way for everyone. For this reason, I will first describe the experiences of others. The clearest example is someone I know well (we met in psychiatry in

1986). He wanted to change his situation fundamentally. So he began psychotherapy, worked intensively on his own history, and tried to organize his life more consciously. In this context he gradually and then completely withdrew from neuroleptics. At first this went well. He felt more intensely and discovered hidden energies, and he confronted his family situation more intensively than previously. But the energies, the tension and the excitement grew constantly. Finally, the pressure, fear and tension became so great that he made a grave mistake while driving, which caused him to lose his license and landed him in a psychiatric hospital. With great effort he was able to pass the medical-psychological examination with the public safety regulators and got his driver's license back. This was particularly important to him given that he is dependent upon his car.

Psychotherapy helped him along his life's path with more clarity and self-awareness. After these experiences he decided to take a small dose of neuroleptics that he could control himself according to his need. He speaks at regular intervals with a psychiatrist or a social worker from the health department. He has found his way by dealing consciously with his limits and his possibilities. He is well aware of all the known harmful effects of neuroleptics, even in smaller doses which are less often problematic.

It was possible for me to withdraw from my neuroleptics and lithium for the long term. I have been involved in psychiatry since 1975 (when I made the transition from school to a profession). After my stays in psychiatric hospitals from December 1975 to February 1976 and from March to August 1976, I had been receiving depot injections of neuroleptics that I gradually tapered off and ended in 1979. Then things went well for me for ten years both psychologically and in terms of my health, despite a serious personal crisis.

When I found myself under immense stress in 1986 (due to important and comprehensive projects in my profession, training for further qualifications, and applying for a new position), my mental illness broke through. My madness, the paranoia and fear that I will be killed, is what I call my "psychosis." I have suffered so much under it that I never want to have to "walk barefoot through hell" again.

That's why I started taking neuroleptics again after a three and a half month stay in the hospital in 1986. After approximately one year I "slipped" into a "psychosis" again and had to be admitted as an inpatient for three and a half months. This time it was because my girlfriend at the time had broken up with me. Without my parents I would have gone under during this difficult period because I would not have been able to live alone and get by without help.

To avoid further "psychoses," I received an additional lithium preparation —one whose mechanism of action is still not understood today but which according to the statistical averages was supposed to abate psychotic crises or make them less severe. My psychiatrist had informed me very accurately both in person and by giving me literature on the side-effects (possible effects on the thyroid, kidneys, possibly life-endangering effects with an increase of lithium in the blood system). I then went to my internist, who is also my regular doctor, with all my medical records and we agreed to do regular comprehensive blood, liver, kidney and heart (EKG) examinations. My thyroid was checked and had become so large that I had to take an additional thyroid preparation.

Because I had been out of the psychiatric hospitals for seven years since 1987 and had been able to get through my psychotic crises as an outpatient, in 1994 I was able to gradually withdraw from the lithium preparation within nine months under consultation with my psychiatrist. Finally I was also able to withdraw from the thyroid preparation.

Since 1987 my psychiatrist has treated my psychotic crises—with my consent—pharmacologically by initially giving me a high dose of Haldol and Melleril, which is then reduced according to my level of stability and tiredness. At first the Haldol dose is reduced and the Melleril remains constant, and then the Melleril is gradually reduced. One neuroleptic was reduced at a time in order to more clearly determine the effects. In the period after a psychotic crisis when I was no longer on medical leave and had to work again, I was constantly tired and slow. It was most important to me, on the one hand, to take as many neuroleptics as necessary to keep my thoughts and feelings from becoming stuck and to avoid great internal tensions, and, on the other hand, to take as few neuroleptics as possible so that I could cope better with my work again.

And so I asked my psychiatrist at almost every visit if there weren't something else we could reduce. The reason I asked this at each visit was that after a certain time the tiredness increased and the neuroleptics dulled me more than was necessary to balance out my inner restlessness and the tension.

Because my last three "psychoses" were terrible, I decided to take neuroleptics again at the beginning of the next crisis. This is a decision that everyone needs to make for him or herself based on complete information and after weighing the risks and benefits. The personal conditions and valuations may differ widely for each individual.

In December 1996 I lost my inner balance because I was asked if I wanted to take on a new position of great responsibility. I struggled with myself for three months and then decided not to apply for the position because the sum of the demands on me would most likely be too much. During this period the problem presented itself vividly to me at night: I awoke at 12:30 or 1:30 a.m. in panic at the thought of the new position and could no longer sleep. This disrupted my equilibrium. In consultation with my doctor, I took a high dosage of Melleril, which we slowly reduced again until February 1997.

Even with slow withdrawal from neuroleptics I am usually very sensitive in the first weeks thereafter and need to take care that I have more peace and less stress than usual in order to work though the impressions of the day.

From 1994 to the beginning of 1998 I undertook psychotherapy, during which the goal was to cope with my inner conflicts and to deal with and solve current problems, as well as to consciously acknowledge my limits and recognize earlier than in the past when I am taking on too much and am granting myself too little calm and quiet. Because my personality is such that I am—despite my good intentions—terribly ambitious, diligent and exact, I tend to do too much and overexert myself in my profession as well as in my volunteer work. In recent years I have tried to organize my life more consciously and—when possible—more to my own satisfaction, and to be more honest with myself. Therapeutic discussions with my doctor at long but regular intervals contribute to this.

For example, I have discovered a sure and easy way to recognize early warning signals. When I have reached the limit of how much I can burden my soul, I feel under pressure and I become extremely sensitive to sound. In this state, even a whisper in my ear or somewhat louder music—which usually doesn't bother me—become torturous. This is the sign for me and also for my partner, who can read it in my face and especially in my eyes, that I have reached my limits. Then it is time to pull the emergency brake, to get some rest, and if necessary to call in sick for a short time in order to quickly restore my peace and tranquility.

In this way I have often been able to restore my balance without neuroleptics. But I always keep a neuroleptic (Melleril) in liquid form at home. If I notice that the pressure has become too great, if I cannot sleep at night and the other measures are not enough, then I take a low dosage of this (the drops are easy to dose). In recent years this has happened very seldom and was only necessary when I was under great pressure. I am still working on finding inner satisfaction, acceptable living conditions (an environment that is positive for me and a healthy way of living) and positive-thinking people around me, as well as recognizing and realizing meaning and reaching my goals in life. All this helps me to live my life with more joy and tranquility and to cope more easily with difficult situations—as far as possible, without psychiatric drugs.

Translation from the German by Christina White

Lynne Setter

Return to Myself

Neuroleptics: Risperdal / Antidepressants: Effexor, Ludiomil, Paxil, Prozac, Wellbutrin / Lithium / Carbamazepine: Tegretol / Tranquilizer: Ativan, Halcion, Mogadon, Valium

The first evidence of mental illness was seen when I was an infant and began hurting myself in the crib, diagnosis however was not made until 31 years later. My "self medication" and substance abuse regime began at age nine when I began smoking cigarettes and stealing my mothers tranquilizers. At twelve years alcohol and marijuana abuse began, and I was prescribed Mogadon to be taken at night and 5mg Valium to take three times a day. I was rebellious and diagnosed as "hyperactive." The medication soon changed to Halcion[1], which I abused severely for over ten years. I nearly do not remember life without benzodiazepines. Antidepressant use has been frequent since teenage years, with anticonvulsants and antipsychotics coming into play by 1995. I am now virtually drug free, concentrating primarily on diet, nutrition and stress reduction as a means to manage my condition. Stability has finally become within my reach.

Going back…

During my first year of school I was put forward into a class with children two years my senior. My parents were told this was because I was "bright." I was expelled from this school three years later for throwing violent tantrums, thus beginning a turbulent school life in which I attended seven different schools, most of from which I was expelled. I began writing poetry at age eleven, and on rediscovering this I am able to identify a very unhappy childhood (memories are limited). Apparently I cried myself to sleep often during school years, and by age 14 had almost stopped going completely. Education Department psychologists insisted on trying to make me put round blocks in square holes, and other equally inane "tests." They prescribed more tranquilizers and antidepressants. I don't remember what all the drugs were or the medication duration. I do know I became consistently more unstable and more withdrawn from life and reality. Suicidal ideation was almost daily, and attempts frequent. I numbed my overactive mind with both legal and illegal drug abuse, my thinking totally focused on killing the pain, and trying to be "normal."

At age 19 I had a grand-mal seizure, which I attribute to the previous ten years of substance use. During my teens I also experimented with LSD, amphetamines and many legal drugs acquired on the street. I tried to withdraw from benzodiazepines many times with little success. The physical and emo-

---

1 Tranquilizer, active ingredient triazolam, marketed also as Triazolam

tional pain of the withdrawal was torturous, the worst time causing me to tear out clumps of my hair in an attempt to deflect the otherwise insufferable pain. During many withdrawal attempts I began smoking more marijuana, which did seem to alleviate some of the withdrawal effects. Marijuana has been my companion for 22 years, and I believe the lesser of all the evils I have consumed. It has calmed me without side-effects, and alleviated the impact of the many withdrawals I have experienced. It troubles me that the use of this relatively harmless drug brands me a criminal.

In my mid twenties I left New Zealand and embarked on a ten year period of what would be diagnosed as "hypomanic and mixed states, with rapid cycling." In my experience, this meant "consistent mania with depression always looming," and often taking over. I worked endlessly, the inevitable crash would arrive, and the cycle would begin again. Cycles would last a few hours, weeks or occasionally months. By 1994 I had landed a high powered job in Washington DC, and six months later I was diagnosed as "manic depressive." Within one year I was a full-time psychiatric patient, following a near fatal attempt on my life that put me in a coma. My family was told it was unlikely I would survive, and if I did the chance of permanent brain damage was high. During that year I had been prescribed lithium, Tegretol, Depakote, Prozac, Paxil, Effexor, Ludiomil and Risperdal[1]. The physical and emotional side-effects of these drugs were intolerable, but when trying to withdraw I became so unstable that out of desperation I would try the drugs again.

I was forced to leave my job prior to the coma episode, and shortly after I was snowed in during the "blizzard of the century." That was the icing on the cake—so to speak. I do not remember the preceding two weeks before I was admitted to hospital, but apparently I appeared "more together" than I had in a long time. I had meticulously attended to my affairs, and researched thoroughly the draws full of drugs I now had. My choice was lithium and Tegretol, which nearly worked. I believe the cocktails of drugs, especially in the previous year had made me lose touch completely with reality, and reflecting back now I feel intense fear of revisiting that place. When I was well enough

---

1 Neuroleptic, active ingredient risperidone, marketed also as Risperidone

to be transferred to the psychiatric ward I was again prescribed Prozac and lithium. I pretended I was fine to get out of the hospital, and spent the next six months hardly able to get out of bed due to drug side-effects and severe depression. I tried to stop taking Prozac, and within three weeks I was back in hospital following another suicide attempt. Then I was prescribed Depakote and Wellbutrin[1], and shortly after I decided it was time to come home to New Zealand. I was too sick to work and couldn't support myself, I was not eligible for any government assistance in the US.

I am very fortunate to have support from family and friends, without them I doubt I would have made it this far. With their help I started to rebuild my life and discover alternatives to mainstream psychiatry. I continued to take Wellbutrin and Depakote until early 1997, when I very gradually decreased the dosages over a period of about three months. The withdrawal was the easiest I had experienced which I believe was due to a combination of the following reasons:

1. decreasing the dosage slowly,
2. use of herbal remedies—hypericum and valerian, and nutritional supplements,
3. diet revision,
4. stress reduction—including avoiding sleep deprivation wherever possible,
5. maintaining routine.

Please note that before discussing the above, I would like to stress that in my experience these factors are essential in management of psychiatric conditions overall, however are especially important during vulnerable periods of withdrawal.

---

1 Antidepressant, active ingredient bupropion, marketed also as Amfebutamone, Bupropion, Zyban

1

It is widely known that slower withdrawal from any drug will produce less severe adverse effects. Cold turkey can be extremely dangerous and sometimes has proved fatal. One of my experiences withdrawing from Prozac found me in hospital from a suicide attempt, and I have heard many incidences of homicidal and suicidal behavior caused by withdrawal, in particular recently from Prozac.

2

Hypericum acts as an antidepressant, so as I decreased the dose of Wellbutrin I compensated with increasing the dose of hypericum accordingly. Valerian acts as a sedative so I also increased the dose of that during the time I was susceptible to withdrawal symptoms. On complete termination of psychiatric drugs I was taking quite a large dose of both, which over time I have gradually decreased.

Extensive research on nutritional benefits directed me towards particular nutritional supplements, which I take on a strict regime. These include multivitamins (excluding choline, inositol and lecithin—these are not recommended for manic depression), additional vitamin C, B complex, B_6 and B_{12}, fish-liver oil, antioxidants, calcium, magnesium, and lots of garlic—fresh wherever possible. Since a few months after the withdrawal period, I have gradually reduced supplements and try to satisfy these needs more through diet.

3

I believe diet is very important. The Chinese have talked about the mind/gut connection for centuries. Where there is a situation of food allergy for example, the lining of the gut becomes compromised and leaks toxins through the gut wall, directly into the bloodstream. I have recently discovered I have celiac disease (gluten intolerance), and on modifying my diet to compensate have found my emotions far more stable, putting me in a better stead (both physically and emotionally) to deal with withdrawal, and ongoing maintenance. I have an added complication of candida in the gut, probably caused because the food allergy has left undigested material lying around in the gut, a perfect environment for yeast growth. All the literature I have read on food allergies and candida state depression and emotional instability (among many other things) as common symptoms.

My original diagnosis many years ago was "irritable bowel syndrome." Many consumers of the mental health "industry" have stated they have irritable bowel syndrome. This diagnosis is very vague because what ultimately causes an "irritable bowel"? This aspect rarely seems to be addressed. In my experience these issues are not addressed as diagnosis can usually only be made through observation and diet revision (which can be a laborious process), therefore the 15-minute consultation is no longer viable. Also drug companies make no profits, as the main way to treat these conditions is through diet.

Along with addressing food allergies, I have also eliminated almost all animal fats from my diet. I rarely eat junk food and try to drink lots of water. These are very simple modifications that I believe have had an impact on my physical and mental health. I can't stress enough how important I believe these issues to be, however long the road may be to finding individual balance.

4

Stress reduction—On analyzing the most difficult periods of my life it has become apparent that stress is the biggest demon. During my last withdrawal I eliminated much of the stress I had previously lived with, by staying with family members who, although creating stress of their own, eliminated financial pressure (I was unable to work at the time) and also the most fundamental issues of food and shelter. I no longer had to worry about paying the rent, or buying food. These most basic worries weigh on everyone, especially when our stress levels and overall health are compromised through drug withdrawal.

Dr. Kay Jamison wrote in her book "An Unquiet Mind" (1995) that "sleep deprivation is both a cause and a symptom of manic depressive illness." I believe this. Valerian taken at night can assist with achieving good sleep, however in my case at times I take Ativan to ensure adequate sleep. Healthy sleeping habits are vital.

5

Maintaining routine—results of studies presented at the Second International Conference on Bipolar Disorder in Pittsburgh 1997, suggested that disruptions in social rhythms may play a role in the onset of depressive, and manic episodes. It was quoted that "for reasons we have yet to learn, people with bipolar disorder seem to have more delicate internal clock mechanisms." I concur, this is an important issue. During withdrawals, and also in everyday life without psychiatric drugs, I have found myself more likely to become unstable when even simple routines are changed. Perhaps I have just become more aware of these previously invisible aspects of life, that appear to quite substantially affect my ability to function. Clarifying "boundaries" with family and friends, standing my ground, and learning to say no, these have all been instrumental behaviors I continue to try and teach myself. There is no doubt improving my skills in these areas has helped me greatly.

In summary

My heart and stomach tell me that being diagnosed as "mentally ill" is a very lonely place to be. I feel even more disillusioned having almost completely lost faith in the medical profession, in particular psychiatry. However, I feel fortunate that I have the ability and resources to learn about my body, my mind, and substances and treatments used to "treat" my ails. Certainly for myself, it has become apparent that psychiatric drugs are detrimental, and the medical profession is unlikely to help me. There are so many aspects to our physical and mental well-being that sometimes I feel overwhelmed at the vastness of the picture, but I sincerely believe the entire picture needs to be addressed. The best thing I can do for myself is to continue to learn as much about me as my simple mind allows. I am the master of my own destiny, and this responsibility I am not alone with.

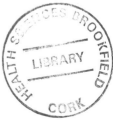

I am now free of all psychiatric drugs except Ativan, which I take on an as needed basis. I would like one day to also manage without these. It is a question of which is more dangerous for me, the mania which inevitably leads to "burnout," severe depression and the danger of suicide, or the confusion, despair and danger of abuse the benzodiazepines seem to promote. It is impossible for us to do everything at once, and I trust I am able to approach this when the time is right. Benzodiazepines have been the most difficult of prescription drugs for me to conquer, however now I am more familiar with the symptoms of addiction, and my mind is cleaner and clearer, enabling me to monitor my usage carefully to avoid beginning the addiction cycle again. Life will always be tough, but finding and maintaining balance in all aspects of being is so far working for me, both through difficult times of withdrawals, and in finally achieving some quality of life.

Professional Acting

Marc Rufer

Creating Fear / Removing Fear
When You Wish to Withdraw, the Opinion of Your Doctor is Dangerous

Neuroleptics / Antidepressants / Lithium / Carbamazepine / Tranquilizers

When withdrawing from psychiatric substances or drugs, a distinction must be made between biological symptoms and reactions which are triggered purely by the psyche. Before I deal with the important psychological conditions when withdrawing, let me first deal with the biological phenomenon of tolerance.

Biologically triggered withdrawal symptoms

The development of tolerance

All biological effects of withdrawal are a result of tolerance. The dose of a psychoactive substance for which users develop tolerance must be increased manifold in order to achieve the initial effect. It is well known that consumers of meprobamate[1], benzodiazepines, barbiturates, opiates and alcohol develop tolerance. Tolerance has a biological cause. The increased breakdown of

---

1 Tranquilizer, marketed as Equanil, Meprobamate, Meprospan, Miltown; component of Equagesic, Meprogese, Meprogesic, Micrainin, Milprem, PMB-200, PMB-400, Q-Gesic

the particular psychiatric substance or drug which can be linked to accelerated breakdown of other foreign substances, or of the body's own substances (hormones for instance) is known as "enzyme induction" (Kuschinsky / Lüllmann / Mohr 1993, pp. 34/61/63/360). Changes at the receptors level can also lead to tolerance: for example, the number of neurotransmitter receptors reduces when the active substance raises the concentration of the transmitter in the synaptic gap (switching point for the neural transmission between two nerve cells); on the other hand new receptors can form if the active ingredient blocks neurotransmitter receptors. These changes certainly still continue in the initial period after quitting and must perforce lead to withdrawal symptoms.

Tolerance is a term associated by psychiatrists primarily with alcohol and opiates. But the formation of new dopamine receptors caused by the neuroleptics leads to the need for an increased neuroleptic dose to achieve the same effect. Furthermore, every psychiatrist knows that neuroleptics must be introduced gradually. The dose which is finally prescribed for long periods is at least double the initial dose. This is all the more amazing, as tolerance is rarely spoken of in connection with neuroleptics. One reason may be that you only find what you search for. Peter Lehmann provides several examples of tolerance (Lehmann 1996b, pp. 428f.). Frank Tornatore and co-authors speak specifically of a possible development of tolerance (Tornatore et al. 1991, p. 53). The question of tolerance is extremely important for a very particular reason. If tolerance has developed then *withdrawal delirium* can occur if the drug is stopped abruptly, causing disturbances in perception as well as disorientation, confusion and hallucinations. Such delirium is well-known following withdrawal from alcohol, benzodiazepines and anticholinergics such as anti-Parkinson drugs. Far too little attention has been paid to the fact that this can also occur when neuroleptics are stopped. Where it is mentioned in the literature it is dealt with under such headings as supersensitivity or withdrawal psychosis. Psychotic symptoms following withdrawal from neuroleptics can be triggered by purely biological or biochemical effects. This is due to new dopamine receptors being formed after the application of neuroleptics (Breggin 1983, p. 143). If the initial dose has been heavily increased indicating the development of tolerance, it follows that the drug should not be abruptly withdrawn. Instead the dose of the active substance must be reduced gradually.

On the other hand, it must not be forgotten that neuroleptics, antidepressants, anti-Parkinson drugs as well as alcohol, cocaine and amphetamines can cause toxic delirium (American Psychiatric Association 2000, pp. 144f.). Disorientation, confusion, hallucinations, and disturbances in perception, therefore, can also be a sign of intoxication with these substances. If toxic delirium results from treatment with high doses of psychiatric drugs, they must be stopped immediately.

Psychologically triggered withdrawal symptoms

Above all, when a psychoactive substance has been taken regularly over a long period its consumption affects the whole personality; it determines to a large extent the life of the person taking it. It is, therefore, easy to understand that coming off the substance is a significant event associated with hopes and fears. Psychological reactions can definitely be expected. The behavior of the doctor determines to a large extent what withdrawal reactions can be expected.

Biologically triggered psychic effects

It is useful to divide the psychotropic substances on the basis of their sedative and stimulating effects. Sedative substances are used to calm, diminish anxiety and induce sleep, while the stimulating (activating) drugs are substances which reduce sleep requirement or cause insomnia. The sedative substances include opiates (heroin, morphine, methadone), carbamazepine, lithium, tranquilizers and sleeping pills (benzodiazepines, barbiturates, meprobamate) and neuroleptics. The stimulating ones include amphetamines, cocaine, Ecstasy and antidepressants. It must also be remembered that standard antidepressants (tri- and tetracyclic substances) are also more or less sedative and that neuroleptics can cause akathisia (feelings of restlessness and hyperkinesia often incorrectly thought to be a stimulating effect).

When the sedation ceases

Psychiatric drugs cannot solve problems. The most they can do is suppress symptoms such as anxiety and despair leading to a situation where the person taking the drugs no longer recognizes their feelings of anxiety or despair. This is true of all sedative substances. The main psychological effect of neuroleptics is the suppression of the ability to be aware of emotions. The effect of benzodiazepine-tranquilizers, sleeping pills and opiates can better be described as a shielding from unpleasant emotions. The example of neuroleptics and benzodiazepines as well as opiates shows clearly the difference between sedation and shielding. Users of neuroleptics complain about the effect on their emotions while users of benzodiazepines and opiates tend to experience their feelings as pleasant. What both groups have in common is that they are far less aware of anxiety.

Anxiety always has a root cause. Often it is the fear of being abandoned by a partner or of becoming unemployed. Other people are afraid of failing during exams or at their job. Whatever the root cause of the anxiety, one thing is clear: the psychopharmacological suppression of their feelings will not make the cause go away. Instead, time is lost: and during this time when nothing is done the situation generally becomes far worse. Anyone who as a result of taking psychiatric drugs has suppressed their own feelings of anxiety for a period, will experience these feelings with even greater intensity when they stop taking the drugs. This is a purely psychological explanation and has nothing at all to do with any biological effects of withdrawal. It is absolutely clear that before taking the psychoactive drugs the reasons were there for the feelings of anxiety. If nothing has been done to deal with the root causes, and—whenever possible—to relieve the situation, then once the drugs are withdrawn the anxiety will return—and usually worse than before.

Regular users, whether of psychiatric or illicit drugs, take their "fix" in the hope of being better able to bear an insecurity, a pain, an unhappiness or a problem. They hope that it will make them feel better. Finally, the use of drugs and of psychopharmaceuticals can be seen as a treatment or an attempt at treatment of an unbearable psychological state. By far the most psychological states of suffering are associated with anxiety—whether as the main or the accompanying symptom. This anxiety, if its causes have not been recognized and altered where possible, will return. At the same time, when stopping the substance the users of the drugs are afraid of losing an effect (for instance the sedation) which they consider to be helpful and essential.

On top of all this, many people are subjected to the persuasive psychiatric message that they are seriously in need of the psychiatric drugs. They are all frightened of withdrawal even if they are not at all happy with the effect of the drugs. They are more than likely to experience real fear if they do stop taking the drugs. In this situation we can definitely speak of anticipation anxiety.

Symptoms of anxiety

Anxiety has direct physical consequences which can be experienced as symptoms. These include: agitation, excitation, shaking, palpitations, raised blood pressure, rapid breathing, sweating, gastrointestinal complaints (stomachache, diarrhea, nausea), insomnia, nightmares.

The greater the anxiety, the more severe the symptoms. It is worthy of particular note that a large proportion of the withdrawal symptoms after quitting psychiatric drugs or illicit substances are the same as those experienced by people suffering from severe anxiety. The symptoms associated with anxiety described above are considered to be the classic symptoms of withdrawal from opiates and benzodiazepines.

Anxiety can on the one hand trigger rebound phenomena, in other words similar psychological problems to those suffered before the start of treatment and on the other hand it can trigger symptoms directly. The direct symptoms of anxiety cannot be distinguished from those of withdrawal.

Not everyone finds sedation pleasant

Users of benzodiazepines and opiates feel as though they have been packed in cotton wool; everything which is torturing them appears to be hidden behind a curtain. This state is by no means pleasant for everyone. Creative and active people always experience any kind of sedation negatively, since it inhibits activity, enjoyment and achievement. Both intellectually and emotionally, sedation impairs real experience. Added to this is tiredness which even during the day can lead to a continuous fight against sleep. Such people feel

relieved when the sedation ceases after they stop the drugs. This is particularly true of those people whose emotions, intellectual capabilities, memory and
abstract thinking had been sedated away by neuroleptics.

End of the increased stimulation

The increased stimulation—judged to be the antidepressant effect by psychiatrists—is experienced by many as unpleasant, even unbearable. This is described
in the literature as akathisia: that which on the outside appears to be increased
activity or as the disappearance of a depressive apathy is experienced by the
users as an unpleasant inner agitation. This is the main reason for the increased
suicide rate among those taking neuroleptics and antidepressants.

What applies to sedation also applies to stimulation. There are two forms
which are regularly experienced by the users as either pleasant or unpleasant.
The stimulation caused by cocaine and amphetamines is preferred to that
caused by antidepressants and neuroleptics. Accordingly, this means the relief following the disappearance of this effect is to be observed in particular in
those people who have used the latter types of psychiatric drugs. Users of
neuroleptics, of course, are also relieved with the disappearance of the impairment of their intellectual capabilities, their creativity, their memory and
their ability to think in the abstract.

The placebo effect

In order to understand the other psychological withdrawal reactions it is
necessary to look a little closer at the placebo effect. Placebos (biologically inactive fake medication) are capable of alleviating or even healing most complaints that people suffer from. Since the 1950s, biological psychiatry has
been carrying out intensive and expensive human trials with psychiatric
drugs. Despite this, it has not been possible to prove that the desired or therapeutic effect of any of the psychiatric drugs is superior to the effect of placebos (Greenberg / Fisher 1989, p. 29).

The placebo effect is based on the belief or conviction on the part of the
patients that they have taken an effective substance and, therefore, they are
strongly dependent on the doctor-patient relationship. Anyone who trusts

their doctor will initially believe in the efficacy of the treatment. (Even drug addicts have a clear idea of the effect they expect before taking their drugs. Therefore, the placebo effect is an important component in the effect of any drug.) It follows that the placebo effect is a purely psychological effect triggered by taking a tablet or injection.

The psychological change observed following the administration of a psychiatric drug always consists of the actual effect of the substance and the placebo effect. The placebo effect must always be expected, while clear proof is always required for the biological effect.

An indication of how important the placebo effect is can be seen in the fact that, among other things, the color and shape of the tablets is important. Injections (the same dose of the same substance) are always more effective than tablets (Faust 1995, p. 55). If the people involved know that they are not taking a biologically active medication, but an inactive fake, then the placebo effect cannot possibly occur.

In "Glückspillen—Ecstasy, Prozac und das Comeback der Psychopharmaka" *("Happy Pills—Ecstasy, Prozac and the Comeback of Psychiatric Drugs")* I described the placebo effect in detail (Rufer 1995, pp. 36ff.). I would just like to point out here: it is extremely difficult to distinguish between the placebo effect and the biologically triggered psychic effect of a psychiatric drug. Even double-blind studies are unreliable; it is not enough that neither the trial subject nor the person administering the tablet do not know who is taking the verum (the biologically active substance) and who is taking the placebo. Because the psychiatric drug has obvious side-effects, it is easy for both those taking the substance and the those administering it to find out who is taking the verum.

Active placebos

Substances with clearly identifiable "side-effects" trigger more, and more obvious, placebo effects. This has led to the use of the term "active placebo" because the users are clearly confronted with the fact that they have taken an effective substance. They have become familiarized with the substance. Antidepressants, which are the best researched group of psychiatric drugs in this respect, cause dry mouth, shaking, clouded vision, dizziness, gastrointestinal complaints and an unpleasant restlessness. An active placebo is thus an active substance with its own clearly determinable biological effect, which has nothing to do with the hoped-for improvement in the symptoms being treated. Because of the side-effects, which are obvious both to the clients and the experts, the psychiatric drugs always tend to be rated too positively even when they are carefully compared with placebos.

Negative placebo effects

Placebos do not only cause desired positive effects; they can also have negative effects (they are then occasionally called "nocebos"). Since the expectations of the users determines the effect of the placebo it is not surprising that fake medication can have both positive and negative effects (for instance dry mouth, nausea, retching, dizziness, constipation, tiredness, headaches and confusion). There are interesting results from a study in which hospital patients who took placebos were told they were being given an emetic. 80% of these patients really did vomit (Albrecht 1997, p. 99). In other words: a placebo—and, it follows, every medication—depending on what the user has been told or has heard, or hopes or fears for, is always capable of triggering, purely psychologically, every possible positive or negative effect. The only prerequisite is that the users are convinced that they have definitely taken a biologically active substance.

In the same manner, stopping a psychiatric drug can trigger effects purely on a psychological level which have nothing to do with biologically induced withdrawal reactions. Because the patients are told, especially by the doctors, that after quitting the psychiatric drug they must expect a recurrence of the complaints and symptoms they had previously experienced, relapses are always possible. These purely psychological relapses (in fact negative placebo reactions) are most likely to occur if the substance has had a strong effect, in other words, if because of the biologically triggered effects (restlessness, shivering, dry mouth, gastrointestinal problems, suppression etc.) it can be understood to be an active placebo. The users very clearly experience the disappearance of these effects, which significantly increases the development of psychologically triggered withdrawal symptoms.

Rituals

The discussion of the placebo effect demonstrates to what extent the effect of the psychiatric drug is linked to the doctor-patient relationship. Anyone going to the doctor expects help and puts their trust in the doctor's knowledge. If the relationship which develops between the patient and the doctor is positive, this in turn can influence the occurrence of positive placebo effects.

Whoever goes voluntarily to a psychiatrist entrusts that person with their emotional suffering. This situation is very similar to that of a believer in the confessional. The doctor who prescribes a psychiatric drug thus exercises a function akin to that of a priest. This applies even more to psychotherapists who use LSD or Ecstasy in their work; they say explicitly that they are performing "rituals" to prepare their clients for the desired effect of the drugs. Even for those who use their drugs among friends, their consumption has a significance verging on the religious or a religious-like experience (Rufer 1995, pp. 40f.).

We are all believers; in the past most people were believers in the religion practiced around them, while today most of us believe in science. One part of our belief in science includes our belief in doctors, including psychiatrists and their words—expressed, after all, in the name of science. Just how unscientific and uncertain these words are is, of course, only clear to those who study this field.

If the psychiatrist or the doctor is a respected expert—as the priest used to be—who can influence the subjective state of the believer's soul with words, and if the doctor is able to convince the believer of the positive effect of the treatment, then the same holds true when the experts use their authority to predict a relapse if the patient stops taking the psychiatric drug.

The relapse—a self-fulfilling prophecy

The following discussion addresses what is told to people hospitalized with the diagnosis "schizophrenia." The influence of the psychiatrist in this case is particularly unfavorable. These patients are told very firmly that they must always, at all costs, take their medication. The rule of thumb followed by

most psychiatrists for the diagnosis "schizophrenia" is that after the first
"episode" prophylactic treatment lasting at least one to two years is necessary
to prevent a relapse, in other words prophylactic treatment with neuroleptics
is prescribed, even if the person is completely symptom-free. From the
second "episode" a minimum period of five years prophylactic treatment is
recommended (Lundbeck AG 1998, p. 10). Herbert Y. Meltzer, professor for
psychiatry in Cleveland, Ohio, goes even further when he writes that "schizophrenia" generally necessitates life-long neuroleptic treatment (Meltzer 1992,
p. XV). Anyone who has been labeled schizophrenic is given high-dosage
neuroleptics in the hospital. This treatment is not prescribed in a simple, cool
and unemotional manner. For the psychiatrist it is of great significance, it is
the most important thing they can possibly tell a "schizophrenic." Their
message is loud and clear:

> "You are ill, you are schizophrenic. That's the way it is, it is your fate. The
> only possibility you have of leading any kind of normal life despite this
> illness, is if you take neuroleptics. You have to realize this, we expect you
> to recognize that you are ill. If you do accept this we will discharge you
> soon. We will see to it that after you have been discharged you will go
> regularly to a general practitioner or psychiatrist who will prescribe your
> neuroleptics. We would prefer if you had a depot injection of neuro-
> leptics every two or three weeks; then we would be absolutely sure that
> you don't forget to take your tablets out of negligence or because you
> don't understand the need for them. If you don't believe us, if you refuse
> this absolutely essential treatment you are making a very big mistake be-
> cause you will suffer a relapse within the foreseeable future and sooner or
> later you will be sent back to hospital. Never forget, you are ill, you have
> the predisposition for schizophrenia in you, you are vulnerable, easily
> hurt. The symptoms of your illness can appear at any time, even though
> at times you'll feel better. Don't ever let yourself be persuaded by any ir-
> responsible people that you are sane, that you can live a good and useful
> life without medication. That would be a great mistake, we know better.
> We have a great deal of experience with this illness. You must believe us!
> You have no choice. You need neuroleptics like a diabetic needs insulin."

For the duration of their hospitalization they are confronted continuously with this point of view. They don't just hear it from the doctor, they hear it from all the staff several times a day. Relatives also play an important role. They hear the same message. Relatives are given the task of making sure that those they are responsible for can live a protected, irritant-free life without excitement. And most importantly, the relatives must see to it that the "patients" take their drugs regularly or go regularly to the doctor to have neuroleptic depot injections. In other words, the relatives are put under pressure by the opinion that the person affected is ill and that the only possible way for them to avoid further hospitalization is to be aware of their "illness" and the risks they face, and above all to keep taking the prescribed psychiatric drugs.

This behavior leads to illness. It creates immense pressure which is almost impossible to escape from. All the more amazing that anyone at all can find the strength to put forward an opinion which contradicts that of the psychiatrist and those closest to them when they come to the conclusion that none of this is true and that they can live far better without neuroleptics (and other psychiatric drugs) which seriously impair their quality of life.

Most of those affected believe more or less all they are told. They identify with the diagnosis. They accept that they are "schizophrenic" and therefore different from the rest of the ordinary members of the society. And along with the diagnosis they accept the "fact" that they are at risk. Put another way: the contact with the psychiatrist causes them to be anxious, extremely afraid of another outbreak of the "illness." But things don't stop there. Not only are they themselves anxious, all those around them are anxious too—both their relatives and the psychiatrist as well as other professional helpers. Those caught up in this scenario—both during their period of hospitalization and after—are surrounded by a climate of fear. They are afraid, and the people surrounding them are afraid. They all fear another outbreak of the "illness," the "psychosis," the "schizophrenia," another "episode" and another period of hospitalization.

This artificial creation of anxiety is absolutely wrong and counterproductive. Anyone who deals with people who have gone through severe psychological crises must not allow their behavior to be determined by fear. Furthermore, the diffuse, stigmatizing and illness-inducing psychiatric terminology

("schizophrenia," "psychosis" etc.) must be avoided. Instead, the circumstances which triggered the undesired state must be examined. What happened before the crisis? What conflicts or unsolved problems existed? These
are useful questions. They help to surmount, often totally, the fear of a merci-
less, relentless biological fate. Thus they learn what they have to try to do:
they have to live their lives so that a similar situation which led to their admission does not recur. The former patient X then knows, for instance, he will
always find himself in a crisis when a woman leaves him. That is far better
then continuing to see himself as the 'schizophrenic X' who can expect, with
great probability for the rest of his life, to have 'episodes' of his 'illness.' He
now has the opportunity to take his life in his own hands instead of remaining
dependent on the help of the psychiatrist who has nothing to offer other than
psychiatric drugs. Nor need he fear another outbreak of his 'illness.'

As has already been said, the behavior of psychiatrists is such that both
they and those with whom they are dealing fear a relapse. It is now easy to
understand what happens when a "schizophrenic" stops taking the neuroleptics against the advice of the doctor. The patient has heard from the doctor
what their relatives "know" as well: without neuroleptics the "symptoms of
schizophrenia" will certainly recur and readmission will follow. The negative
prognosis that psychiatrists present to their "schizophrenics" thus proves in
the majority of cases to be correct. Unfortunately, it convincingly illustrates
the term used by the psychologist Paul Watzlawick of the "self-fulfilling
prophecy" (Watzlawick 1984). The doctor and the most important contact
people expect a return of the "psychosis" which the person himself is afraid
of. It really would be astonishing if the feared "psychosis" did not in fact regularly appear.

Anyone who has been diagnosed as "manic" or "manic-depressive" goes
through much the same as the "schizophrenics" except that they are told that
they absolutely must take lithium or carbamazepine for years.

A brief summary of considerations when withdrawing

If tolerance has developed, the dose of the substance being used must be reduced gradually. This is particularly important with the benzodiazepines,

which should always be tapered off very gradually over a period of several weeks or even months.

At the same time the following should be considered: How is the person? Do they really want to quit? Are they convinced they can live without their psychiatric drug? Are they uncertain or afraid of quitting?

Many people are in fact ambivalent about quitting. On the one hand they complain about the impairing effects of the psychiatric drugs, on the other hand they are afraid that the symptoms they originally suffered from will return if they withdraw. This could lead to renewed psychiatric hospitalization, which would be terrible for them. Great care must be taken with people like this. They should—whenever possible—try to establish a clear understanding of the situation which led to hospitalization and treatment. Only by doing so can they arrive at the important knowledge of how to avoid further admissions. And only by doing so can they then take full responsibility for leading their own lives. Otherwise they will spend the rest of their lives dependent on psychiatry. They remain at risk as long as they still believe in even the smallest part of the message telling them their diagnosed illness could break out again if they don't take the psychiatric drugs. The fateful prophecy of the psychiatrist can become true at any time—in other words: the relapse happens.

Anyone who is ambivalent or afraid of withdrawing from neuroleptics must on no account stop abruptly. It is important during the period of withdrawal to get sufficient sleep. Anxiety can cause insomnia leading to exceptional states of consciousness (Rufer 1995, pp. 216f.) which in turn can be interpreted by psychiatrists, the individual withdrawing and their relatives as a recurrence of the psychosis. In this situation the lesser evil may be a short course of a benzodiazepine sleeping pill (a few days and never on two successive evenings). However, for people who are convinced they have been incorrectly treated and that they are better off without the psychiatric drugs, withdrawal generally presents no problems—at least in my 20 years of experience in providing support during withdrawal.

Translation from the German by Mary Murphy

Josef Zehentbauer

Who is Afraid of Withdrawal?

Medical Advice and Psychotherapeutic Counseling During Withdrawal from Sedatives

Neuroleptics / Antidepressants / Lithium / Carbamazepine / Tranquilizers

Never have there been as many psychiatric drugs available to people as there are today. The spectrum includes agents to calm psychological complaints (tranquilizers such as Valium etc.), agents which can suppress the personality or even destroy it (e.g. potent neuroleptics with long-term effects), or drugs that are meant to ease depression (e.g. antidepressants) or which can minimize severe mood swings between euphoria and melancholy to a gray mediocrity (lithium), and much more.

If psychiatric drugs are taken over a long time, the microstructure of the brain changes gradually. A particularly drastic example of psychiatric drugs taken over a long period and which can lead to such changes are neuroleptics, haloperidol, for example. These psychiatric drugs block the receptors at the brain cells for the chemical messenger dopamine; this is responsible, among other things, for fine motor movements, imagination and mood. However, the brain reacts to the neuroleptic-blocking of the receptors by producing more dopamine molecules. If the neuroleptics are stopped from one day to the next, the excess of dopamine molecules floods the freed receptors resulting in chaos in the brain, a chaos of thoughts and feelings. Unspecific fears can develop, resulting in paranoia, depressive despair or a hopeless emotional chaos. When someone stops neuroleptics abruptly (sometimes even at the dangerous advice of the psychiatrist), there is a risk that the brain will react with completely chaotic panic.

If sedating and tranquilizing pills—whether Haldol (neuroleptic), Saroten (chemical antidepressant *[active ingredient amitriptyline]*), Valium (tranquilizer), lithium or carbamazepine are suddenly withdrawn after one week or even months of taking the medication, among others, the following symptoms of withdrawal can occur: vomiting, nausea, gastrointestinal problems, outbreaks of sweating, racing pulse and blood pressure problems, trembling, inner agitation, insomnia, depression, states of anxiety or confusion and even paranoia. Anyone who has been taking long-term and/or high-dosage psychiatric pills and wants to withdraw must, therefore, approach this carefully and take a series of rules to heart. During the withdrawal period, in particular from long-term medication or high dosage, the supervision of a trusted doctor is very useful.

Psychiatric drugs are not a remedy, but at most an aid in dealing with mental difficulties, psychological disturbances and crises. But psychiatric drugs—especially in the hands of most psychiatrists—are also a means of enforcing conformity: conformity to the ruling norm. Anyone who resists the pill that leads to gray mediocrity and who has the courage to display a unique psychic state is not suffering from "hallucinations" but has unusual perceptive abilities; they are not suffering from "paranoia" but are living their own visionary selves; they are not sinking into "endogenous depression" but are experiencing deep, peaceful melancholy or are in a period of deep existential experience… and: not all suffering is illness.

General points when withdrawing

Below are some general points: withdrawing from psychiatric drugs means, among other things, a willingness to accept more responsibility for oneself. The treatment of psychological suffering and acute conflicts is not put primarily in the hands of doctors prescribing psychiatric drugs: responsibility is taken for one's own personality.

Apart from conventional psychiatry there are other, quite controversial alternative approaches in the area of psychosocial care, just as there are, in addition to the proponents of nuclear power, also experts for solar energy. Professional counter-information to the concepts of conventional psychiatry is required. Thus, for example, neither the so-called psychosis prophylaxis through neuroleptics, nor has the apparent prophylactic effect of the chemical antidepressants been convincingly proven with statistics. And if the neuroleptics have a positive effect on some people this must also be weighed against the serious risks of long-term treatment, for example.

The time to start withdrawing should be well-chosen to avoid periods of particular stress.

The crisis which led to long-term medication needs careful consideration and must be worked through with the aid of psychotherapists, for instance. Following the withdrawal from psychiatric drugs, a natural perception should be re-established and the desire to modify sensory perceptions with chemicals should subside.

It can be useful to draw on the practical experience of others, for example gradual dose reduction, possible alternative medication, or other treatments that aid withdrawal.

A basic restructuring of approach is also helpful: any moods which occur should be lived out in so far as they are not damaging for oneself or others. In addition, tolerance for one's fellow human beings who are also "living out" their feelings should be practiced. Tommaso Losavio, a psychiatrist in Rome, has expressed it as follows: the off-balanced should be a little more normal and the normal a little more off-balance.

As already mentioned: whoever has taken psychiatric drugs and now wants to withdraw must do this carefully and take heed of a number of practical hints.

Milestones when withdrawing

The fear of withdrawal, in particular from neuroleptics, but also the fear of withdrawing from tranquilizer dependency can be immense:
• Fear of acting against the advice of the attending psychiatrist who may have called long-term treatment with neuroleptics a psychosis-prophylaxis (a "prophylaxis" with no guarantee of effectiveness)
• Fear of the reaction of one's family
• Fear of the reoccurrence of mental disturbance or crisis after stopping the apparently curative medication
• Fear of ending up in a psychiatric hospital again as a result of a recurring crisis.

In the face of so many fears, it may make sense not to initially withdraw completely, but rather—as a preliminary target—to only aim for a marked dose reduction and to maintain this dose for an extended period. Especially with neuroleptics, it can be helpful for people with numerous fears when gradually withdrawing to be given the chance of switching to another "chemical crutch" instead of neuroleptics, tranquilizers for example, but only temporarily (!). However, the real aim is to make this last crutch, in this case tranquilizers, superfluous or to reserve them for emergencies. Everyone should decide for themselves if they wish to aim for a life completely free of drugs.

When withdrawing from neuroleptics it may occasionally be necessary to use stronger (including chemical) sedatives, the tranquilizers just mentioned for example; in this case, regular consultation with a doctor is absolutely essential. Dependency on tranquilizers can be avoided if certain rules are observed: tranquilizing medication should only be used temporarily, the dose should never be raised on one's own volition, one should be informed about the potential for dependency, the tranquilizers should be withdrawn as soon as the psychological state has improved, etc. Overall, less side-effects result from tranquilizers—despite the risk of dependency—than from neuroleptics. Opium tincture or morphine can be used as natural medications—briefly!—to treat the side-effects of neuroleptics (the same applies here to tranquilizers concerning the risk of dependency).

What should be done if there are signs of a new mental crisis during or after the withdrawal? The measures to be taken are numerous and have in part already been mentioned. They should not only be dealt with in individual therapeutic consultations but also with the respective partner or well-disposed family members and friends. The problems of a recurring crisis must be dealt with in supporting psychotherapy in order to reduce diffuse fears and to increase self-confidence. In addition, it may also be useful, in case of an emergency, to choose a more or less acceptable psychotherapeutically oriented clinic (consult health insurance companies, general practitioner and especially self-help groups!).

The fears briefly outlined above can be taken beyond the specific examples during psychotherapy sessions and used as a basis for learning to recognize and deal with one's own structures of fear.

Keeping well-informed

I am only in the position to offer a consultation to very few of the many consumers of psychiatric drugs who come to me for advice. I advise the majority
to negotiate with their attending psychiatrist (in so far as the psychiatrist is
not a hopeless case) or to seek a constructive dialog with their general practitioner. But before doing so the person using the drugs should access information through books and videos which adopt a critical stance on psychiatric
drugs (e.g. Breggin 1991; Lehmann 1996a, 1996b; Rufer 1995, 1997; Zehentbauer 1989, 1997b, 1998). They should be clear about their objective and
then put their case vehemently yet with charm ("fortiter in re, suaviter in
modo"; *"decisive in action, friendly in tone"*). For example, the gradual reduction
of a neuroleptic … or … the switch from a chemical to a herbal antidepressant (St. John's wort) … or the careful withdrawal from a lithium or carbamazepine long-term medication and the request instead for a homeopathic
treatment (from a specialist) and/or psychotherapy … or … an outpatient
withdrawal from tranquilizer dependency…

The degree of success that a direct and demanding attitude has on physicians, especially general practitioners, continues to surprise me. Because it is
not only clients who are helped in their aims. The physicians, too, have been
helped to understand the subject better, so that to a certain degree both have
received help.

Take precautions

The understandable fear of readmission to a psychiatric hospital can be reduced if a half-way acceptable clinic is found which does not work within the
strict limits of conventional psychiatry. Some (but by no means all) so-called
hospitals for psychosomatic medicine are mainly oriented towards psychotherapy and are rather restrained in their use of psychiatric drugs. Your health
insurance company or general practitioner can provide a list of hospitals for
psychosomatic medicine.

The understandable fear of readmission to a psychiatric hospital can be reduced if a half-way acceptable clinic is found which does not work within the
strict limits of conventional psychiatry. Some (but by no means all) hospitals

for psychosomatic medicine are mainly oriented towards psychotherapy and are rather restrained in their use of psychiatric drugs. Your health insurance company or general practitioner can provide a list of hospitals for psychosomatic medicine. It is usually pointless asking a psychiatrist because they generally react in a simplistic, dogmatic manner: "psychotics," "the severely depressed" and "schizophrenics" belong in large regional psychiatric hospitals or university psychiatric clinics, the "mild neurotic cases" can go to the hospital for psychosomatic medicine. In many countries, such as Germany for example, hospitals for psychosomatic medicine are generally private clinics; however, the health insurance companies usually cover the costs of a stay. It is difficult to gain admission to a hospital for psychosomatic medicine for someone who is already in a state of acute crisis. But during periods of mental calm, a stay in such a clinic can be helpful in gaining insight into the psychodynamics and biographical roots of crises and to reduce or withdraw from existing levels of psychiatric medication. Although many hospitals for psychosomatic medicine have quite a distinct approach from psychiatric institutions (whether regional or university hospital), the person caught up in psychiatry will not always find it easy to assert their ideas with respect to withdrawal from neuroleptics for example.

Don't rush things but withdraw slowly if necessary

There are users of psychiatric drugs who withdraw abruptly from long-term high-dose regimens without any reflection. This can work out, but one must expect—especially when withdrawing suddenly from neuroleptics—to suffer a withdrawal psychosis: hallucinations, paranoia, anxiety and panic attacks, insomnia, confusion, depression… The conventional psychiatrist interprets such withdrawal psychoses arbitrarily: the patient did not behave, did not take the medication and now we have the anticipated psychosis. (Most conventional psychiatrists deny the very possibility of withdrawal psychosis when neuroleptics are abruptly withdrawn, even though they see this happening in "rebellious" patients and even though it has been reported in international specialist journals.)

A withdrawal psychosis can be avoided if a careful, step-by-step withdrawal is chosen. After use of long-term medication, gradual, step-by-step withdrawal using the 10% formula can be used: the original daily dose (e.g. 100 mg of a psychiatric drug) is reduced by 10% (thus in our example to 90 mg). While this is easy to apply with drops, the 10-percent rule often has to be modified in the case of tablets. If there are no withdrawal symptoms such as sleep disturbances, inner agitation or depression after two weeks, the dose can be reduced by a further 10% (to 80 mg). The subsequent dose reduction then continues in steps of one to two weeks until zero dose is finally arrived at.

The following are a few remarks on the individual groups of medication:
• Neuroleptics (e.g. Haldol, Neurocil *[actice ingredient methotrimeprazine]*): if serious psychological and physical damage has already occurred following the use of long-term medication (e.g. high-grade suppression, depression, dyskinesia, Parkinson syndrome, hormonal disturbances, other internal and neurological syndromes), it may be advisable to reduce somewhat more rapidly, possibly with the aid of a tolerable alternative medication. A change from classical neuroleptics (like Haldol) to atypical neuroleptics (like Leponex *[active ingredient clozapine]*, Risperdal, Solian[1] or Zyprexa) might also be helpful, even if a complete withdrawal is planned in the long-term. (As it seems, some side-effects, for example muscle disorders, are less often to be seen with atypical neuroleptics.)
• Synthetic antidepressants such as the classic older Saroten and Anafranil or the newer so-called selective serotonine-reuptake-inhibitors (SSRI) such as Prozac, Trevilor *[active ingredient venlafaxine]*, etc.: if the expected antidepressant effect does not set in, or if the effect is too mild, the long-term medication can be reduced using the pattern given above, but the pace set can be faster. If there are serious side-effects (which especially with the classic antidepressants can be numerous, ranging from urine retention to a paradoxical depressive mood), a rapid, even immediate withdrawal may be considered.
• Lithium: this is usually taken for several years. In this case withdrawal should be effected over several months, in other words, special care must

---

1 Neuroleptic, active ingredient amisulpride

be taken. (In any case, because of the serious risk and the danger of poisoning, lithium should only ever be taken by people who have suffered several episodes of severe depressive or manic crises and are thus significantly endangered. But those affected must decide for themselves, having been properly informed of the risks of treatment, whether they are prepared to accept long-term lithium medication. During long-term lithium medication, the extreme highs and lows of human emotions are cut off so that both great joy and deep sadness are only experienced in reduced form. Some of those affected experience this narrowing of their emotional spectrum as a very unpleasant chemical manipulation; so they would rather choose not to take lithium thereby accepting the risk of a renewed psychological crisis.)

- Carbamazepine (e.g. Tegretal): this agent, known primarily as an antiepileptic drug was approved by the former Federal Health Office for psychiatric use only "if lithium treatment has failed or if lithium cannot be used" (Benkert 1995, p. 80). The so-called prophylactic effect of long-term carbamazepine treatment is clearly markedly less than that of lithium treatment. Careful withdrawal is also advisable in this case.

- Tranquilizers (e.g. Valium, Adumbran *[active ingredient oxazepam]*): these pills have subjectively pleasant effects (calming, vegetatively harmonizing, antidepressant, carefree and euphoric, anxiolytic, sleep-inducing, etc.), making them potentially addictive. In contrast to neuroleptics, which are often taken under direct (e.g. under legal guardianship) or indirect force (e.g. through whipped up fear of another episode of psychosis) tranquilizers are usually consumed "voluntarily," although often in ignorance of their effects. In the case of low-dose, long-term medication, immediate withdrawal is possible, whereas in the case of high-dose long-term medication, inpatient withdrawal in a suitable clinic is recommended. The symptoms of withdrawal result from the sudden absence of the positively experienced effects of the tranquilizers described above: inner agitation, states of anxiety and confusion, depression, insomnia, vegetative disturbances such as outbreaks of sweating and a racing pulse. Supportive measures as described below during withdrawal are advisable.

Support during withdrawal

It is difficult to deal with people who have been taking relatively high-doses of neuroleptics and tranquilizers as long-term medication and who are not willing to withdraw, even though medicinally induced disturbances have become obvious (in the case of neuroleptics, for example, dyskinesia, akathisia, depression; in high-dosed long-term use of tranquilizers sleepiness, apathy, flattening of personality, etc.). Sometimes there is a false trust in a new, apparently tolerable medication and a resulting reluctance to withdraw. (At this point the new, atypical neuroleptics should be mentioned again. These have less dramatic side-effects than the old neuroleptics, but they are nevertheless still associated with horrendous risks and can pave the way to massive personality changes.)

When there is great uncertainty in the face of withdrawal, sometimes a whole potpourri of supporting measures must be considered as a replacement for long-term medication in order to at least prepare the way for a certain willingness to live a life free of psychiatric drugs. Some sensitive psychotherapy sessions can create a degree of trust enabling the gradual withdrawal.

The step-by-step withdrawal using the 10% formula represents—apart from a few exceptions—a quite careful procedure and takes quite a long time. Rapid withdrawal is possible, if alternative parallel medication (e.g. a herbal remedy) is taken, or trust-building psychotherapeutic support is provided, if necessary with several sessions per week or a stay in a suitable friendly psychotherapeutic clinic or in a hospital for psychosomatic medicine.

It is important to inform a partner, friends or possibly family members of the intention to "withdraw" from psychiatric drugs.

Sufficient relaxation and sleep is essential. Sedative teas and warm baths may be necessary. Autogenic training or other relaxation exercises such as yoga or meditation techniques are definitely to be recommended; however, these should be learned during a crisis-free time.

The supportive administration of B vitamins (especially B_1 and B_6) and vitamin E can help reduce neuroleptic-induced disturbances; in the case of the vitamin B complex, intramuscular injections can sometimes be more useful than tablets. Other concomitant herbal remedies can be useful: St.John's wort for depression or velarian, hops, balm, etc. (so-called phytotranquilizers) for pleasant sedation and a mild release of anxiety.

Diet and the psyche

A brief reference to the large subject of "diet and the psyche": a balanced, vitamin-rich diet is to be recommended during the period of withdrawal and, in addition, above average amounts of fluids (e.g. mineral water, herbal tea) should be drunk, as this encourages a reduction in body fluid and the excretion of psychiatric drugs.

For mental stabilization it is advisable to completely avoid meat, sausage and fish: in other words, not to kill or eat any animals.

Unfortunately, only very few of those affected by psychiatry are willing during withdrawal from psychiatric drugs or during the treatment of mental suffering to accept ideas regarding "diet and the psyche." In fact a radical change in diet can often bring about amazing success, as demonstrated, for example, by the concept of "clinical ecology" or "orthomolecular medicine" (to mention just two approaches among many).

Put simply, clinical ecology assumes that individually intolerable substances, for example in food stuffs, can trigger not only physical allergies, but also a "mental allergy" (which is then expressed in the form of, among other things, depression, paranoia or anxiety attacks). Using a—quite complicated—testing method of individually intolerable diet constituents, it is finally possible to find a diet which can lead to a marked improvement or a disappearance of psychic disturbances. During the psychiatric drug detoxification process such a "psychic diet" can be a useful support (see Calatin 1995; Pfeiffer 1988; Randolph / Moss 1980).

Orthomolecular medicine (as developed by the double Nobel prize winner Linus Pauling) tries to achieve mental and emotional well-being by making sure that the right ("ortho") substances ("molecules," e.g. vitamins, trace elements) are in the body in the right concentrations. It has long been known that a relative deficiency of certain vitamins can lead to severe mental disturbances. Thus in the case of a vitamin B_1, deficiency can lead to a severe mental disturbance classified (incorrectly) as "schizophrenia" by the conventional psychiatry and wrongly treated with neuroleptics. Orthomolecular medicine emphasizes that the correction of a substance deficiency, as determined by complicated laboratory investigations, can alleviate or cure mental complaints. Furthermore, orthomolecular medicine examines the effects on health of toxic metals such as lead, mercury, aluminum, copper or cadmium, which get into the human organism through pollution and which can tip mental balance (see Pauling 1990, pp. 123ff.).

Mobilizing the body's own drugs

Most people only know exogenous drugs, in other words usually in the form of pills introduced from the outside, for example morphine or Valium. But very few realize that the body produces its own psychotropic drugs. The discovery of the body's own drugs is a sensational success story in human science at the turn of the millenium. Unheard-of possibilities have opened up. Every human being has their own morphine-like substances which have a strong calming and antidepressant effect, its own anxiolytic substances (e.g. the body's own Valium), diverse antidepressants (e.g. noradrenaline), substances which stimulate the imagination, motor activity and sexuality (e.g. dopamine). The body's own pharmacy provides far more possibilities than the pharmaceutical industry can.

But it is easier—at least initially—to swallow the psychiatric pills prescribed by the doctors than to stimulate the body's own drugs with the help of mental or somatic techniques. Endorphins (the body's own morphine-like substances) can be targeted and mobilized; the effect of this endogenous drug is calming, antidepressant, and analgesic. The body also has drugs which activate our intelligence, imagination and drive, and others which are sleep-inducing and mood-lightening, sexually stimulating, etc. (for more details see Zehentbauer 1997a). The mood-lightening, joy-creating noradrenaline increases rapidly during trampoline jumping, bungee jumping, fast ball games or cheerful music (to name only a few examples) and noradrenaline makes us happy or makes us laugh whether we want to or not. During a marathon we express large amounts of endorphins. A similar effect is brought about by lullabies by Sufi dancing or when these images are called up in our imagination; when the high of the body's own endorphins make depression, agitation and anxiety disappear. Muscle relaxing, autogenic training and relaxing music stimulate the body's own Valium, which makes us happy without the need for any prescription drugs. An off-balance life (as manifested, for instance, by painting faces not only at carnival, dancing naked on the street) floods dopamine through our brains and drives us to the limit between genius and madness; whoever can more or less steer this off-balance will not land in the prison of psychiatry… Experimenting with wild or harmonizing 'endogenous drugs' is a fascinating area of research which demonstrates astonishing aspects of the self-regulating powers of out souls!

Useful additional information

When withdrawing, one must remember that some psychiatric drugs have very long half-lives (i.e. the time they spend in the body). Withdrawal symptoms or the recurrence of symptoms which have previously been suppressed by medication can only be dealt with after one or several days or after only one or two weeks, or even later.

Heavy consumption of coffee and nicotine weakens the effects of neuroleptics, especially the deadening tiredness and disturbances in personality. If during the step-by-step withdrawal coffee and nicotine are also seriously reduced, even a reduced dose of neuroleptics can have a strong effect.

Some people take a combination of several psychiatric drugs (for example a high-dose neuroleptic such as Haldol during the day, and evenings the tranquilizer Adumbran, the antidepressant Saroten or the low-dose neuroleptic Neurocil). In this situation it is usually recommended to first withdraw the neuroleptic step-by-step (see above); the tranquilizer should be reduced last (also step-by-step) to zero.

Psychotherapy and self-help

Participation in self-help groups can provide a valuable exchange of experiences and emotions and establish the feeling that one is not alone with withdrawal difficulties. A prerequisite for this is, however, that the person affected is ready to free themselves from their life-long belief in doctors and to confront the mode of action and effects of psychiatric drugs and to take responsibility for themselves.

Psychotherapy can be an important support when withdrawing from psychiatric drugs. By "psychotherapy" is especially meant in this case a supportive relationship in which dealing with day-to-day problems is a central issue.

Whether the method used is talking therapy, Gestalt or behavior therapy is of little relevance. Regardless of the method used, it is crucial to establish a trusting relationship between client and therapist. During the withdrawal phase, one to two sessions every two weeks (which may only be of ten minutes duration) may be useful; afterwards, depending on how things develop, one therapy session (50 minutes) every one to three weeks may follow.

The aim of psychotherapy is not to alter the person affected and make them conform to normality, but to accept them as they are. Even the most imbalanced forms of behavior can be understood (or at least accepted), if we view the statements and actions of someone who stands out psychologically as a dream or nightmare. The initially strange ideas-world of an imbalanced person can be understood in terms of symbols.

Giovanni Jervis, a psychologist from Rome, distinguishes between psychotherapy by "specialists" (psychologist, psychotherapists, etc.) and psychotherapy by "non-specialists" (porters, bartenders, bar owners, etc.). Psychological support from sensitive friends, empathetic acquaintances or ordinary people who can listen, empathize, and are also affected but not fully occupied with their own experiences are "natural helpers" who are unfortunately not always available in crisis and emergency situations (and if there were more of these types of helpers, perhaps fewer crises would come to a head).

Psychotherapy is not a value-free method. In the hands of conservative psychiatrists and therapists psychotherapy becomes a correspondingly conservative procedure. Psychotherapeutic psychiatrists often want to suppress mental disturbances with all means at their disposal and to change the personality structure to that of an apparently desirable normality. If psychotherapeutic measures do not succeed in doing this, neuroleptics and antidepressants are often used thoughtlessly and there is even the threat of admission to a psychiatric unit. However, it should be added that there are situations in which psychiatric drugs, tranquilizers or antidepressants for example are helpful. Each person must decide for themselves.

The American psychotherapist Carl Rogers developed a view of psychotherapy which—although this was not his primary intention—ran in the face of conventional psychiatry. The patient, whom Rogers called the "client," is to develop his/her personality during the course of "therapeutic meetings."

Therapists are expected to empathize with the clients without evaluating or analyzing, and to provide human warmth and respect for the clients as they are. None of this is intended as a therapeutic facade or technique but should really reflect the attitude of the therapist, i.e. this must stem from real interpersonal feelings. If a therapist is not able to empathize with the client and cannot accept the client unconditionally as they are, therapy should not begin or continue. Psychotherapy means for Rogers the setting up of a certain kind of relationship which enables the client to discover the ability to change and develop. Thus, more self-realization, self-development, responsibility for oneself and autonomy are achieved.

As already mentioned, psychotherapy in the hands of conventional psychiatrists can be a medium for non-medicinal suppression and for enforcing conformity to the ruling norms. However, psychotherapy with an antipsychiatric and humanistically-based therapist can be a major help in withdrawing from psychiatric drugs and can also be a support in the attempt to develop one's own philosophy of life and to gain more freedom. It is important, as I have already said, that a relationship of trust develop between client and therapist and that psychotherapy becomes an aid to self-help. Sometimes a few therapy sessions are sufficient, and other times a therapeutic process develops only after several weeks or months. Sometimes there is a low-frequency supportive psychotherapeutic relationship (i.e. therapy sessions only take place every three to six weeks). Sometimes group therapy is necessary and on other occasions individual sessions are more useful for the client.

And do not forget: one can be dependent not only on psychiatric drugs, but also on psychotherapy. Careful avoidance is required here, especially on the part of the therapist: after stabilization of the client, the lowest possible frequency of therapy sessions (e.g. one session every one to two weeks) should be established. As soon as possible there should be breaks in treatment (one to several weeks). Some "psychotherapeutic methods" of self-help can be offered and practiced where appropriate (e.g. relaxation exercises and breathing exercises, reflection on dreams, keeping a diary, living consciously, biographical work and self-analysis, exercises from Gestalt and behavior therapy, etc.). Despite empathy, human warmth and respect the therapist must always be aware of maintaining a friendly distance (clear timing, definite clarity on the "artificiality" of the therapeutic relationship and its time limits). Self-esteem and self-confidence must be encouraged and a respectful manner towards oneself and others; one's own philosophy of life, to discover the meaning of life…

Summary

Special psychological moods such as depression, excessive desire for activity, euphoria, painful emotional disturbances, changes in perception or vision can be normalized though the use of chemical drugs. These special emotional states can, however, be lived through ("acted out") after the withdrawal from psychiatric drugs and thus contribute to important individual, but also socially relevant understandings and experiences. Psychological crises can in fact be an opportunity to view one's life and general social situation critically, to question it and to possibly search for changes and new paths.

  Have the courage to stop taking emotionally limiting psychiatric drugs (but be sure to observe careful rules of withdrawal). Have courage to expand the sound of your soul.

Translation from the German by Mary Murphy

Martin Urban

"Am I Really Still Disabled?"
Psychotherapeutic Support During Withdrawal from Psychiatric Drugs—A Case Report

Neuroleptics: Fluanxol

I would like to introduce Eva. She is a good-looking woman of 38 years who appears youthful, friendly, eager for contact with others, and perhaps a bit too open-hearted. She has creative talents and until recently she attended a fine arts school; she earned a modest living as a part-time clerk in a health food store. She may soon get married, as she is for the first time in her life in a relationship that is good for her and in which she feels she is treated as an equal partner.

Sounds like a very normal woman? I would definitely say "Yes!" Sure, sometimes it would be better if she had a little more self-confidence, for example when her art professor gives individual comment on her colleagues' drawings yet walks by her without a word. Honestly speaking, it should be an easy thing to pull the professor aside and say to him the following sentence: "Excuse me, I would like some comments from you. After all, that's what I pay my tuition for!" We came up with this sentence together and practiced it in her group therapy, but when it came time to use it in a real context, she couldn't.

A very normal woman? I said she was a bit too open-hearted, sometimes telling others what she has experienced with too much emotional rapture. She doesn't always check to see if the listener is able to or willing to follow her. She has a very great need to share herself with others and to receive attention—but isn't that rather human, indeed, normal?

Eva has decided, in any case, to view herself as normal in the future rather than as a chronically ill psychiatric patient. And this also entails her decision, 17 years after her first severe illness, to withdraw from a constant dose of neuroleptics—despite her own doubts about this. For fourteen years she went to the doctor every two weeks to receive a depot injection of Fluanxol. A few days after these shots she had always felt especially uneasy, both physically and mentally, and often had panic attacks. She doesn't want this anymore. Now she would like to marry and have a baby, i.e. to just live a normal life—and not, you should be aware, to live like a cripple, dependent upon a crutch for the rest of her life. That's what she felt like every two weeks when she heard from her psychiatrist once again that she has a chronic mental illness which she will always have and that she will have to take neuroleptics her whole life long in order to battle it.

Of course, she had been very ill. By the time she finished her high school exams, she had already developed anorexia and lived in a dream world. She felt misunderstood by her parents; her father was strict, detached, achievement-oriented, and never spoke about personal things or feelings. In his presence Eva felt small, useless, worthless, and guilty. The mother was very anxious and usually stood in the shadow of her husband. Following her example, Eva tried hard to conform and be a good daughter. When she was 21, doctors discovered a malignant thyroid carcinoma that had to be operated. Eva was not afraid; instead, she was rather high strung and fled further into her dream world. One day she declared herself the virgin Mary and experienced extreme states of fear, and she was admitted to a psychiatric hospital.

This was a set-back in her life. She had to drop out of the graphic design program she had begun. In the following years she experienced a second psychosis and was admitted to the hospital again. After that she started a relationship with a man with a difficult personality whom her parents rejected. When she became pregnant, the problems only accumulated. Her parents pressured her to have an abortion, and she yielded, only to experience extreme guilt that brought on another psychosis. Then came a third hospital stay and a course of rehabilitation, which was interrupted by another hospital stay due to further extreme states of fear. After this she was in a transitional home for two years, and then in a guided residence for three years. During this time she trained to be a florist, an occupation that did not suit her and that she never practiced with success for very long.

Nonetheless, ten years after her first psychosis she had been able to stabilize herself throughout these different stages enough to live alone and to move into an apartment her parents had bought for her. She tried out various jobs and decided to begin training in a painter's workshop. Perhaps she was too sensitive in her associations with others, perhaps as the only woman in the program she should have been better able to withstand the coarse jokes of her male colleagues. In any case, she wasn't able to hold out. Is this the distinctive vulnerability that the schizophrenia experts speak of?

Despite many failures, she did not give up. One day she came to me and asked if I would offer her psychotherapy because she had heard that I was one of the few therapists who took on clients who have a psychosis. I agreed, and thus began our work together five years ago.

At the time she had not had an acute psychosis for years. But she suffered from extreme states of fear and panic that appeared precisely within two to five days after she received her depot injections of Fluanxol. She was otherwise also anxious in the presence of her colleagues and her superiors, and above all when she was alone at night in her apartment. The fear of being alone is related to a child's fear of not being able to survive on their own. Behavior therapy and gradually learning to cope with fear fear are very useful, but above all Eva had to learn to experience herself as an independent, capable individual with a right to an opinion and a life of her own. And she had to develop a sense of her own value as a person. It is the role of the therapist to help those who seek help on their journey out of their dependencies, yet without making the patient dependent on the therapist.

For two years Eva had a boyfriend who was an idealist and belonged to a religious community. He unfortunately had a character trait that did not serve Eva well at all: he was constantly instructing her on how she should strive for perfection and on what God wanted from her. The consequence was that she felt worthless, yet she could not imagine being able to live without him. She needed another two years before she could break herself free of this dependency and, after several preliminary attempts, finally make a final break with him. She had grown, but he had not changed at all.

Making a break from her parents was equally difficult for Eva. Though she had not lived with her parents since she was twenty-five, she lived only an hour's drive from them. Even at this distance she was still trying to be a good daughter. The parents meant well and supported her financially, but each time she returned from their home she was unhappy. She felt they did not understand her and could not accept her the way she was. She felt like a sick daughter who had not made anything of herself for whom they constantly had to care. This caused her feelings of guilt and anxiety. (This has only begun to change in the past three years.) It is difficult to make a small bud grow up confidently given such an environment.

Eva's deep doubts about herself and her environment also affected our therapy sessions. For example, after I had personally handed her the form for extending her therapy in order to expedite its arrival at her health insurance company, her guilty conscience led her to confess to me the following week that she had opened and read my confidential assessment of her intended only for her insurers. She had greatly feared that she had mistakenly judged my character and that I in fact, deep down, despised her. I was so moved by her suffering and doubt that I spontaneously reacted in an appropriate way—without anger and without a reprimand. This made her feel relieved. Incidentally, she also agreed with everything I had written in the assessment. She was pleased to see that I had not written anything that I had not already said to her in our sessions. I had passed her test in trust.

After two years of individual therapy sessions I suggested to Eva that she take part in a group session. This was a necessary further step on her route to recovery because she needed to learn to represent her opinions and her feelings to others, indeed, to first become aware of them and respond, rather than withdrawing out of disappointment when others did not share her thoughts and feelings.

She had come a long way—one day she was even able to tell her mother something that had tormented her for years, namely, how terrible it was for her when at age twenty-three her parents had made no attempt to understand her and had pressured her into having an abortion. Contrary to her fear that she would insult her mother, the mother was instead very moved and sympathetic.

After separating from her boyfriend Eva suffered from feelings of loneliness, but she did not panic anymore. When she attempted to take her exams for graphic design school fourteen years after having dropped out, she was rejected because—despite her good marks—she was deemed to be too old. This was quite a blow for her. But she didn't capitulate—to the contrary, she decided to apply at a private fine arts school. She had saved the money herself at her job as a salesperson. A new relationship brought about a final change: she now felt mature and desired to start a family. She wanted to become a mother and work part time in her husband's office. Art remains a hobby for her.

The bimonthly depot injections of neuroleptics no longer fit into her life. The idea of needing a crutch to avoid another psychosis—the thought was a hindrance that put a damper on her zest for life. Two years ago she had attempted to make a plan with her psychiatrist for gradually withdrawing from the medication, but without success. She only managed a minimum reduction of the dosage. The doctor was strictly against a complete withdrawal because she felt it was too risky. All the signs of progress Eva had made, and the fact that she had not shown the symptoms of a psychosis in thirteen years were of no avail. The doctor spoke of scientific findings on her illness that indicated she would be helpless without constant medication.

At that time Eva was too fearful to challenge her doctor or to take things into her own hands. But today she no longer accepts this judgment and she has made her own mature decision. In order to avoid the same old debates, she quickly decided to find a new doctor. The new psychiatrist generally agreed to her wishes to withdraw from the neuroleptics, but insisted on a careful, gradual withdrawal plan. Instead of depot injections every two weeks, she now takes one tablet daily—a dose that she holds in her own hand! Eva feels that this is immense progress and she is relieved. When she once had a bad day, her old fears crept back again. She asked if this were the consequence of—or the punishment for—her attempt to come free. But she soon was able to trust herself again.

Once more she experienced another setback when she spoke with her gynecologist about her desire to have a child. It was the idea of becoming pregnant that had given her the last bit of strength to carry through with withdrawal; she did not want to endanger the pregnancy with any drugs. But her gynecologist told her she must keep taking the neuroleptics to avoid another psychosis that would most surely come—particularly with the pregnancy. Once again another god in a white coat had given her the feeling that she was a cripple who could only hold herself up with a crutch—the medication—without which she would fall apart. Then her protest found a voice: "How could he possibly know that for certain?" And: "Does he not trust me enough to know that I would go to a doctor if my condition became bad again?"

Eva still needs support. The group therapy has been good for her; she gains from the exchange of ideas with those who are similar to her and from the trusted and trust-building guidance of the therapists. One day she will no longer need this. Since moving into group therapy she has worked on reducing her (unavoidable, temporary) dependence upon her therapist. She will accomplish the goal of independence and she will be a very normal woman—as capable, independent and healthy as we all are: relatively, that is!

That is Eva, whom I wanted to introduce. For me she is living proof that psychiatric illnesses, even chronic psychoses, can be overcome—not without leaving traces, but also not such that anyone affected is a lesser person at the end of an illness or a crisis. To the contrary, I am convinced that Eva is more mature and grown up than before. Maybe she got lucky in the midst of her ill fortune and found the right conditions in which she could recover from a severe illness she had suffered with for years. No doubt there are other cases in which the same success was not possible. We don't need to expound on them (or do we, in order to find out why they did not succeed?). This example shows that a normal life and good mental health are attainable goals (even if the patient does remain vulnerable).

Eva's comments

It is possible to recover from psychosis, but not without working on oneself. That has been my experience. An internal orientation toward self-confidence and belief in myself are the goals. Sometimes I can't attain this very well, but often I have been able to. It is important that I allow myself to receive help and remain open to help, especially that of psychotherapy. I think a lot of those who were my fellow patients end up falling back into psychosis or they get stuck in it because the illness is more familiar to them than the difficult process of healing, and because they can't take a good look at themselves, make changes, and take responsibility for themselves.

Medication? What I always hear from the doctors is that they are in favor of patients continuing to use these crutches for their own security. "Don't do anything without a doctor," they say. They are right about this, I need to work with a doctor, but does that also mean that once you have a psychosis you'll never be healthy again? The fear of falling back into a psychosis is still with me. Instead of giving me courage to face this fear, the doctors only strengthen the fear because they trust their text books more than individual people.

I know that I can not outwit my fate. But I am on the right path now and I'm trying to be true to myself.

I read through the above text by my therapist and made improvements three times in order to insure an accurate picture was conveyed. In particular, it was important to me that my parents not be represented in a bad light.

Translation from the German by Christina White

Roland A. Richter

Supporting Withdrawal with Orthomolecular Medicine

Neuroleptics / Antidepressants / Lithium / Carbamazepine / Tranquilizers

What happens when you tell your neurologist or psychiatrist that despite treatment with psychiatric drugs, you still have hallucinations, fears, and suicidal thoughts? Usually your dosage is raised or you are committed to a hospital. Some of my patients who were taking neuroleptics, anti-Parkinson drugs, antidepressants, lithium and tranquilizers yet were still experiencing mental problems saw no sense in continuing medical treatment and the psychoactive drug-induced numbness it caused. In this situation, I could either convince them to take Risperdal, Truxal *(active ingredient chlorprothixene)*, Haldol, Dipiperon[1], Dogmatil[2], Eunerpan[3], Neogama *(neuroleptic, active ingredient sulpiride)*, Neurocil *(neuroleptic, active ingredient methotrimeprazine)*, Taxilan *(neuroleptic, active ingredient perazine)*, Tegretal *(mood stabilizer, active ingredient carbam-*

---

1 Neuroleptic, active ingredient pipamperone, apparently not currently marketed in AU, CA, GB, NZ and US

2 Neuroleptic, active ingredient sulpiride, marketed as Dolmatil, Dogmatyl, Sulpiride, Sulpitil, Sulpor

3 Neuroleptic, active ingredient melperone, apparently not currently marketed in AU, CA, GB, NZ and US

azepine), Fluctin *(antidepressant, active ingredient fluoxetine)* etc., or I could take their wishes seriously and offer guidance and support as they attempted to realize them.

I asked myself what kind of concrete help I could organize or offer myself because withdrawal from psychiatric drugs can bring on unbearable fears and hallucinations, including those that may lead to a suicide attempt. Occasionally withdrawal causes sleep patterns to be severely disturbed for several weeks, so that it is nearly impossible for the patient to get the necessary rest and relaxation they need.

Unfortunately, I have come to understand that doctors favor in particular the prescription of neuroleptics because sedating people in psychiatric wards and hospitals—by putting a chemically-induced damper over a disturbed or disturbing consciousness—is the easiest way to guard and control them.

My patients' withdrawal attempts demonstrated to me that they never identified with the treatments they received and instead wished to live their lives without neuroleptics or other psychiatric drugs. They in fact could only imagine a free and self-determined existence without the influence of psychiatric drugs. With this recognition, I could no longer see my task to be that of exerting pressure on patients in order to enforce psychiatric drugs at the wishes of neurologists and psychiatrists.

My experience has shown me that the pharmaceutical industry, via medical schools, determines the treatment of all psycho-social problems that are considered by many to be "mental illnesses." There are no influential social or political authorities that seriously consider whether or not there are alternative forms of treating those with mental problems. Money plays a large role in this. For example, an "optimal" neuroleptic prescription of Risperdal can cost approximately 2500 Euro per year (this includes only the cost of the psychiatric drug). The doctors recommend what the pharmaceutical industry has told them. Why would the medical industry make the effort to find meaningful alternatives to prescribing psychiatric drugs if these alternatives are not paid for by public health insurance plans, or perhaps only after a patient has gone to court?

My practical experience has been that orthomolecular medicine can aid in withdrawal or fighting unwanted psychological symptoms—but the patient must pay for this him or herself. (Linus Pauling, the American Nobel prize winner for chemistry and the founder of orthomolecular medicine, described the treatment as maintaining health and treating illnesses by changing the concentration of amino acids, enzymes, vitamins, vitaminoids, trace elements, minerals, fat and protein which are normally found in the human body and which are necessary for good health.) If, for example, an orthomolecular treatment cuts the 2500 Euro cost in half, shouldn't it be a point of honor that health insurance cover the cost? Hardly.

The power of the pharmaceutical industry can only be understood if one knows that the greater part of doctors' further training lies in the hands of this sector. Even the health insurance companies are not in a position to consider alternatives to orthodox medical care as a part of their services. In general, after the administration of psychiatric drugs no one is interested in a patient's biography anymore. This is particularly true for those people taking neuroleptics. No one will help you to develop strategies for coping with your frustrations, aggressions, mourning, disappointments, expectations, or problems negotiating closeness and distance in relationships, nor with finding constructive ways of integrating these into your personality.

Before I describe my experiences with orthomolecular medicine, I would like to say a few words about the dangers of an uncritical appropriation of this report. This is important to me because it will help you little to idealize this information. If you have been taking psychiatric drugs for several years already, it should be clear to you that you may have developed a habit and a dependence on the drugs. Withdrawing abruptly from psychiatric drugs or substituting orthomolecular medicine for the drugs will hardly yield success.

When withdrawing, it also makes sense to make a definitive change in your diet; I will briefly say something about this. You can receive support from psychologists and social workers or other people in your most immediate environment who stand by you and whom you trust can help you.

A successful withdrawal

The first time one of my patients withdrew from neuroleptics on his own without giving notice and almost entered a psychosis, he really did not want to wind up in a psychiatric ward. He was almost crying when he asked me to keep him out of the closed ward. I asked him if he had ever tried taking vitamins. He answered that he would take anything that would help him get out of a cycle of moving in and out of closed psychiatric hospitals. I gave him some (non-prescription) vitamins, which he took right away, and then I accompanied him while we drove to a doctor who gave him an intravenous infusion of vitamins. His condition improved immediately. These measures were enough to avoid having him committed. When he began taking very high does of vitamin C in the form of nitrite ascorbate, his condition improved even more. A magnesium and calcium preparation was additionally helpful. An antihistamine, which is known in the medical profession to be effective, had a stabilizing effect. A dose of tryptophan[1] made it possible for him to rest through the night. Positive feelings resulted from eating meals with saffron in them. With passion flowers and peonies, he was better able to sleep through the night. Further progress in the central nervous system was achieved with a high dose of magnesium. A change of diet to one based on raw vegetables brought further relief.

A change in diet

One of the most important observations I have made is that orthomolecular medicine is much more effective for people with psychiatric diagnoses if they choose a natural food diet. It has already been shown that incorrect nutrition can cause illness, for example the book "An Alternative Approach to Allergies" by Theron G. Randolph and Ralph W. Moss (1980). A further aid in treating my patients has been the information presented in the book "Nährstoff-Therapie bei Geisteskrankheiten" ("Nutritional Therapy for Mental Illnesses," 1988) by Carl Pfeiffer.

For people who are willing to make rather large sacrifices in order to improve and optimize their mental and physical well-being, I would like to recommend the book "Großen Gesundheits-Konz" ("Konz' Big Book about Health," 1995). My observations of several patients have been that Franz Konz's teachings in combination with orthomolecular medicinal treatment

---

1 Antidepressant, marketed also as Optimax

(Dietl / Ohlenschläger 1998) have contributed in some cases to an increased sense of psychological well-being. For example, after one of my patients was able to get her alcohol addiction under control by using tips from Konz, information from the Canadian Schizophrenia Foundation, and a treatment recommended by orthomolecular medicine, I discovered that the unusual approach of Konz to heal via a natural diet is not out of place for people with mental illnesses. I cannot judge whether or not it would help everyone. Nutritional advice particular to orthomolecular medicine can be found in "Burgersteins Handbuch der Nährstoffe" *("Burgerstein's Nutritional Handbook,"* 2002) by Lothar Burgerstein.

Another successful withdrawal

When one of my patients, a young alcoholic man diagnosed with "paranoid schizophrenia," came to me several weeks after being discharged from a psychiatric ward and was about to be committed again (he had withdrawn from Haldol and Truxal within six weeks), I recommended a raw vegetable diet and an orthomolecular medicine treatment. He was able to abstain from alcohol for about a year without taking psychiatric drugs. With pedagogical support he became healthy enough to attain an almost normal capacity for work. The orthomolecular medicine consisted of a high dose of B-complex vitamins, calcium, magnesium, zinc, beta carotene juice (1 kg carrots daily, freshly juiced is best), folic acid, manganese, paba, biotin, selenium, chromium, vitamin E, vitamin C (as sodium or calcium ascorbate in high dosage), an additional high dose of vitamin B_1 and injections of high doses of vitamin B_1, B_6, and B_{12}. With a strong concentration of peony and passion flower tea, he was able to sleep soundly. Vitamin C powder, magnesium, and calcium had a further sleep-inducing effect. With tryptophan he was able to fall asleep after about 90 minutes. He was later able to withdraw from tryptophan.

A failed withdrawal attempt

A thirty-four-year-old patient of mine was tortured by hallucinations and thoughts of suicide. Again and again he received various psychiatric drugs and/or higher doses. Having recently adjusted Risperdal, which had severe side-effects, he wanted to withdraw from it. When I warned him not to suddenly withdraw from it, he decided on an orthomolecular treatment with a psychiatrist. Within four months he was thus able to avoid having his dosage raised. The Risperdal dose could not be further reduced because the higher monthly costs for an orthomolecular treatment (50 Euro) were more expensive than the patient could afford. After the orthomolecular treatment ended, his Risperdal dosage had to be increased by two and a half times again. If the a public health insurance company had taken over the costs for the orthomolecular medicine, approximately 1000 Euro could have been saved annually.

This example shows that the health insurance company has no real interest in saving money. It is important that groups and experts who question conventional medicine and its practices and who engage in attempts to have effective alternative methods of treatment should be heard. But the federal ministries and the authorities are deaf to everything but the interests of large pharmaceutical companies (who have a monopoly on expensive psychiatric medical care).

This costly state of emergency in patients' care is a political problem that is not being taken seriously by any of the established parties. Because it is obvious that politics and the interests of pharmaceutical companies were always closely tied, it should be easy for those affected by mental health problems to see through this quandary and its structural causes.

Concrete steps

If you are seriously interested in gaining control over your mental problems and their treatment, I recommend joining a self-help group. You can find the relevant addresses in the internet on the website of the European Network of (ex-)Users and Survivors of Psychiatry ("www.enusp.org" with links to groups all over the world).

If there is no self-help group near you, you could found one yourself (it is part of the job of social workers, education specialists and psychologists to help you with this). You will soon recognize that you are not the only one who is making an attempt to (re)gain responsibility and self-determination in your life.

If you are of the opinion that you need to use some kind of medication to treat your so-called mental illness after withdrawal, a further step would be to take a part of the medical treatment into your own hands. Orthomolecular medicine sets out to utilize nutritional substances as building blocks and as alleviating substances during withdrawal, as well as to fight against symptoms of a so-called mental illness. A practical utilization of the recommendations of Burgerstein in his "Handbuch der Nährstoffe" *("Burgerstein's Nutritional Handbook")* could lead, for example, to the following line of questioning: Should I buy some of the vitamins and trace elements listed here? Should I look for a doctor who can help me and advise me in taking vitamins, trace elements, minerals, amino acids (for example tryptophan)? Because vitamins and trace elements are not prescription drugs, I could buy them on my own and take them in order to find out if they improve my condition.

Will it help me to go off nicotine, caffeine, alcohol, refined sugars and illegal drugs? Will raw foods help me? Should I find a new neurologist/psychiatrist? Why shouldn't I try experimenting with herbal teas? Do I need a medical doctor at all?

Further experiences

My experiences have shown me that avoiding all kinds of addictive drugs increases a sense of well-being after a successful withdrawal. What is true for all other people is also true for people with psychiatric diagnoses. Regular exercise in fresh air, regular sleep, constant social contact, a supportive circle of friends or acquaintances, and if necessary psychotherapy can all have a positive effect on the course of psychological problems.

In one case I observed how a misdiagnosis led to a patient being psychiatrically treated with neuroleptics. When the patient, who was also my client, complained of increasing bouts of forgetfulness, I recommended that he consult with a specialist for internal medicine or radiology. The specialist discovered that he had a thyroid disorder. The dosage of replacement hormones, the specialist put him on, was able to be lowered by combining it with a dose of trace elements. Such a treatment is not usually recognized by conventional medicine. In another case (the diagnosis was "borderline disorder with an alcohol dependency"), a multivitamin preparation with trace elements (Viomin N), a daily dose of the antidepressant L-Tryptophan, and a healthy diet were able to make a prescription of neuroleptics superfluous. By visiting and calling my patient on the telephone, I have been able to ward off his suicidal thoughts during crises. Certainly a closed ward would also have been an easy way to cancel the risk of suicide—but the only one this would have made it easier for is myself, given that neuroleptics and antidepressants often contribute to suicide and that suicide rates are very high in closed wards.

Finally, I would like to recommend to all those who have been diagnosed as having "psychiatric illnesses," they should not passively resign themselves to traditional medical treatments. They should look critically at such treatments and not give up their autonomy. In this context I would like to mention that it was above all the insights of humanistic psychology that allowed me to develop the capacity for remaining free of fear in extremely stressful situations. This was also true for all problematic situations that resulted from withdrawal attempts. My Christian beliefs were also a source of support.

The publications by (ex-)users and survivors of psychiatry and their supporters are in my opinion very helpful in countering a whole world of ignorance and prejudice created and administered by (some but not all) psychiatrists and neurologists. Orthodox medicine, unfortunately, still persists as an odd world that stubbornly contradicts common sense. A lack of meaning, orientation, or stability in life cannot be dealt with by psychiatric drugs nor the traditional school of psychiatry, which has proved to have little relationship to reality. Instead, such problems must be solved in dialog with oneself and with others. It is the task of psychiatry to devote itself not to the pharmaceuticals industry but to individuals who need help in developing a productive idea of who they are, where they stand, and where they are headed.

Instead of this, psychiatric drugs are being prescribed and individuals are being steered into institutionalized forms of care. The institutions that exist are the ones organized by social and political forces that are tied to the pharmaceuticals industry and the traditional schools of medicine that support the industry. Neuroleptics and antidepressants can temporarily mask life-endangering psycho-social problems and thus seem to solve them (although sometimes they are the cause of the problem in the first place!). In my opinion they should be used, if at all, as a temporary form of crisis intervention and only with the informed consent of the patient. After witnessing the withdrawal attempts of my patients, I have come to see neuroleptics and antidepressants as a dangerous crutch. Whoever uses a crutch longer than is necessary will eventually become used to and dependent upon it. In my opinion, living in a responsible way that is respectful to oneself means living without the long-term use of neuroleptics and antidepressants. Because the pharmaceuticals industry and traditional schools of medicine have political forces watching out for their interests, they will offer no initiatives that would give psychiatric patients the kind of help they are seeking. I can only recommend to all (ex-) users and survivors of psychiatry as well as their friends, family, and supporters that they should turn to all possible forms of help that can avoid a long-term stay in psychiatric hospitals or after-care institutions.

Translation from the German by Christina White

Constanze Meyer

"Withdrawal from Dependence on Medication…"
Thoughts About Withdrawal from Benzodiazepines and Analgesics Among Women

Tranquilizers / Analgesics

Dependence on medication among women is a silent and secret addiction that no one speaks about. Consequently, no one ever hears about withdrawal among this group either. In the context of my work in continuing training for professionals and educators in the field, I have repeatedly referred to the possible complications of benzodiazepine withdrawal. And I am often surprised how little the public is informed about this issue which has remained the special knowledge of interested workers in the medical field.

For good reason, attention has been paid to the symptoms and complications that may occur during withdrawal which are potentially quite dramatic; they must be taken into account when planning a withdrawal, particularly if it is done on an outpatient basis. Beyond a description of possible symptoms, the following will also address impressions and evaluations gained through clinical experience in order to construct a comprehensive picture of the process of withdrawal.

Most of the women who come to our counseling center with heavy dependencies experience the process of withdrawal as very threatening, while those who are dependent upon lower doses generally have an easier time withdrawing—despite a few cases that have been dramatic among this group as well. The conditions under which women receive guidance during withdrawal must also be taken into account because this also has an effect on the success of the withdrawal.

Before taking a closer look at the withdrawal problem, I will first briefly detail the different classes of medications to which I am referring.

Benzodiazepine (sleeping pills and sedatives)

Excluding those who self-medicate and those with private insurance, 1.4 million people are dependent upon medication in Germany (Remien 1994). In other countries the essence of the situation is probably no different. Because there are always discrepancies between the numbers of prescriptions written within the public health system and the numbers of prescriptions actually sold, it can be assumed that the number is in fact much larger (cf. Glaeske 1997, p. 55).

Sleeping pills and sedatives containing benzodiazepines make up the class of medications that are most often misused. Even at low doses this group of drugs has a high potential for dependency. Their effects are relatively unspecific: they reduce anxiety, calm nerves, relax muscles and induce sleep. The indications for benzodiazepines are that they should be prescribed for a limited period of time (for example during an acute crisis), because, regardless of the dosage, dependency may develop even after only two to three weeks of regular consumption.

A distinction must be made between a low-dose dependency with no increase in dose and a high-dose dependency during which the daily dosage increases rapidly. In addition, a multiple dependency must be differentiated in which other addictive substances such as alcohol or illegal drugs are taken in combination with benzodiazepine. This is important because different complications may arise during the course of withdrawal.

A characteristic specific to benzodiazepine dependency is its iatrogenic character, that is, the fact that the medication is prescribed by a doctor. Because two-thirds of these medications are prescribed to women, we can describe this as a gender-specific pattern of prescibing.

Pain killers (combination preparations)

It is difficult to estimate the number of people who are dependent on pain killers, because, only 25% of these substances are prescribed and paid through public health insurance plans. A small portion are prescribed privately but the majority are consumed via self-medication (cf. ibid., pp. 61ff.). Pain killers are the most widely sold medication in Germany, and it can be assumed that the level of abuse and dependence is as high as with benzodiazepines.

I am referring here to the combination pain killers available without a prescription that are used to fight light to moderate pain which can potentially be misused and cause dependency. With the help of mass advertising for pain-killing medications, a social climate has been created in which people are led to believe that well-being, freedom from pain, and productivity can be accomplished at all times through the use of medication. Information about the potential for abuse and the side-effects are not given ("Ask your doctor or pharmacist about possible side-effects and risks…").

I am not referring to the strong analgesics (pain killers) or opiates and opioids that play a role among illegal drug users. In contrast to other European nations, they are seldom prescribed in Germany even for patients with very serious pain.

One of the most popular analgesics available without a prescription are combination pain killers. They sell particularly well because a psychotropic substance such as caffeine is added. The pain killing effect of caffeine has not been determined, but it acts as a stimulant and increases productivity. The chemical change accomplished by this combination adds to a sense of well-being yet also creates a high potential for misuse. Non-prescription mono-preparations, i.e. drugs that contain only one active substance such as aspirin, have a very low potential for misuse because they have no additional psychological effects.

Preparations containing codeine must be prescribed; the euphoric effect of codeine makes this substance potentially addictive. Long-term abuse of such substances—depending upon the combination of active substance—can create side-effects such as constant headaches, stomach problems, and possibly kidney failure leading to the permanent need for kidney dialysis. The European Association for Dialysis and Transplants estimates that the kidney problems of 10–25% of dialysis patients can be traced to the abuse of analgesics (Hautzinger / Janssen 1994). In such cases women constitute the majority of users.

Why women?

More than two-thirds of those dependent upon medication are women. For the over-40 age group ca. 75% of those prescribed psychiatric drugs are women. These figures indicate that women are specifically at risk for dependence upon medication. Why are women prescribed these drugs more often and/or what makes them more likely to seek medication?

Symptoms such as exhaustion, pain, sleeplessness, restlessness, nervousness, tension, marital crises, guilt, loneliness, and isolation are often named as the reason why women seek out a doctor or pharmacist. Often, women have an unspecific multiple complex of symptoms when they first seek out a doctor. This has been confirmed by both the women themselves as well as the literature. These multiple complaints and lack of well being are often diagnosed as neurosis, vegetative dystonia, depression or psychosomatic dysfunction.

In comparison, the same symptoms in men are less often diagnosed as psychiatric disorders. They are more thoroughly examined and attributed to problems at work or to organic illnesses (cf. Cooperstock 1976). Thus, men are less likely to be prescribed psychiatric drugs.

The Berlin psychologist Doris Latta has hypothesized that the gender specific discrimination in which women are more often prescribed psychiatric drugs can be traced to a social matrix that makes women more likely to become dependent upon medication (Latta 1994, pp. 80ff.):

- gender-specific socialization that ascribes to women a general principle of dependency
- gender-specific division of labor that creates a conflict of roles for women as professionals, housewives and mothers ("One is too little, both too much.")
- suffering caused by structural and individual relations of violence (for example traumatic childhood experiences)
- self-destructive relationship structures in which "giving love" is often confused with giving up oneself and thus leading to extreme self-sacrifice and illness.

Many women react to their social conditions with complaints such as headache, dizziness, fears, restlessness, insomnia, etc. In addition, crisis situations, a partner's addiction, divorce, unemployment, illness and many other factors may contribute to the development of women's dependency on medication.

A closer look at the psychogenesis of our female clients shows that many have come from families that were emotionally and often materially lacking. The family climate was often influenced by addiction, a greater neediness on the part of the care-giving generation, a lack of boundaries and frequent ruptures in relationships. Daughters are often functionalized early on in the role of caregivers, which has an immense effect on their psychological development and above all the development of a stable sense of self.

In their adult life they are then forced into a conflicting position of repressed need and attempts to stabilize their desolate sense of self by "helping others"—a situation that leads over time to an increasing self-depletion.

Women who come to our Berlin information and counseling center "Schwindel-Frei" *("Head-for-Heights")* often describe how they feel very alone with their problems in life and how even within the context of a family they receive rather little support. Those who have already attempted a (more or less successful) withdrawal—often as a self-experiment—report that their experience has been very depressing. They feel even more alone with their symptoms which have meanwhile become further aggravated.

My clinical experience has shown that very few attempts at withdrawal are undergone in a situation of support and/or with adequate professional guidance. People with an exclusive dependency on medication are underrepresented at withdrawal clinics. Very few statistics are available, but reports from clinics and our experiences at the counseling center corroborate this. For example in rehabilitation clinics (cf. Hüllinghorst 1997, p. 131) far fewer patients have received treatment for dependency upon medications in comparison with those being treated for alcoholism. According to the "Jahrbuch Sucht '98" *("Addiction Yearbook '98")*, in those parts of Germany which made up the former West Germany, only 296 patients were approved for treatment of medication dependency, while 24349 were approved for rehabilitation from alcoholism (ibid.).

Where does withdrawal take place?

Often, those with a medication dependency begin a withdrawal unintentionally and unconsciously and thus are unable to understand the developing withdrawal symptoms. Depending upon the varying half-life period for benzodiazepines, the symptoms may not appear for several days after initial withdrawal.

Here are a few typical examples of how withdrawal has been carried out unintentionally or in an unconsidered way and in which medication has been withdrawn suddenly and the effects of withdrawal have not been properly recognized or realistically calculated.

- Self-experiments in withdrawal are carried out such that the first day or two seem fine because of the drug's half-life, yet when they finally appear, the withdrawal symptoms are so intense that the attempt is broken off.
- A patient winds up in the intensive care unit of a hospital due to illness or an accident. Her dependency is not known and she thus experiences an abrupt or "cold turkey" withdrawal so that in addition to the original problem she experiences withdrawal symptoms that are not recognized as such by doctors.

- Patients often describe vacation situations during which their luggage has disappeared or they have run out of pills.

The classical course of withdrawal through health and social services with professional guidance such as a counseling center, a rehabilitation clinic, or a supervised reduction plan is rather rare.

What makes for a successful withdrawal?

Looking at the literature on the subject, one notices that the descriptions of withdrawal and rehabilitation are limited to an isolated list of withdrawal symptoms such as muscle aches, the shakes, intense sweating, stomach problems, accelerated heartbeat, weakness, anxiety (fear of going insane), pain, thoughts of suicide, restlessness, hallucinations, insomnia, cramping, headache, etc. We have noticed in our clinical work that there are often massive psychological effects as well. Few diagnostic criteria have been established that can predict who is at risk for a particularly difficult course of withdrawal. Our experience has yielded the following list of factors that influence the course of withdrawal and the way in which it is experienced by the patient:

- dosage and how long a substance has been consumed
- how quickly the withdrawal occurs
- the patient's general psychological state and health status.

The following conditions make withdrawal easier:

- information about possible withdrawal symptoms
- the conscious decision and preparation for a withdrawal
- a supportive and calm environment
- in- or outpatient guidance and/or the aid of a physician
- a build-up of resources in the motivational and preparatory phase
- other supporting measures (for example alternative medicine).

These factors can, of course, be expanded. In our work we aim to support women with information and counseling such that they are in the best possible starting position, thus opening up the realm of possibilities, building their confidence, and encouraging them to actively seek change. We offer regular individual counseling, telephone counseling, a contact center, and participation in an after-care group during the course of a clinical rehabilitation.

Beyond the above description of what patients suffer during withdrawal (or perhaps as a result of a sharp increase in suffering), the phase of withdrawal represents a break in the life of the patient—sometimes constituted by a low point, but often also a changing point and the start of a new orientation. This aspect will become clear in the following fictional examples of typical biographical patterns. I have chosen this form of representing the possible course of withdrawal in order to make the process easier to understand and to frame it within a larger context. I have differentiated between types of dependency in order to avoid overgeneralization.

Typical biographies as seen from the perspective of a professional counselor

High and low dose benzodiazepine dependency

If a woman responds to her current life situation with restlessness, nervousness, and anxiety, and if she never learned to actively change her situation or if she sees no possible way out of it, she will likely seek the help of her family doctor. It is possible that she will experience on her own body the previously-described gender-specific patterns of prescribing at the physician's practice. Because she is unable to help herself and is under pressure from others around her, she will describe and complain about her situation and insist that she must be able to function again very soon. If she is lucky, the doctor will not give in to the pressure but instead send her to a counseling center, list a number of options where she can receive psychological and social counseling or will take the time to listen to her story. The women who come to our counseling center were usually not this lucky. Generally, they left their doctor's office with an unspecific diagnosis and a short-term prescription for a psychoactive drug.

In the beginning the sedative has the promised effect: The woman is calmer, more relaxed, her anxiety has subsided, and she is able to function again in her daily life. Her conflict-laden situation has been repressed and she is once again able to meet her own expectations and those of the people around her.

Quite possibly she lives with a partner who has a substance addiction for whom she has taken over responsibility, or in addition to her job she takes responsibility for a family member in need of care. If her situation remains the same, it is very likely her short-term use of a substance will develop into a mid-term or ultimately a long-term use.

The effect of the sedative proves to be limited, she may develop a tolerance and may increase the dosage. The original complex of problems is not solved, and instead the woman has become detached from her own experience of it; the problems are not solved but merely veiled. Thus she begins over the years to suffer from depression, loss of interest, and isolation due to her retreat from society. The permanent medicating not only turns the original problems into chronic problems, but it also creates a further problem, namely a physical as well as a long-term psychological dependence.

In the meantime over the past ten to fifteen years the woman has changed doctors several times ("doctor shopping") and is now taking a high dose of benzodiazepines. Her addiction is quiet and hidden, only her immediate family and friends know. Others may suspect that something is not right with her or for example, that her personality has changed. Her family has slipped into a new balance of relations. She has perhaps tried several times on her own to quit the substance around which she has somehow organized her life. Because the withdrawal symptoms do not necessarily appear immediately due to the half-life of the substance, she may misinterpret the initially delayed symptoms when they finally appear in extreme ways (e.g. anxiety, shaking, restlessness). A relapse to the pills is almost programmed.

Pain killers

If she tends to chronic fatigue, tension, and headaches as the result of her problematic situation, or if she suffers from migraines (possibly as did her mother), she may first go to the pharmacy and buy a pain killer. Generally, she will quickly start using a combination preparation because additives such as caffeine initially effect an increased productivity in addition to the pain killing effect, thus making her able to function again. Being productive and functional are so important to her identity and her self-esteem that she cannot bear losing them. Over time she increases the dosage because she has build up a tolerance to them. She does not actively change anything in her stressful life; her strategy for coping will only create a chronic pain problem.

After several months she suffers dull headaches daily. Due to the continuous use of combination analgesics she now also has a headache caused by these substances. If she is a migraine sufferer, then this has by now developed into a permanent migraine for which she also takes migraine medication daily.

In the meantime she now has sought out several doctors who prescribe her additional pain killers. Perhaps she has been through an intensive diagnostic examination in which "nothing has been found." Now and again she requires an emergency doctor's visit because pain killers have only a limited effect. She also suffers from depression and loss of interest, she has isolated herself and developed a guilt complex because "something is not right with her." If she is unfortunate and unable to find an alternative solutions, after years of medication abuse she may end up with chronic kidney problems and possibly the need for regular dialysis.

Searching for help

Women such as this will typically come to our counseling center after ten to fifteen years of drug abuse. They are between 35 and 45 years old, their children have just left home and their lives seem bleak. Perhaps their relationship has recently ended, or they have professional difficulties that seem more and more difficult to tackle. Often they work in the health and social services and thus have easy access to medications.

If a woman is dependent upon benzodiazepines, then she inevitably knows about her own dependency even if she does not want to admit it. She is afraid of withdrawal and can no longer imagine a life without medication. The pills are invested with emotion, and before every vacation she stocks up "because the pills may be unavailable later."

Her thoughts permanently revolve around the pills, yet she also has a great desire to finally leave them behind her. Her fear of withdrawal is compounded by her unsuccessful experiences with withdrawal (that caused, for example, jittering as well as the feeling of being completely vulnerable). This combination of feelings creates an inner state of high tension and pressure. She worries too much about her relationships with the doctors who have prescribed her medications for so many years. With each new prescription she had felt a sense of relief. She has meanwhile also discovered the pharmacies where she can buy medications without a prescription, but this route makes her feel ashamed. She even feels a pang of anger at her doctors for having done this with her for so long. She has lost all trust in the public health care system.

If she is still on a low dose, she will at first have difficulties acknowledging her dependency. She may have an intact social context and in no way resemble the typical image of an addict. If she can rely on the support of her social environment, normally she would seek out a doctor to undergo a gradual withdrawal on an outpatient basis.

She regularly attends supportive counseling and seeks additional forms of help. She needs to talk about her experiences, find support, and be calmed. A gradual withdrawal can stretch out over weeks or months. She may not be able to accomplish withdrawal in this way and thus chooses to enter a residential clinic.

With a low-dose dependency the withdrawal symptoms can be delayed a few days after quitting, and they may last for quite a while. She is restless, irritable, vulnerable, perhaps she suffers from insomnia, and conflicts build up in her immediate environment. She hears from her husband or partner that she is no longer the same person. Old memories come back to her, the original problems that led her to take the medication return to occupy her. Sometimes she is flooded with feelings that she does not understand, and this may lead to overwhelming fears. In addition, physical withdrawal symptoms such as a racing heartbeat and shortness of breath may occur. Explanations and information on withdrawal are important at this point because they can calm anxieties and relieve tension. The last crumbs of benzodiazepines she takes will mark a historical moment and a break with her former life. She will note the date and celebrate her "clean birthday" every year.

If she is dependent on a high dose, we recommend withdrawal on an inpatient basis because severe, threatening symptoms may develop with this type of dependency. In this case the patient requires medical supervision around the clock. Symptoms may occur at the psychological level as well as vegetative, motor system and/or nervous system disorders, but they cannot be predicted in advance. She has reached a point in her life where she knows things cannot continue as they have been. At this point, she lands with us and receives information about the process of withdrawal and what kinds of changes she can expect in her life at this point.

The factors that influence someone to begin withdrawal can be very different. It can be a spontaneous decision or one that is accelerated by certain events, but it may take a long time before the decision is final. If she really wants to take this step then she will prepare herself with professional help. She inquires at the clinics whether it should be done "cold turkey" or gradually.

Looking back, many women who had high-dose dependencies describe the process of withdrawal as a nightmare and as a time in which they felt themselves at the mercy of their symptoms or of the institution in which they sought help. An immense loss of control is threatening in particular to women who experienced trauma in their childhood. Rehabilitation clinics that offer intensive psychological and social counseling can offer women a supportive setting in which they feel safe and protected.

Patients are vulnerable in the period after they have initially stopped taking the medications and after being released from the hospital particularly because they fear a relapse. Their thoughts still revolve around the pills, even after they have experienced success with their withdrawal and were able to clear all remaining pills from the house.

Their unrealistic hopes soon confront them; the illusion that the problems will have gone as soon as the medication is gone proves itself wrong. On the contrary, the patient is confronted with overwhelming, frightening symptoms which she experiences with great immediacy as she is unable to distance or protect herself. She is confronted with her own neediness which she had numbed with the drug and which now suddenly seems endless. Normally she will still have to struggle with withdrawal symptoms for a long time (up to two years), though they will lessen over that time.

Women with a benzodiazepine dependency corroborate in their description of feeling very different without the medication, "as if a veil had been removed," as if they had previously been "padded in cotton" or "swimming in a fish bowl," or as if "the wall around them is now gone."

After initial detox, many women choose to apply for an inpatient rehabilitation course in order to create a larger span of time for intensive therapy in a safe place where they are better able to work on themselves with distance to their usual environment.

Withdrawal from a dependency on pain killers takes a different course. Take for example a woman who suffers from a constant headache induced by her medications. If she comes in for counseling, she will have a hard time admitting her dependency. "I only have a headache, which would be cured by obtaining the proper medication that has not been prescribed yet." Recognizing the psychological and social context of her problems may be very difficult for her. The fact that feelings of being burdened, overworked, and depressive may manifest themselves in the form of headaches and migraines does not fit into her biomedical model of explanation. She cannot accept that beyond a predisposition and family history, migraines in particular are in part caused by inner conflicts and behavior patterns, and that they can thus be actively influenced. In addition, her dependency disgusts her and makes her feel guilty. This is particularly the case if there has been an addiction problem in her family's history.

In such a situation, providing information is the first step, allowing her to recognize that regardless of a predisposition for migraines, the headaches are more immediately triggered by psychological and social problems. She must also be aware that treating dependency successfully first requires withdrawal. For this, it is very important that she work together with doctors who have been sensitized to the issues involved and who medically confirm the presence of psychosomatic symptoms.

If a woman decides to withdraw—normally after a long period during which she has become motivated—she will most likely want to do so on an outpatient basis because she fears the possibility of landing in a rehabilitation clinic with others who have drug and alcohol addictions. She will need much support because she may develop an unbearable headache during the detoxification phase over the first week. She may also suffer from nausea, vomiting, circulation problems, the shakes, sweating, and other vegetative symptoms.

In this case it is also important that she receive appropriate information in order to calm her.

Detox usually takes seven to ten days; the constant headaches may only subside after four weeks, but thereafter the original headache still remains. After that she will have to decide if she will confront her problems and be completely clean in the future, or if she will continue taking pain killers on a controlled basis. If she decides to remain clean, then she will look for alternative means of healing which are not addictive such as alternative medicine, physiotherapy, relaxation techniques, sports, psychotherapy, or a self-help group.

Women who decide to treat headaches with the controlled use of monopreparations must exam the sources of tension in their lives in order to avoid falling into old patterns. Experience shows that the women best able to succeed at this are those who have not suffered an addiction over many years, those who do not have a history of addiction in the family or those who are motivated to change their lives. Even if monopreparations do not cause physical addiction, the psychological association of headaches, medication, and a lessening of symptoms becomes a risk factor for women with a history of addiction.

Concluding remarks

Finally, I would like to make reference to the almost epidemic dimensions of women's dependency upon medications. Next to the other "big" addictive substances such as alcohol and illegal drugs, the effects of which are known and the withdrawal from which takes a shorter period of time, dependency upon medication is a problem that has remained mostly hidden. Because of this, there is an even greater need to provide public information and to take action in order to create more possibilities for women (and men) to step forward with their problems and to begin withdrawal under optimum circumstances. "Optimum circumstances" means having access to a course of withdrawal tailored to the specific character of medication dependency and which takes psychosomatic illnesses and addiction equally into account. It is high time to develop an offensive policy of disseminating information and practical knowledge throughout the health system such that existing cases of medication dependency can be recognized early and new cases can be prevented.

Only then can treatments for this form of addiction be individualized and the specific negative consequences mentioned in this article be tackled. In addition, it is necessary to promote the kinds of supporting preventative treatments such as those offered at our counseling center for women who are at risk. These women must come to recognize the problems in their lives and then adopt drug-free health strategies for coping if they are to avoid falling into a dependency upon medication.

These solutions have in common that they normally need much time and an active confrontation with one's own situation attitudes and patterns of behavior. They are anachronistic within today's zeitgeist ("For every problem there's an appropriate pill!"), but they do offer a more gentle means of preserving the body and the soul.

Translation from the German by Christina White

Klaus John

Withdrawal and Detoxification from Psychiatric Drugs from a Naturopathic Point of View

Neuroleptics / Antidepressants / Lithium / Carbamazepine / Tranquilizers

Science is divided on the old question of humanity: what came first, the material or the spiritual. The one pole is the materialistic idea of neurology and psychology which assumes that consciousness, psyche and mind are located in the brain and can be freely modulated with chemicals: humans may believe they have a soul but that this is just a product of their nerve cells; it is a fiction and is quenched when the nervous system ceases to function. The opposite pole is of the opinion that consciousness, mind and psyche are anchored in morphogenetic structures and that the brain functions like a holographic receiver establishing access to experience: the soul is primary and immortal while the perception of solid reality is a pure projection, a material illusion.

Both positions can be supported by the most modern research findings and we will have to learn to deal with this paradox. At the very least we would do well to remember Socrates' words: "I know that I know nothing." Having arrived at the gates of our individually different perception, we should observe and treat creation with respect. This particularly applies to our fellow human beings who don't consult us for help only to have us destroy their nervous system.

A clarification of the risks and damage caused by psychiatric drugs may create a desire in patients to withdraw abruptly from the particular drug they are using. This abrupt withdrawal can have disastrous consequences. Depending on the general circumstances, individual disposition, preparation, dosage and duration of usage, a gradual reduction is to be recommended.

Problems are especially caused by those substances which create physical dependence. Withdrawing too rapidly causes disturbed sleep, anxiety, vegetative disturbances, pain, (cerebral) convulsions and severe disturbances in blood pressure as well as deliria and psychotic symptoms. In the case of psychological dependence it can happen that the previous psychological symptoms return, sometimes even worse than before. There is always a risk that the symptoms which led to treatment with psychiatric drugs and have long been suppressed by these drugs will emerge in a psychotic episode or loss of control. The therapy of the patient's abuse of psychiatric drugs, alcoholism, drug addiction or a combination of these can be complicated by a possible tendency toward repression. In addition, it is often very difficult to find a doctor who not only prescribes psychiatric drugs but also provides help in withdrawing from them. The search for such a doctor should be continued with the support of self-help groups or by inquiring at the State Medical Boards and naturopath professional associations.

General principles of naturopathy

The principles of naturopathic treatment which can apply when withdrawing from psychiatric drugs are 1. to stimulate the body's own self-regulation; 2. to remove blocks and toxins which inhibit this self-regulation or to eliminate them by stimulating the body's detoxifying organs such as the kidneys, liver or intestines; 3. to provide support for the regeneration of the organism using natural substances and medication, as well as homeopathic and phytomedication (herbal remedies) etc. Blocks can be the result of scars, sites of infection or inflammation, environmental and consumer product poisons, allo pathic medication, geopathic or electromagnetic disturbances as well as toxins from diseases that have not been fully healed. The psyche can also play a blocking role as a result of stress, feelings of guilt or repressed trauma. The purpose of treatment always is to see the person as a whole physical, spiritual and social being and to achieve harmony of all their energies.

Before the psychiatric drugs are withdrawn, the patient and therapist should look at the possible consequences and discuss appropriate responses. Naturopathists should try to co-operate with the patient's doctor. Unfortunately, this is often not possible due to inappropriate professional pride on the part of the doctors or because the patient does not wish it. If this situation prevails it makes treatment more difficult and the naturopathist should encourage the patient to involve a doctor whom they trust, especially if the course of withdrawal is likely to be difficult. The inclusion of partners, family and friends can be helpful in handling a crisis. Before beginning the treatment, the therapist should ensure that the patient is fully informed and fully understands their responsibility. It is absolutely essential for the therapist to consider carefully the possibilities as well as to be aware of what the limitations are, and in cases of doubt to pass the treatment on to a colleague with the patients permission. The therapist must be aware if the patient is in any way at risk of committing suicide.

Medical alternatives to psychiatric drugs

Phytotherapy

Worldwide, there are approximately 80,000 plants containing psychoactive substances many of which have been in use since the early days of human history. The knowledge of these plants used to be guarded by shamans, medicine men and wise women and is in danger of dying out in our ethnocentric culture. Science, in the shape of the pharmaceutical industry, is trying to obtain some of this knowledge and to patent it. If a substance proves to be of value it becomes the property of the industry. The industry does not even stop at patenting human genes from indigenous people (the Amazonian Indians for example).

Most drugs come from plants or are chemical variants of their compounds. Nowadays, attempts are being made to bring every possible variant of an active ingredient onto the market without long trial periods which might allow competitors to corner that portion of the market. The proof of any possible damage is left conveniently with the patients. Even Contergan (active ingredient thalidomide) is again on the market and of course it is no fault of the manufacturer if women in the so-called third world countries cannot read the package insert.

Among recommended remedies from various manufacturers are the following:

- St. John's wort / hypericum (hypericin). It has a mood-lightening and anti-depressive effect but it must be taken for a long time for the effect to unfold.
- Valerian root / valeriana (valepotriates). It relieves tension and encourages sleep.
- Hops Humulus (lupulin). Helps with falling asleep. The plant and its constituents are closely related to hemp and its psychoactive compound THC.
- Passion flower / passiflora incarnata (different alkaloids and flavonoids). Alleviates nervous sleep disorders.

In Germany until June 2002, kava (kavain)—a plant for consumption and healing, which has been used in the South Seas for 3,000 years—could be purchased unlimitedly in different proffered forms. It has no potential for addiction and relaxes the muscles by lowering the nervous impulses without casting a cloud over the consciousness. To treat stress-induced states of tension, kavain was a good alternative to psychiatric drugs. Apart from reversible eczema or yellow coloring of the skin under very high doses, side effects were unknown. Because of the suspicion of serious liver-damaging effects from kavain, on the recommendation of the pharmaceutical industry, the former approval of the German Federal Drug Administration has been withdrawn.

More and more now, hemp and its active agent THC in hash and marijuana are discussed as a more important alternative, too, which can resolve stress and cramps. Due to the current ban on kava, THC has reappeared with its age-old use as a cultivated and healing plant. The discovery of the ananda-mide-receptors explains the calming effect of THC, kavain and chocolate, as does diazepam, too. To create a market free from alternatives, to delight mankind with the dubious blessings of the chemical industry, should finally even chocolate become forbidden?

The subject of phytotherapy is discussed extensively by Anna Ochsen-knecht in her article "Die seelische Balance—Pflanzenheilkunde Unterstüt-zung bei psychischen Problemen und beim Entzug von Psychopharmaka" (Ochsenknecht 1993; *"Mental equilibrium—naturopathic help with psychological problems and the withdrawal of psychiatric drugs").*

Homeopathic remedies

The founder of homeopathy, Samuel Hahnemann summarized his healing principle in the sentence "Similia similibus curentur" ("like cures like"). Hah-nemann made the discovery that if a poison is given in low doses it can heal symptoms which it would cause at a higher dose.

Following this discovery Hahnemann started to create a medicinal profile of substances by testing them in higher doses on healthy subjects and then catego-rizing the resulting symptoms. Sick people with symptoms similar to this medi-cinal profile were then given the most suitable substances in low doses.

What chemists see as being a less active dilution of the starting material is for homeopaths the potentiation: a strengthening of the healing effect using an energetic shaking process. A 6 X, for instance, would be a one millionth part. From 23 X, arithmetically, one liter of the medication only contains one molecule of the starting substance. Nevertheless, a 1000 X dose is still effecti-ve, which can only be explained by the fact that during the step-by-step po-tentiation of the substance the magnetic field of the solvent as carrier of the information is changed.[1]

---

1 "X" means "decimal potency." One part of the mother tincture is mixed with nine parts of solvent (alcohol / water) and then vigorously shaken to become potentized. That makes a 1 X of the mothertincture. The 2 X derives from one part 1 X mixed with nine parts solvent and shaken again. This means the "decimal" steps. (K.J.)

Today we understand how this information can be transported electro-magnetically and filtered according to potencies by using computers. This technique is used in the AcuPro-System per remedy-test. The classic homeo-path would chose the most suitable individual preparation (or complex pre-paration made up of several substances) by a personal consultation with the patient and prescribe it in a certain dosage and potency, drawing on training and experience. The symptoms may initially worsen. This indicates that the remedy fits but not the potency. Earlier symptoms may return in milder form for a short while and are then discussed with the therapist.

Acupuncture

Classic acupuncture, especially ear acupuncture (auriculotherapy), can also have a regulating effect on body and mind. Ear acupuncture is recommended for all conditions affecting the central nervous system and the psyche which are expressed in episodes of anxiety and depression. It is thus possible to in-fluence a large number of functional disturbances which are not helped by classic procedures. These include fear, claustrophobia, neuroses, poor con-centration, dyslexia (difficulty in reading), dizziness, stuttering etc. Detoxifi-cation via liver, kidney and intestines can easily be stimulated by needle, elec-trical stimulation or laser. This technique may be necessary when withdraw-ing body-blocking substances. Success with pain therapy and treatment of addiction is of particular interest here. Disrupted hormone and nerve func-tions can be effectively treated using acupuncture. However, neuroleptics (as well as cortisone) can weaken or even block the effects of ear acupuncture. Despite this, it is still of use both for withdrawal and for abstinence treat-ment. All this knowledge and information is provided worldwide in courses by the National Acupuncture Detoxification Association (NADA Acupunc-ture) and is used in many institutions for outpatient treatment of addiction.

Following an initial patient interview, recording the case history etc., the therapist examines the ear of the patient in various ways using pressure sen-sors or electrical measurements of the acupuncture points and then applies the needles or laser to the selected points. The needles, made from sterile dis-posable material and which are applied with almost no pain remain in place for 10 to 30 minutes to take effect. The patient experiences a sense of relaxation along with the healing impulse and an energetic equilibrium. The laser treatment carries absolutely no danger of infection since the skin is not damaged during treatment. This has the advantage that the points can be monitored after the treatment without any pain allowing even very sensitive patients to be treated with.

Psychological help when withdrawing

In total, there are about 30 different schools of psychology, all comprising important aspects but contradicting each other in important points. Psychology, therefore, is not a science like mathematics, where it would be unthinkable for the result of 1 + 1 to be somewhere between 1 and 30. Science is unthinkable without clear definitions. If one looks at which school of psychology is more successful we discover that the criteria for successful therapy lie primarily in the attitude of the therapist towards the patient as well as in the relationship of trust which may develop. This requires time and attention. Finally, about 20% of the therapists are comparatively more successful no matter what school they belong to. If a person becomes aware of being dependent on an addictive substance, and then realizes that instead of receiving attention they are being fed psychiatric drugs, it will take a number of steps to regenerate.

In the case of alcoholism the movement Alcoholics Anonymous (AA), which uses a twelve-step program to achieve abstinence as well as personal and spiritual development, is an excellent example of functioning self-help. Many people who wish to withdraw from psychiatric drugs need to learn gradually to understand that they had problems prior to taking the drugs or were in difficult relationships which led to their usage. If the causes and symptoms have only been covered up by psychiatric drugs, the symptoms will reappear when the drugs are withdrawn. Also, new psychological problems, which were created during times of usage of these drugs, could surface during withdrawal or after.

Since psychiatric drugs severely inhibit the ability to actively deal with problems of the psyche, on "waking up" and afterwards there is much to do to reestablish physical, emotional and mental equilibrium.

Meditation, autogenic training, etc.

In these methods patients learn how to achieve tranquillity in everyday life by allowing themselves to achieve a state of relaxation. By concentrating on certain contents of the mind and on physical processes, the self-regulation of body and mind is supported. Practiced over a longer period, a planned correction of behavior and deeper self-discovery is achievable.

Color therapy

The basis of this therapy is an empirically proven correlation between organs, colors and emotions. The colors allow—beyond direct questioning—a broad overview diagnosis of the actual attitude of the patient to certain life issues. The resulting color patterns show a personality pattern which can be discussed and reflected on with the patient. The color therapy itself uses the colors of a desired pattern which has been previously determined, for instance using electro-acupuncture (Electroacupuncture according to Voll—EAV / Electrodermal Screening). Various applications of these colors can facilitate a re-orientation of the patient in attitudes to certain life issues.

In-depth psychotherapy

Commonly used in therapy are psychoanalysis according to Sigmund Freud, analytical psychology according to Gustav Jung and behavior therapy methods. Since many mental disturbances are not approachable or easily approachable with these methods, it is sensible to broaden the theoretical context and to integrate logotherapy according to Viktor Frankl or other approaches from humanistic psychology. Or key experiences and blocks can be searched for in the unconscious or in the transpersonal area. Nonordinary states of consciousness become accessible and can facilitate the integration of incomplete elements of the psyche. Long-standing psychological symptoms can come to be understood as part of self-healing and disappear as soon as the appropriate key events have been relived. Deep reaching approaches such as hypnosis-supported regression procedures and methods such as Holotropic Breathwork™ should be mentioned.

Holotropic Breathwork™

Holotropic Breathwork™ is an experimental method of self-discovery, developed by Christina Grof and her husband Stanislav, a psychiatrist from the former Czechoslovakia who emigrated to the USA. It is the result of 40 years of research into human consciousness using modern and classic spiritual methods (C. Grof 1993; S. Grof 1988; S. Grof / Bennett 1992; S. Grof / C. Grof 1989, 1992). The term "holotropic" (from the Greek: holos = the whole, and trepein = to move in the direction towards…) means to move towards wholeness. The method of self-discovery and self-healing is based on the mobilization of the spontaneous healing potential of the psyche in non-ordinary states of consciousness induced by intensive breathing. Evocative music, supporting body work, mandala painting and group sharings are other important elements in the holotropic process. The psychoanalytically oriented research into nonordinary states of consciousness using psychoactive substances such as LSD, DMT (dimethyltryptamine), MDMA (3,4-methylene dioxymethamphetamine, Ecstasy) and psilocybin finally led Stanislav Grof to develop the completely drug-free Holotropic Breathwork™. Its theoretical framework bears many similarities to the observations of C. G. Jung, Roberto Assagioli, Joseph Campbell, Fritz Perls and the cartographs of many spiritual traditions. Important elements are taken from the twelve-step program of Alcoholics Anonymous.

Holotropic Breathwork™ provides a safe and supportive framework within which the participants can discover the wide range of experiences found in every human psyche. It enables access to all levels of consciousness and the experiences which facilitate personal growth and spiritual development. Events and phenomena from all areas are understood as normal and natural elements of the psyche, and are accepted unconditionally as they occur.

A key principle in this process is that solutions and answers to existential questions are hidden within all of us and with a little support and unconditional acceptance they can be facilitated. The following can be achieved with Holotropic Breathwork™:

- abreaction of stress and tensions, release of old psychological and somatic blocks

- integration of unresolved biographical elements before, during and after birth
- bringing memories, systems and matrices which control perception and psyche to the surface of consciousness
- working through life's problems and traumatic sequences
- dissolution of inappropriate destructive structures of the psyche
- letting go of addiction and dependency
- returning to drug experiences which had been incompletely integrated and have therefore caused complications
- release of suppressed zest for life and creativity
- emergence of spirituality, trust and mental growth
- integration of transpersonal phenomena such as mystical peak experiences, contacts with archetypes, space and time transcending experiences, understanding of karmic patterns, spiritual experiences, awakening of Kundalini
- deepening of interpersonal relationships and communication, better understanding of others

Dramatic changes ensue when a previously suppressed zest for life is released or when old pain and tension is released and leaves space for a balanced lifestyle.

These and other equally intensive approaches are not suitable for everyone. Co-operation, acceptance, dedication, letting go and insight are required. The application of such deep-reaching approaches following the psychopharmaceutical suppression of mental problems can lead to a severe and long-lasting reaction. Therefore, weekend workshops or other outpatient structures are not recommended. Because of the possibility of severe somatic and mental stress during confrontation with critical situations, the method is also contraindicated in the presence of cardiovascular disturbances, glaucoma, epilepsy, pregnancy and shortly after surgery.

Spiritual emergency and psychosis

Spiritual development is a inborn evolutionary ability of every human being. It is the movement in the direction of wholeness, the discovery of one's "true" potential. It is as normal and natural as birth, physical growth and death—it is an integral part of our existence. However, for some people the transformative spiritual emergence leads to a crisis during which the changes are so fast and inner states take such a toll that for a time it becomes difficult to cope in day-to-day reality. Triggers of spiritual emergency may be: illness, accident, surgery, physical exhaustion, long-term sleep deprivation, giving birth, miscarriage, abortion, intense sexual or emotional experience, loss of a relationship, death of someone close, separation, divorce, loss of a job, material loss, experiences with drugs, meditation, yoga, spiritual practices and much more. Spiritual emergency can be experienced as a crisis of meaning, as Kundalini-awakening, an experiencing of an awareness of unity ("peak experiences"), as psychological renewal through activating the central archetype, as a crisis of a psychic opening, as past life experiences, as communication with spiritual leaders and "channeling," as near-death experiences, as UFO-encounters, as possession states or going on a shamanic journey.

Many people experience phenomena from these areas as a crisis. While other cultures accept them as completely normal, they are labeled by our western medicine as psychotic or schizophrenic. If during such a crisis there is support from friends, family or therapists, the crisis can finally be perceived as a gentle experiential process that does not overstretch one's ability to integrate even though it may put it under pressure. The event which is experienced as a crisis is then seen as a cleansing process and an opportunity for growth. A willingness to cooperate and gain insight into the process is arrived at.

The distinction Grof made between spiritual emergence, spiritual emergency and psychosis is helpful in answering the question of whether the method can be generally applied. The term "psychosis" is limited by Grof to states resulting from organic brain damage caused by tumors or diseases as well as injuries which severely damage cerebral matter. Sometimes physical illness can cause altered states of consciousness. In cases of doubt careful examination is required to rule out such causes before the concept of spiritual emergency is applied.

If organic damage is such that intellect, memory and consciousness are disturbed to the extent that basic orientation problems ensue where the patient cannot remember name, time and place and there is confusion and disorganization, and if intellectual functioning impairs communication and cooperation, in-depth psychotherapy is of no benefit. Psychological criteria are important during evaluation because patients who are not willing to face their problems, are aggressive towards themselves and others, constantly confuse inner experiences and the external world, and practice extensive projection and blaming cannot benefit from this approach.

By limiting the often discriminating term of psychosis to a clear physical cause, many symptoms can be re-evaluated as "normal." Nonetheless, traditional medical therapists find themselves confronted with diagnostic problems and must be liable to those who finance treatment and insurers. It becomes preferable to diagnose a psychosis rather than running the risk, should complications arise later, of being accused of professional negligence or of being made liable for compensation for withholding treatment. Thus, therapists are often caught between financial interest and mainstream knowledge on the one hand and new understanding on the other.

In the meantime, an international Center for Psychological & Spiritual Health (CPSH; former: Spiritual Emergency Network) has been formed. This network brings together people in crisis, lay people and professionals creating opportunities for providing encounters and care. Following the US model ("Pocket Ranch"; cf. Bragdon 1990, pp. 198f.), centers are to be founded in Germany which will provide round-the-clock care where patients can live, work on themselves and return to health. However, in this time of cutbacks in the welfare state and with the serious lack of nursing personnel, implementation will be difficult. Idealism is called for if people are to work on a voluntary basis for organizations such as CPSH.

Detoxification from psychiatric drugs

Each therapy should be preceded by as accurate a diagnosis as possible. Following a long odyssey through diverse hospitals and practices, patients bring along with them diagnoses and doctors' letters which sometimes provide some useful laboratory findings but often are questionable. In my practice a combination of bioelectronic functional diagnosis and electroacupuncture (electrodermal screening) has proved useful in obtaining an overview of the patient's condition. These and similar procedures are continually being developed and at present there are many variations. What they all have in common is that the electrical measurement of the acupuncture points is undertaken mainly on the head, hands and feet. This allows the recording of the energy status of the individual points and the corresponding organs.

The detection of toxins using electro-acupuncture according to Voll and Leber and using bioelectronic functional diagnostics (BFD) according to Schimmel

In the 1950s the physician Reinhold Voll created the basis for the electrical measurement of acupuncture points (EAV). He conducted research into the classic Chinese acupuncture points and meridians and assigned the points already known, along with new points and meridians he discovered, to their corresponding organs. As a result, the significance and classification of up to 2000 points have now been explained so that the documentation of the measurements taken at these points provides quite an accurate picture of energy distribution in the organism.

BFD as developed by the dentist Helmut Schimmel is a variation of EAV with the aim of shortening the measurement process and simplifying it. The electrical resistance varies at acupuncture points due to the different electrodes. While in EAV a strong indicator increase followed by a drop is evaluated as a sign of weakness, in BFD the drop of the needle is seen as unimportant, and only the endpoint is recorded. Both schools arrive at astonishing results.

Using the AcuPro-II-System according to Leber it is possible to make a comprehensive diagnosis and documentation. The rapid screening of 40 control measurement points on the hands and feet enables an initial view of the body's energy balance.

The diagnosis made using these measurements is refined and verified by the remedy test. This test is another major discovery of Voll. Following the detailed measurement of different points, the patient is brought into contact with test ampoules. Depending on whether the substance is tolerated and can help the body, the acupuncture points respond accordingly. If, for example, the patient shows a high measurement at an allergy measuring point and if this can be corrected using a homeopathically prepared toxin, it can be assumed that it was this toxin which led to the allergic irritation as a primary substance. The same applies to low measurements. If, for example, a degeneration of the jaw is found and the homeopathic preparation for "ostitis of the jaw" is found to balance this point, it can be assumed that this ostitis of the jaw exists (inflammation of the jaw bone) or existed and has led to inflammatory foci of disturbance. Determining the effective individual potencies allows an estimation of the severity as well as the duration of time it has been active and the approximate time of intoxication. It also indicates how far the toxin has invaded the cell.

There are an enormous number of test substances available. The classic procedure using glass ampoules has been further developed with the Acu-Pro-II-System according to Douglas Voll into a virtual remedy test; this means that the information from approximately 7000 substances in diverse individual potencies can be simulated per computer. This corresponds to approximately 500,000 single ampoules which can be combined with each other. This list of substances includes heavy metals as well as a large collection of allopathic, homeopathic and phytotherapeutic preparations.

If it has been discovered that a toxin, in this case a psychiatric drug or one of it's metabolites, is capable in homeopathic form of stimulating an energetically disturbed organism to self-regulation, it can be assumed that it was exactly this toxin which was initially involved in the disturbance. The next step is to draw the toxin out of the body using the correct potencies. This can be done by using homeopathic remedies which usually do not represent the original substance but instead balance the energy using the principle of similarity. Diagnostically it is interesting to test nosodes (prepared from pathological products and used in higher potencies to treat the same disease) and special remedies in order to determine the substance by the patient's reaction. It is not only possible to stimulate regeneration with organ preparations but it is also possible to determine which organ preparation will regulate a disturbed point. This then provides a hint of which organs should be regenerated.

Preparing patient-specific virtual remedies

The substances determined using the AcuPro-System and their potencies can either be obtained at the pharmacy or be prepared as a virtual remedy using the imprint procedure. Unfortunately, many psychiatric drugs are not available in the program. However, if a sample of the original substance is available, it can be used to prepare the remedy by "reading" the information and imprinting it onto media like water in small bottles or ampoules containing physiological saline solution. Other methods such as bioresonance or MORA therapy use mechanisms similar to the AcuPro-II-System. The advantage of this virtual remedy is that the particular toxin is not administered in molecular form but only stimulates the immune system to respond to the toxin. This is particularly useful if there is a danger of allergic reactions.

Administering the chosen remedy

The virtual remedies relating to toxic stress should then be tested at the disturbed measuring points and lead to a balancing of energy. The simplest way to apply the remedy is, for example, by rubbing a few drops on the skin every day. It is also possible to inject the imprinted ampoules with physiological saline solution. If a patient is severely affected, a radical procedure with too high a dosage could lead to an initial homeopathic aggravation. In this case the dose should be reduced and the parallel elimination with lymph, liver and kidney remedies should be intensified. As already mentioned, acupuncture is also recommended. As an adjuvant, organ preparations of the affected organs from HEEL or WALA (see above) can also be prescribed.

Checkup

The following criteria are used to evaluate the course of treatment:

Subjective condition

The detoxification improves the patient's subjective sense of well-being. This can be accompanied by supportive psychotherapy, if the patient does not prefer individual self-help or active involvement in a self-help and encounter group. The improvement must be observed over a longer period because it has been observed that many disorders progress in phases.

Regulation of the measured energy

By using suitable homeopathic remedies and nosodes, the energy of the acupuncture meridians arrives at an equilibrium. The balance of the measurements indicates positive developments in the healing process. But because
this occurs with the aid of medication, as soon as aberrations occur or at the
latest after four weeks, the remedies must be adjusted again. The patient is
considered healed when a subjective sense of well-being is reestablished and
the measuring points have been stable without medication over a longer period of time. Following this, half-year checks should be conducted.

Successes and failures when withdrawing from psychiatric drugs

Success and failure depend heavily on the expectations of the patients and
therapists. Sometimes a patient has already withdrawn from a drug or had
taken one a long time prior to the consultation. The diagnosis with electro-
acupuncture may link existing discomfort and symptoms to the earlier use of
the drug. The success of the therapy is then seen in the alleviation or final disappearance of these complaints. Often a patient has been prescribed a psychiatric drug without having had any mental problems, for example for pain
resulting from a neuralgia of facial nerves or for sciatica. Once the cause of
the pain, e.g. a dental abscess or amalgam, has been found and dealt with, a
gradual, step-by-step withdrawal can be started and a safer pain killer such as
ASA (acetyl salicylic acid, e.g. Aspirin) or a homeopathic remedy can be given
until the cause of the pain has been completely removed.

It is more problematical if dependency on a psychiatric drug has developed
and a rebound effect or withdrawal symptoms can be expected. If there is a
good relationship of trust between therapist and patient, these problems can
be coped with. Failures are seen by the therapist, among other things, in discontinued therapy which can have a number of causes:

• The doctor prescribing the psychiatric drug convinces the patient that
  withdrawal is far "too dangerous."
• If there is a recurrence of symptoms similar to those which led to the prescription of the drug in the first place, the patient becomes distrustful or is
  not willing or capable of working on these symptoms in therapy.

Addresses

Grof Transpersonal Training
PMB 516
38 Miller Avenue
Mill Valley, CA 94941
USA
Phone: +1-415-383-8779
Fax: +1-415-383-0965
gtt@holotropic.com
www.holotropic.com

Klaus John
Healing Practitioner
Alte Wache 15
D-21481 Lauenburg
Germany
Phone/Fax: +49-(0)4153-53828
mail@klaus-john.de
www.klaus-john.de

Douglas C. Leber
Wellness Center of Grapevine
230 S. Park Blvd. Suite 103
Grapevine, TX 76051
USA
Phone: +1-817-481-4116
Fax: +1-817-329-3385

National Acupuncture Detoxification
Association (NADA)
P.O. Box 1927
Vancouver, WA 98668-1927
USA
Phone: +1-360-254-0186
Fax: +1-360-260-8620
Toll-free telephone from within the US
at 1-888-765-NADA
nadaclear@aol.com
www.acudetox.com

NADA UK
PO Box 208
Oldham OL2 8FL
United Kingdom
Phone: +44-(0)161-2327564
nadauk@btinternet.com
www.nadauk.com

Center for Psychological & Spiritual
Health (CPSH)
(former: Spiritual Emergency Network)
1453 Mission Street
San Francisco, CA 94103
USA
Phone: +1-415-5756299
cpsh@ciis.org
www.senatciis.org

- The family of the patient, who lives in dependency, refuses their support.
- The institution involved abuses their position of power to pressure the patient not to try to withdraw.

Some patients do not want to reduce or withdraw. This can be interpreted as a failure by the therapist if they know that taking the drug is harmful for the patient. In this case the only course is to offer advice. Some patients are satisfied if they achieve a reduction in the dosage, while others consider it a failure if they cannot live completely without the drug or cannot withdraw fast enough.

The basis for a trusting, responsible cooperation exists if therapist and patient know that they can learn from each other. This basis is all the more solid if the therapist is experienced and the patient knows that they can rely on the therapist if there is any trouble.

Translation from the German by Mary Murphy

Kerstin Kempker

Withdrawing from Psychiatric Drugs in the Runaway-House

Neuroleptics / Antidepressants / Lithium / Carbamazepine / Tranquilizers

In 1998, after two years of practical experience at the Berlin Runaway-House, I collected the experiences of the members, occupants, staff and interns in a book, "The Flight to Reality—The Berlin Runaway-House." The following text is an excerpt from the chapter "Statistics" that begins:
    "Statistics lie. They mask the particular, the remarkable. They indifferentiate. They look for the appropriate questions to suit the answers they already have." (Kempker 1998, p. 271)

Considering that the main interest of a runaway-house is to offer a place beyond the reach of psychiatric labeling and methods, then a discussion about psychiatric methods—about the prescribing and administering of neuroleptics, antidepressants and tranquilizers—takes on an important role in a runaway-house. It may be astounding at first, but with a second look less so: taking pills is a subject not often discussed at the Runaway-House. There is a lot of fighting, suffering, yelling, destruction—but little is ingested (pills, alcohol), though there's a lot of smoking (tobacco). There's a lot of tea-drinking, various herbal teas, and sometimes coffee. The punching bag in the basement is used, even more than the wide fields that stretch from the end of the street to the next village. If you can't sleep at night, you stay up and talk with us or those staying here or with yourself, take a bath, listen to music, read, cook something for yourself. The staff and/or the occupants love to take long evening walks.

The usual reasons for reaching for a pill, with which many who have spent time in psychiatry are familiar, are not found here. This is hard for some to take at the beginning of their stay here, because as much as they want to come off these psychiatric drugs, the drugs also serve as a "last crutch"—as something which is there for them when nothing else is there any more. It has proven valuable to offer a place in our "safe" at such times. We reserve a supply of drugs there for these moments when nothing else works, as a last resort. Just having it on supply is usually enough to ward off its use. On route to the "safe," we make ourselves available not as staff who must be bothered for access to prn *(pro re nata; when required)* medicine, but as people who want to understand what is wrong, and who think of many things besides releasing the burden, bridging the gaps, or finding solutions—and least of all doling out pills. And because most people living here for more than two weeks are not taking psychiatric drugs (60%) and/or withdraw completely or gradually while here (40%), there is a lot of experience that gets shared concerning how one can "do without," and all that one can do again "without" the drugs.

Ninety percent of those living here are on welfare, the others receive either unemployment or a pension. About 80% have had no job training, many lack a high school diploma. All of them have been under psychiatric treatment at least once, most (over 80%) more than once (3 to 48 times) or for a long period of time (one-half to ten years). As to the reproaches when we opened the house that we would only cater to the elite, it was in fact the case that those who came were those who had been dealt a good hand in life: young, motivated and active students.

Back to withdrawal: those who came to us using psychiatric drugs mostly came straight from a psychiatric ward and had been there either a long time or repeatedly. Of the 21 occupants who withdrew while here, two-thirds were successful, that is, they did not relapse into psychiatry again.

That means that one-third landed in psychiatry again, at least temporarily. We have long wondered why this is. Our observations, experiences and discussions have led to the following conclusions as to what caused this:

* the assumption that running away from psychiatry would solve all problems.

* the conviction that all past suffering could be traced to the maliciousness and lack of understanding of others, and that one was not required to make changes in one's own behavior.

* withdrawal problems caused by the psychiatric drugs themselves that can make one crazy, for example receptor changes, rebound phenomena, and the supersensitivity of the nervous system.

* an unfavorable choice of time to withdraw: too many wounds (for example memories of abuse, experiences with violence in psychiatry) or unresolved problems.

* the lack of (long-term) financial coverage, the lack of money, friends, work, or personal space, or inadequate support in the Runaway-House.

* lack of experience among the staff in the early stages of the project, and a lack of doctors to give support and guidance for gradual withdrawal and to minimize fears of withdrawal.

* the freedom of occupants to behave "wrongly" and or disregard advice, including our advice.

On the other hand, most were successful in withdrawing. Those who were previously unsuccessful in their attempts to withdraw—alone or with the grim prognosis of their psychiatrist—were now able to do so with the stabilizing support and the sense of community available in the Runaway-House.

Translation from the German by Christina White

Elke Laskowski

Biodynamic Body and Aura Work
with Bach Flowers, Stones and Colors

Antidepressants / Tranquilizers

I have been practising naturopathy since 1991. Frequently, patients searching for an alternative to psychiatric drugs come to me for help. The following are two examples of such patients.

Case 1

Approximately three years ago I received a call in my practice from a young woman asking me whether I would be able to treat her with Bach flowers as an alternative to a psychiatric drug. She had been prescribed an antidepressant by her doctor but was adamant that she did not want to continue taking it as she was afraid of becoming addicted.

The following day she came to the practice as arranged. She was accompanied by her husband as she was afraid of driving alone. The woman, who had just turned 40 and was the mother of three daughters, was extremely anxious and made a very apathetic impression. She told me that after stopping a thyroid medication she had suddenly developed strong but diffuse fears and finally became depressed. Her doctor had then prescribed her an antidepressant. This made her feel as if she were drunk and dead inside. She had the feeling of no longer being able to take in her surroundings and of no longer being herself. The patient was determined to stop taking the antidepressant and to try an alternative remedy.

We discussed the mode of action of Bach flowers. These 38 flower essences, discovered by the English doctor Edward Bach about 60 years ago, act on negative emotions. By taking the various healing essences we are able for example to transform insecurity and impatience thus becoming more secure and more patient. They affect the state of our souls and we learn to understand ourselves better. Because of the resulting self-knowledge we are in a position to alter our behavior and our actions. The flowers do not work on a physical level but instead affect our "aura." This in turn has a number of levels. The aura is usually represented as the "egg surrounding the body." The energy it contains is for example the emotions and thoughts of a person. The Bach flowers act on these feelings, in other words on the emotional body and therefore have no direct effect on our physical body and so there are no side-effects.

The couple agreed to the treatment, although the husband was extremely critical. He had no idea at all what his wife was going through and was of the opinion that all she needed to do was pull herself together. He wanted to know how long the anxiety state would last. Of course it was impossible for me to predict that. We discussed how the family could show understanding for the patient, particularly for problems designated as constituting a psychiatric illness as well as how they could provide support in every possible way and how they could show her that she was still loved and needed, or that they might simply be prepared to be there to "hold her hand."

I prescribed the woman the first Bach flower mixture. We arranged for her to contact her doctor to withdraw the antidepressant. In addition, we also agreed on biodynamic therapy as developed by Gerda Boyesen (Boyesen 1987, 1995; Boyesen / Boyesen 1987).

The contact between us was established. This aspect of my work stands out again and again in my mind. I must establish contact with my patient on a non-verbal level for successful treatment to ensue.

We ended our first meeting agreeing that she could call me any time she or her family needed my support. The patient gradually stopped the medication over the following weeks. She only took it for a total of fourteen weeks. At the beginning she felt somewhat worse and the anxiety increased. She came to me every four to five days and I treated her with biodynamic therapy. First I used a method called "emptying the aura." By this is meant that the aura is cleansed and the energy can start to flow. At the same time I changed the Bach flower mixture. I also selected a stone, to act on her mental state or on her thoughts. This has the advantage that the patient can hold onto something, in this case a stone. I chose a turquoise to which she clung avidly.

The Bach flowers are strong-acting on an emotional level while the stones act more intensively on the mental level. This does not mean that when using Bach flowers or stones only one level is addressed, but rather that these are starting points and that both levels are influenced.

Her family gave her support so that she was never alone, there was always one family member close by. The patient recovered slowly. She told me that she slept little during the nights after our sessions and that she was emotionally very upset. But on the days immediately after and on subsequent days she felt better than she had before the treatment. Her progress was steady despite outbreaks of impatience.

We often discussed the fact that healing is a process and that things that have become gradually bottled up can only be dealt with gradually. We recognized that the whole of her childhood had been marked by anxiety. For six months she came regularly on a weekly basis and after that every 14 days. We had many discussions. She had married at the age of 18, had children and had accepted a subordinate role to her husband who ran the business which they owned jointly. She slowly began to recognize her own needs. With the help of biodynamic aura work old childhood dreams which she had to confront came to the surface. She continued to talk to her husband who kept maintaining that he did not understand her. She finally mastered her severe depression and started her own business where she found an independent role for herself. She continued taking the Bach flowers for approximately 18 months and I changed the mixture at regular intervals. Now she only comes occasionally, sometimes because of an acute illness or because of feelings of anxiety, although these are never as severe as they used to be.

Case 2

The second patient I want to talk about was a student of veterinary medicine at the start of treatment and was suffering from severe exam anxiety. She came to our appointment which I had arranged with her friend and sat tensely in front of us anxious and hiding behind a smiling facade. She said that she felt totally blocked whenever she thought of the next exam. She would be totally overcome by panic and her head became absolutely empty. Sometimes it was so bad she was unable to speak and felt that she would die if she had to open her mouth. She was then unable to go the university and had to stay at home where she became overwhelmed by despair. She told me that she had been to several doctors who had all prescribed psychiatric drugs. She had taken various medications (Lexotanil *[tranquilizer, active ingredient bromaze-pam]*, Tavor *[tranquilizer, active ingredient lorazepam]*, doxepine), although usually only for a short while around exam time. But she couldn't and wouldn't swallow any more as she could not study under the affect of antidepressants. Furthermore, the depression and anxiety she suffered when she stopped taking them worsened each time. I prepared a mixture of Bach flowers for her as I usually do following the rules of the track procedure developed by Krämer (Krämer / Wild 1989). We arranged the next appointment for the following week and I told her she could call me at any time if she found herself in an acute situation.

In my experience this gives the patients a great sense of security. In fact, the patients rarely call me but they frequently tell me how important it is for them to know that they can call should the need arise.

At our next meeting I discovered that both her parents had died at an early age, her father following a long and difficult kidney condition and her mother from cancer. Her two siblings, an older brother and a younger one, are both successful business consultants and my patient had an extremely bad relationship with both of them. She lived in her parents' house with her 83-year-old grandmother, with whom she had a very cool relationship, living in an upstairs apartment. In fact there was little communication in her family and they certainly did not discuss problems. Nobody in her family knew about her anxieties and depression, including her aunts who lived nearby. They all noticed that she had been studying a long time but no questions were ever asked.

One of her biggest problems was establishing contact with people around her and this was made even more difficult when under the influence of psychiatric drugs. I prescribed her an appropriate mixture of Bach-flowers. Our meetings were mainly spentalking. I started to work gradually with color and meditative cleansing exercises so that her aura and body were flooded with white light. During this time I became aware that she could access color easily. She learned to calm herself with an imaginary blue cloud. I find it important to work with a variety of methods in order to give each patient the one that is individually right for them. To be able to imagine a coat of blue or a blue cloud can be very important during exam stress. She sometimes found the work, i.e. constantly having to confront her problems, very difficult and very different than when under the influence of psychiatric drugs. She required a great deal of gentle encouragement. In the period between exams she recovered somewhat, but the symptoms increased the closer it was to exam time and she came more often then. The fact that she had few friends and no support at all from her family exasperated the situation. But she did have friends who accompanied her to exams or we talked on the phone shortly beforehand and conducted some relaxation exercises.

She learned autogenic training in one of my courses. At irregular intervals we spoke at great length and we worked through the situation with her brothers, her grandmother and her parents. She had completely suppressed her parents' death and felt responsible for keeping the family together. She therefore felt unable to make any changes in the house or to decorate it because she felt an inner compulsion to keep the memory of her parents alive. Her brothers did not want any changes at all, although they did not even live in the house. The house belonged to the three of them and she lived in one room. Although her parents had been dead for over ten years the house was exactly the same as when they were alive. All of this was only admitted with the greatest of reluctance.

The major difference between the consumption of Bach flowers and a psychiatric medication lies in the fact that the Bach flowers do not cover up problems as psychiatric drugs do but, instead, uncover them and help develop awareness. This uncovering requires the patient to be actively involved and to be willing to change. Bach flowers regularly help to clarify the situation we find ourselves in and to pinpoint the errors we make in dealing with them thus enabling us to initiate change.

A further problem was that the patient asked far too much of herself. She tended to be a perfectionist so exams had be passed with good marks otherwise they were not worth anything. Because of this way of thinking she felt worthless, that her life was worth nothing and that she was not even worth loving or having as a friend. The Bach flowers had a comforting effect and helped her recognize her own intrinsic value. As with the patient in my first example I again used the various biodynamic methods of Gerda Boyesen: exercises to cleanse the aura and to activate her life's energy. The patient has since passed her exams and is now working in a veterinary clinic.

I am convinced that Bach flower therapy applied together with biodynamic work offer a good alternative to using psychiatric medication. Of course, talking about problems and offering the patient the opportunity to call at any time have an incomparable therapeutic effect. The observations described here have been confirmed in my experiences with many other cases.

Translation from the German by Mary Murphy

The Time After

Regina Bellion
After Withdrawal, the Difficulties Begin

Neuroleptics: Haldol

Each individual must make their own decision regarding whether or not they wish to withdraw from psychiatric drugs. It would never occur to me to tell someone else they should withdraw.

I have the tendency to react psychotically in certain situations. Neuroleptics (apparently) protect you from psychosis.

The first time I withdrew from neuroleptics, I didn't yet know that I would have to find something else—something that no one can sell me or that I could buy at the pharmacy.

Now I know what that something is. I have to work hard and exert myself if I want to stay in reality. I constantly have to check myself to make sure that I am reasonably balanced. I must recognize if I feel hurt and find out what has hurt me. I have to notice if I feel sad. I cannot pretend that everything is okay if I have a bad feeling. And I am allowed to have bad feelings. I can trust my own feelings more than the words of others. I cannot act as if I were not a very sensitive person. I cannot conform if something doesn't feel right. Etc.

Since I stopped taking neuroleptics I now have other problems. I am doing better with these. I cannot recommend them to anyone else, however. Everyone must decide for themselves what he or she can handle.

I will write here about my experiences. Of course, I hope that they will be of use to others. That would make me happy.

One can learn something when patients sit together in the hospital ward and struggle with the same questions again and again. I learned the following truism: Whoever has been taking neuroleptics for a long period of time must not just suddenly quit. Otherwise the symptoms will likely reappear quickly. Often even on the first day. And whoosh—you are back in the closed ward. Neuroleptics must be gradually withdrawn.

Just released from the clinic. The doctor said to me that for the foreseeable future I should take neuroleptics, other forms of therapy are not to be considered, and I shouldn't experiment with anything.

Alone at home. Three times a day I count my Haldol drops. I don't do much else. I sit on my chair and stare in the direction of the window. I have no sense of what is happening outside. I find it difficult to move. Nonetheless I am able to get up everyday. I don't notice that the apartment is getting dirty. It doesn't occur to me that I should cook something. I don't wash myself. I don't even ask myself if I stink. My misery progresses—but I don't even notice.

I vegetate behind my neuroleptic wall and I am locked out of the world and out of life. The real world is further from me than Pluto is from the sun. My own secret world is also gone—my last refuge, and I had destroyed it with Haldol.

This is not my life. This is not me. I may as well be dead. An idea has begun to take shape. Before winter comes I will hang myself.

But before that I want to try and see if my life would be different without Haldol. I reduce the number of drops. I take less and less until I arrive at zero.

After one month I am clean. Then I begin to notice how unkempt I am. I wash my hair, make the bed, clean the apartment. I prepare a warm meal. I even enjoy doing this. I can think again.

Of course, I am afraid that I will become psychotic again without medication. So I get some relevant books. In them I find the standard recommendation: For psychotics in the recovery phase it is important to have a clearly structured daily routine in which little emotion is involved. A life on the backburner protects one from further psychotic episodes.

Something so lukewarm that looks halfway like a daily routine cannot be my life. I don't want a life on the backburner. I don't want to get locked in a hospital again. Psychiatric drugs are not what I want either.

How can I organize my life such that I don't run the risk of becoming psychotic again? And in case I do: How can I avoid letting my neighbors find out and having them call the police?
I have to clear up these two questions first—and quickly. Thank goodness I have friends who are crazy like me. They help me clear this up.

My friends report to me on their psychotic experiences. They talk about fears, dreams, desires. I am afraid to reveal myself. If my friends know more about me they won't want to have anything more to do with me. The others are much more open than I am. I establish a boundary. Beyond this boundary I only have conversations with myself. I let no one look past my boundary. I fear that I will destroy the image others have of me. The furthest corners of my soul are accessible only to myself. There's not supposed to be any far corners. I don't take anyone there to see.

If only I had early-on taken my friends to see the depths of my soul. During my next psychosis when my automatic censor was out of commission, they found out anyway what moves me and what I wanted to hide. Words, images and actions bubbled forth from me uncontrollably and inundated my perplexed friends. A miracle happened. They didn't turn away from me with horror when they glimpsed the anger in me, but instead they organized emergency care so that I was not alone during the psychosis.

When I had been off Haldol for four months the next psychosis began. At that time I did not yet know under which circumstances I react psychotically. I didn't see the psychosis coming and so was unable to prevent it.

One can survive a psychotic phase without a doctor, a hospital, or neuroleptics. I have done it. And I have watched friends do it. I am only describing my experiences. I can only discuss that which I know first hand.

Without medication and without a doctor, the acute phase of my psychosis can be overcome in about a week. After a maximum of ten days the world is familiar again and I grope my way back into reality. At this point I cannot yet handle conflicts with others. But the most necessary daily tasks can easily be accomplished again. Sometimes I am even able to enjoy myself again.

In order to get through a psychotic episode I need:
* a room in which I will not be bothered by others
* a mattress, a cover, an occasional sip of water, a little something to eat (if anything at all)
* a friend who understands my fear because he knows me well and who doesn't resent me for my condition, who stays calm and stands by me until—in my experience after eight to ten days—the world has regained its familiar contours.

An acute psychosis without psychiatric drugs

When my relation to reality becomes shaky, usually it is already too late to prevent the psychosis—I have to get through it. I can no longer observe my situation with a certain distance. A spiraling movement has begun that follows its own laws and cannot be influenced from without. Usually at the beginning the situation is still interspersed with little islands of reality. Standing on one such island, I can still make myself understood. Sometimes this happens unconsciously, without my intention. If one is not heard at this point, or not understood or rejected, then the whole process is accelerated and the islands sink.

A prompt call for help is important. My friends and I have now reached the point where we can ask each other for help. But we still do this too late. By "late" I mean when the person calling can hardly be understood, when he has already swallowed a bunch of sleeping pills, when he is hindered in calling (most likely due to hallucinations), when he is panicking because he realizes that he has hurt himself, or when relatives are there who have become over-excited.

Once my psychosis has reached the acute phase, then I am locked into my own reality. Only occasionally is it possible for me to perceive the actual reality around me for short moments, though it seems to me to be unreal or unreliable.

In this state I can be very active and do things that I later regret. (I am describing this briefly in case any of the readers do not know what it looks like when someone is having what is called in psychiatry an "acute psychosis.") Violence against others and against oneself cannot be ruled out. The greater the fear is, the more the aggressiveness builds. The destruction of things and oneself are common in my experience. The person experiencing the psychosis no longer knows that he had asked for help, or for other reasons he may not be able to open the door for those who have come to his aid.

Of course he would like to share what is happening inside him. In the last few hours or days he has participated in extremely important and strange things. Perhaps he will tell of intrigues against him and their origins, which he has finally grasped. Or he has just experienced something incredible that would take your breath away. He is in a type of time centrifuge in which experience happens at high speeds and nothing is predictable. He can go on about this for hours. We try not to encourage him to do so. He can tell all about it later, but now is not the time.

But you have to take him seriously. Answer his questions so that he can orient himself and approach reality again. You won't help him by pretending that everything is just fine.

The most reasonable thing to do is to radiate calm. It is very important that the person begins calm, steady breathing and finally lies down.

It must be determined if and when the person has reestablished a connection to reality for short moments. Those are the moments in which he listens and understands what we say to him quietly and calmly. At this time his behavior can be influenced. Such moments are the best time to encourage steady breathing. This is important because only then can the panic subside. (Panic can bring on hallucinations.)

These short moments of clarity are the islands of reality in the sea of a psychosis. One can rely on these islands of reality. One can make use of them (something that apparently only a few people are aware of). These islands of reality always return. No matter how bad the situation is, the next reality island is on the horizon! It is the sole responsibility of the helper to see if and how the islands can be used. The more comfortable and anxiety-free the person feels on his reality islands, the more the islands grow in size and number. Reality islands appear even to those who have raged for days and nights without sleep and ransacked the apartment and thrown dangerous objects. It is good if someone helps him to step up onto these islands. Even the most terrible psychosis has reality islands. Once arrived at such an island, one asks a question or recognizes someone nearby. Even those who speak schizophren-ically can be conversed with occasionally.

We have never seen a case where it has taken more than a few minutes for a so-called acute psychotic to accept an embrace or the suggestion of lying down. Lie down next to him. Make sure your body is very close to his. But be absolutely sure that this is what he wants. Avoid any obtrusiveness. Your calm, steady breathing will make him calm. If you are not that intimate with each other, just sit down next to him and hold his hand. That alone can work wonders.

Above all, the person needs peace and quiet, a reliable and kind environ-ment, and the assurance that the helper will stick to the agreements made. It may be that the helper or close friend will occasionally not be appreciated or even suffer physical assault. It is possible that the helper will be rejected. An appropriate helper is someone whose presence does not make the person un-comfortable and who is currently at peace with himself and can keep calm.

The alternation of periods of tumult brought on by the person with a psy-chosis and the periods of calm effected by the helper can last eight to ten days. In my experience, the psychosis is over after this period of time. It may be two or three weeks until the psychotic associational thinking has faded away. Whoever gets to the bottom of his psychotic experiences afterwards obviously does not run into the next psychotic phase all too soon.

During my acute phases it is senseless to try to bring on sleep with sleeping pills. They don't do any good during this time. Even a high dose of prescrip-tion sleeping pills do not induce sleep. A psychosis that has reached the acute phase seems to have its own dynamic, like a dream that may be influenced by outside circumstances but still has to be dreamed to its conclusion.

A relaxing deep sleep is not possible as long as the psychotic "film" is run-ning. If I am able in an acute phase to lie down often and relax my body then I am sometimes able to fall into a light sleep (like most dogs) that allows me to recover a bit. Once you know from experience that sleep will come again af-ter a week or so, then this topic is no longer so disturbing.

To avoid misunderstandings, let me differentiate the terms. An "acute phase" is not the time during which a world of delusions is being built up, during which I am still well able to grasp the reality around me. An "acute phase" is the relatively brief period during which I can only sporadically perceive reality.

Just as a person can fall back into a psychosis, it is also possible for him to look toward reality if this seems worthwhile. The tendency to one or the other of these possibilities can be influenced by the person himself or his environment, though not at all times nor to the extent we would hope for.

During the acute phases of my psychosis, it was not good for me to be alone. Constant presence quiets not only the person experiencing the psychosis but also the fears of the helper.

The fear of the helper is not without reason. Even after ten episodes that ended fine, a bad ending could be next. In certain grim, long moments hope evades us because no one can guarantee that a so-called borderline patient will fall asleep each time within six hours. Any one time it could be different. For *me* as an acute patient, not calling a doctor means a lapse in getting the appropriate help. If I am left alone even briefly I may slit my wrists during my madness.

The helper's fear will often be hushed by the person suffering the psychosis. He will suddenly want to know what day of the week it is. He has landed on a reality island for a moment and says: It's good that you're here. He asks: How long did it last for you last time? Then the voices come again from the corners of the room, and the person doesn't recognize you any more. He thinks he has to kill himself or you, or he thinks he is a baby or that the world is breaking in two. You should lie down next to your friend and breath deep in order to calm him.

The experiences you have now will give you confidence during the next psychotic phase—even your own. That is, if you have another at all. Who can prophesy this?

For months I had not taken any more neuroleptics. I had stopped visiting the psychiatrist long ago. I dared to leave the questionable care of traditional psychiatric institutions. My friends and I tried to help one another. But we weren't sure that this would work. It was just the beginning for us. We were afraid when we arrived to help each other. We had little experience and we were not familiar with the dynamics that lie at the heart of every psychosis.

Each one we got through together was like a strange, dangerous, solitary journey outside the law. We would not have been able to explain to anyone what we were doing. We didn't even know ourselves. We hardly spoke about the exceptional circumstances that we experienced together.

But I knew approximately what I was risking with this solitary route. I could wind up committing suicide, or I could land in a closed ward by accident, or in a ward for chronic patients, or I could become so aggressive that I end up as a hopeless forensic case. Or I could quickly begin taking psychiatric drugs again and avoid all that. Or I would have to use my own strength to stay balanced. I decided upon the last option. At least I wanted to try it that way.

A psychotic episode doesn't just fall from the sky. I began to understand this. I had observed it in my friends. This must surely be the case with myself as well, but I could see it more immediately in others. An episode has its causes, it builds up. The course of its building up can be retroactively reconstructed. Therefore, it must also be observable at the time.

I drew conclusions. The circumstances prior to a psychosis lead into the psychosis and must therefore be interpreted as warning signals. The earlier these circumstances are detected, the earlier the warning can be taken seriously, the better the prognosis. Today I know that it doesn't always have to come to a psychosis.

I have to keep an eye on my condition and to name that condition so that I know how I'm doing and what I need to change. If I am questioning whether or not I can trust my perception it is probably already too late.

I try to observe myself from a certain distance in order to track those disquieting changes in myself early on. If I become sensitive to noises, for example, that is an alarm signal. If I am up all night working on something, that's also a sign. If I feel like I want to withdraw from the world for a long time that is less a sign of being balanced than of being on the way to an extreme position. If I am constantly on the move and cannot be alone, that's just as bad. I try to stay in balance. I struggle with it every day. And sometimes I have little time for anything else.

An example: Excitability and activity, paired with euphoria, can be diminished or stopped. If I don't take account of my excitability, activity and euphoria, this condition can grow into a mania. And then I am no longer in a position to determine how I am doing or if things are alright. Mania can seamlessly evolve into a psychosis. If my excitability has reached a certain degree, the wise thing to do is to lie down on the sofa and to think about my situation. I try to account for the condition I am apparently in. I breath calmly and deeply and remain lying down. I don't answer the phone. I do nothing or after a few hours of peaceful rest I take a walk. (This kind of self-treatment doesn't help anymore with a well-developed mania. I must recognize immediately how I am feeling.)

There are techniques (gymnastics, breathing exercises, posture) for influencing and changing your condition. Everyone must discover the techniques appropriate for him or herself. This is not something that can be done quickly in one's spare moments. It takes time and energy to develop one of these techniques into an aid that can be promptly utilized.

An example: As quickly as I can bring myself into a stressful state with quick, short breaths, I can also bring myself into a peaceful state with calm, deep breaths. Or if I constantly slink around with my head low, then it is no wonder that my mood will become depressed. Such simple things are not a panacea. But they have effects that I can make use of.

When I was trying out new things, I came upon a catalog of preventative measures. These measures are nothing special. But they are of use to me. Many of my friends have also been able to help themselves with them.

Taking precautions

We have found it useful to create a partially structured daily routine that is not full of duties and boredom. Regular meals are important, enough sleep, and—if necessary—fragrant baths. Many people who occasionally react psychotically are night people. If I find myself being a night owl for a long period of time, I can more easily fall out of reality. At night it is important to keep breathing regularly and not to breath too flatly or to hold your breath unintentionally. Abdominal breathing can be very painful at first or induce a fit of crying. It is important to avoid situations that become hectic. I am now in a position to walk away from situations that are too stressful for me.

When emotions whirl around me, I am in danger of a psychosis. You can't avoid twists of fate. Instead of giving in to temptation or withdrawing in an emergency situation, we need contact with friends more than ever. Contact with people who take us seriously, but to whom we have no great emotional relationship, is also important. With their help we can test whether or not we still have one foot in reality. This is a touchy subject that we constantly have to watch out for. Many people who occasionally react psychotically have been so hurt that they have become over-sensitive. They withdraw from others.

One must particularly watch out when falling in love. In a love relationship there is a great danger of my being hurt in the way that I was earlier as a child. If early traumas are called forth again, I can easily react with a psychosis.

Of further importance is having a task, some kind of work, an activity that we experience as meaningful. Each individual must find their own appropriate type of activity. (It is irrelevant what others think of this activity.) It is important and very freeing to let go of the idea that one must represent an image of normality. It is important to live out one's individuality and give expression to it—even if it is unconventional.

It is never wrong to ask oneself on relatively healthy days what it was that spurred the recent hallucinations. Ways in which we can work against tricks of the senses are described in a book by the psychotherapeutically-oriented psychiatrist Silvano Arieti (Arieti 1979, pp. 109ff.).

And of course everything possible must be done to establish and to stay in contact with one's own body. Foot reflex zone massages, jogging, T'ai Chi, belly dancing—everything can be of use, or not. (Caution: T'ai Chi can be dangerous for people who have knee problems.) It is worth it to keep searching and experimenting until you can feel you own body again. This feeling has to be reestablished every day.

Particularly important to me has been to avoid building up networks of associative ideas, but instead, if necessary, to ask others from the waking life to describe from their perspective the relations that seem suspicious to us. We people with the diagnosis of a "psychosis" apparently did not have the chance to develop a basic feeling of having a satisfying identity and a corresponding self-confidence. Thus we must care for ourselves particularly well and devote much attention and time to ourselves. It is not enough to finish one's studies or to achieve some kind of success that is universally admired.

These are the common maneuvers of self-deception that have little to do with inner satisfaction. The feeling of being worthy comes to me more readily when I take time to dream and lie in the bathtub. Others find their peace by playing guitar or writing in their diaries.

The most important thing is to recognize altogether contradictory behavior (so-called double-bind situations) early enough and to back away. Absurdities, disrespect and double-bind messages hurt us and make us crazy.

An assertion: my psychosis is not senseless

There are important points in life that make changes necessary. Or a change in your attitude to life becomes necessary. Sometimes a new orientation is called for, a new beginning with largely unknown starting conditions cannot be averted. The fact that things have gotten to a critical point is often preferably swept under the carpet.

A critical point can be for example entering adulthood. Or an exam period. If a person we love leaves us, a crisis can ensue. There are few rituals in our culture that help us to regain strength during a crisis or at least give us the feeling that we are not alone.

People who react psychotically in such situations are usually given psychiatric drugs and kept in the loony bin until they can create the impression that they are once again conforming. Then they are released back into the same unchanged situation that had brought on the crisis. Thus the next "episode" is already programmed. For some the situation is different. But this is exactly what my experience has shown me. Established clinical psychiatry does not grant the experience of psychosis much regard, and it doesn't find that a psychosis can be of use. "It's all chaos without any meaning," said the doctor at the state hospital.

I am of another opinion. When I have gotten through a psychosis, I cannot pretend that nothing has happened. I have to work through my psychotic experiences; they hold meaning for me. The psychotic "films" are grounded, they relate to me and my life. They are a mirror and a message for me, like my dreams at night. I must take my psychosis seriously just like others do with a heart attack. I must pay attention to the signal that my psychosis emits. If I don't want to do this, if I can't or don't, then I shouldn't be surprised at the next "episode." (Of course I can only speak for myself. If someone else sees this differently, then he or she has their reasons.)

In a psychosis there are more or less encoded images of destruction and new beginnings. That is no secret. Someone who does not see the possibility of change and a new beginning after a psychosis, or who cannot reorganize their life, does not want to develop into a new phase of life, or who first becomes depressed—he or she could possibly be helped through these stages with alternative psychoactive medicine. This is exactly what I did earlier—take psychoactive drugs, that is, psychiatric drugs—and I could do it again.

Once again I was done with this world. This time it was clear to me that I had nothing to lose. I had skidded past death and through insanity—what else could possibly happen? I felt I could risk something new. What that new thing would look like, I certainly did not know.

I still don't know. But since October 1993 I haven't had another psychosis, I haven't killed myself, and since the summer of 1993 I have done well without psychoactive drugs. That is not such a long time. It is hardly worth mentioning. But for me it is amazing.

Translation from the German by Christina White

Erwin Redig
A Mental Struggle
How I Stopped the Use of Psychiatric Drugs

Neuroleptics

When I was in the psychiatric hospital, there was an old man who was always drawing birds with colored pencils. He did this on his own, in a corner at a table, after the hours of therapy. I believe that the therapists did not even notice this little expression of his creativity. One day I went to the man and asked him if I could buy one of his drawings. These were not perfect, but to me they were of great value. He was rather amazed, but consented and I gave him 300 BF *(about 6 US-Dollar)* for it. What I in fact did was say to this man: what you do is good, I like it, there is vital creativity in you that can develop. This little act, unnoticed by the crew of psychiatrists and their servants, gave the man a great kick of self-esteem. Now, eight years later, his drawing is still on my wall in my apartment. I did not buy it out of hypocrisy; I bought it as a sign of living hope, human creativity and a silent struggle against the suffocation of psychiatry.

How to get rid of neuroleptics might be a technical problem, with withdrawal-effects and post-neuroleptic syndromes, it is also a mental problem. I have been treated with neuroleptics against my will. These drugs left me in a condition with temporary paralysis, which was explained by the doctor to my family as a catatonia as consequence of feelings of guilt. Until now I have not been able to sue this doctor for bringing me to this dangerous condition.

I have understood that neuroleptics do not heal, only subdue the individual, his creativity and life force. It may well be that they make symptoms disappear. I believe they make mental growth impossible and the cause of suffering remains. This is my opinion and I can accept other opinions as long as they are not based on the desire to make money or ignorance. Psychiatrists now claim that it would be unethical to refuse these drugs to for instance so-called schizophrenic patients. But what about exposing people to risks such as tardive dyskinesia and malign neuroleptic syndrome, even without warning them? This seems more unethical to me. The practice of treating people against their will with dangerous drugs that can cause death and always have a series of very unpleasant side-effects must be looked upon in a number of cases as a form of torture. This is well known by people who suffered this treatment. Officially, it is medical treatment. Because the concept of mental sanity can be used as a means to oppress people it makes me think about the heretics of the middle ages. The church formulated truth then, and whoever opposed the church were liars and a danger to society. We now learn in our schools that the persecution of people with other views on religion, the torture and death sentences were a mistake. We do not learn that the concept of mental sanity can become a kind of religion with its own inquisition.

If someone with free will accepts the propositions of his doctor about his mental state and the advice to take neuroleptics, we should respect this free will. For others, who want to get rid of the use of these drugs it is different. Some people can have lived for years using these drugs. When they stop, the same old problems might occur. Where is this mental distress coming from, what does it mean?

If you stop the use of neuroleptic drugs it means the confrontation with yourself again. You were probably asked to take these drugs to function as other people. But what if you are not exactly as other people? What about strange moods, desires, ideas, wishes? Great sensibility?

Salvador Dali was probably someone who had hallucinations. He called his method of painting the paranoid-critical method. In his work you can see forms change under the influence of the hallucinatory power. This man never went to a doctor to say: "I have hallucinations," whereupon the doctor would have answered: "You are a paranoid schizophrenic, I will give you neuroleptics." Instead this man with his strange gift became one of the greatest painters of our time. In this way, he turned what might be called "insanity" into power.

Signs of mental pain and distress can make sense and be useful, as long as one is not overwhelmed. What you feel is real, and must be taken seriously. Maybe it is human to be in mental pain in a society such as ours. Maybe the others are not human, only normal. You have a riddle in yourself that must be solved. You know the doctor's solution. You are a person with a disease, a bit less than the healthy people. So you can chose as the people in Aldous Huxley's "Brave New World" did, to take Soma, which makes the pain disappear.

To live with your particular states of mind will be difficult. But there must be a way to turn this confusion into power and balance. Strangeness and sensibility I see as a gift, one must learn how to use it. If I can find the force to say: "This is how I am, I love myself and am friend of myself," I would have regained the autonomy that psychiatry denies me.

Neuroleptics will not give you the power to love yourself, and knowledge of your own self. Psychiatrists are partly afraid of you, because they know if there is honesty in them that the madness that you have taken on your shoulders is also in them. People live on the verge of madness. Being immortally in love is like being mad; therefore people did not like what Romeo and Juliet did, until they were dead, and then people were sorry.

When we take the example of so-called schizophrenia we see that people that have this mental state do not always experience unpleasant sensations. Their sensations are out of the common but can be benign. Experiences or sensations that bring you good can hardly be called symptoms of disease. I ask myself if the dramatic decay in persons, treated with neuroleptics, with the diagnosis of schizophrenia has not to do with the prolonged use of neuroleptics. I have found that what is called "catatonic schizophrenia" in the DSM III code is similar to a syndrome caused by neuroleptics, with muscle rigidness which leads to strange poses.

I think that I have made myself clear in saying that the altered states of mind can lead to other solutions than becoming a mental patient and taking drugs. Your personal experience might be hard to live with, it can be a richness too. As the Belgian psychiatrist Karel Ringoet puts it, we have in our cities an effect of "overcrowding." This combined with pollution and noise creates an unhealthy atmosphere. The link with nature is lost. You are forced into an unhealthy way of life; someone is leading this game, but you do not even know who or where; your environment is becoming harsher and uglier every day; you must live in concrete cages close to each other; this is the normal insanity. Then you develop a disease, and you are punished for it with diagnosis and orders to take neuroleptics. The goal is to make you adapt to this life that has made you sick. "There must be some kind of way out of here," as Jimi Hendrix sang, "there is too much confusion I can get no relief."

Is the so-called disease not the resistance of your organism against circumstances that are dangerous to you but which you cannot overcome? Many of us know the theories of Ronald Laing and how he tried to estimate experiences out of the common. This is in fact what Freud did also. Instead of calling patients "neurotics" and "fools" of several kinds, Freud started to talk with his patients and he sought what was behind their madness. This resulted in his theory of the unconscious and one might say that Freud has learned a lot of his madmen, and he has made the healthy people listen.

With more or less success these two doctors have tried to learn from the experiences of their patients. In both cases, they developed a philosophy, and they have both attacked society. This kind of courage we must not expect from all psychiatrists. Neither can we expect from all people living in the psychiatric institution to take their strangeness as a gift and to resist the pressure to take neuroleptics. But there is a way to stop the use of these drugs, it may take time and patience and support. This support will not come from the people that declared you ill. This support must be sought amongst people that look upon you with other eyes that have honest appreciation and true interest; the hypocrisy and nine till five attention in psychiatry will not much help.

Honest appreciation from people that look at you with other eyes than mental health professionals can make you realize that the image they made of you in psychiatry is false or not whole. There is more in you than the doctor's diagnosis.

You should ask yourself why you are taking neuroleptics, and part of the answer might be that you take these under pressure of others. If you do not take them, your behavior becomes embarrassing for the others. If this is the case, you must realize that you are taking these drugs for the pleasure of others, because they find you unpleasant when you do not take them. How far can the demands of the others go? They ask you to take dangerous drugs, because they feel better if you take them. Is it not your right to reject their demands? It may be that when you are not on these drugs, people find you hard to live with. There is something unclean in you, something that the others do not have, and they ask you to hide it. And you take drugs to hide it. I want to become as the others, etc. You are afraid, afraid of losing their love and attention, even if the quality of this love and attention is bad. You are afraid to become a lonely person, powerless against the devils in his own mind.

I do know for whom this article is written. It is not only written for the people who have chosen to build a career as mental patient. It is not only written for people who want to escape jail by going into psychiatry, although this might turn out bad as the film with Jack Nicholson has shown us. Particularly it is written for people that have not played games, but were only in serious mental distress, have looked for help and became trapped in diagnosis and drug taking. For these people I say that there is hope. You are not alone. There is an international survivor movement now. Some of us understand that the mental patient movement, like the homosexual movement, is an important sign in this time. In both cases people want to affirm their identity, break their fetters and emancipate.

The use of neuroleptics is not restricted to mental patients, elder; prisoners, children are treated with them as well. Even in the former USSR dissidents were treated with neuroleptics, as Amnesty International has reported. This massive use of dangerous drugs on the population is an assault on freedom. I do not want to live in a drugged democracy. And yet people are working hard to make more forced use of neuroleptics possible. Some of us realize that the real problem of a part of the psychiatric population is a social problem. When you live in certain circumstances, your behavior changes. When you live for four years on the street, for instance, and you meet people of the higher classes, they will find your behavior strange. Maybe they will find you a dangerous person. But you have lived in poverty and misery for years, and this has changed you. This circle of poverty and isolation from society may end in psychiatry. A part of the population of the hospitals is what Victor Hugo called "Les misérables." In psychiatry, they receive medical labels. It is, it seems, easier for society to say that there are many schizophrenics these days than to say that there is much poverty and misery amongst people. In this way, psychiatry hides social misery and can in future become even more important in dealing with social injustice. You can stop the poor from revolt by calling them "mentally ill" and giving them neuroleptics. Proposals of this kind have even already been made, as is reported by the American survivor movement, where a psychiatrist proposed preventive treatment for possibly dangerous (black) persons. This raised protest, but nevertheless psychiatry is already treating social problems as medical diseases. It is in that way a political instrument.

I have experienced that neuroleptics diminish the sexual potency. This "side-effect" is important. Sexual energy is vital energy. It is clear to me that if neuroleptics diminish sexual power, they diminish vitality. And it is vitality that is needed to overcome problems. As Freud has shown us, sexual power is the source of many works of high culture. I think that it is unjust to give people drugs that damage their sexual potency. I believe that the sexual power is source of creativity and imagination.

It is precisely creativity and imagination that you need to get off neuroleptics—imagination to see other possibilities, creativity to make your own world. The advice I give to people taking neuroleptics is to ask themselves if they feel whole and free with it. If not, if it seems a hindrance to freedom, one must draw conclusions.

To find balance without psychiatric drugs will take time and there will be pain. This pain will maybe last, but on the other hand there will be a raising of consciousness. I do not know a kind of life without pain and darkness. Yet I have found that there is light also, happiness is possible. Some of the people I met in psychiatric hospitals I still remember, for they were beautiful people, with rare gifts, that cannot easily be found in society. Maybe their fault was a too great openness, a kind of childishness. These people deserved a better life.

I have revived much of my balance in nature. Psychiatry is eight years behind me now; I still spent at least an hour a day in the field or in the wood. I think that I have never returned from nature's arms without force and refreshment. These hours I spend in nature are maybe the best of my life, while I sit there and do nothing, I am in fact doing very well, listening to the rhythm of the great mother. It is she that can soothe the mind of the restless.

There was reason in my madness. I have found this reason and do not see why any other shouldn't. I have nothing to do with psychiatry any more. Once in a few months I see a psychiatrist. We walk together in the fields. I discuss with him things that can be hardly spoken of with other people, like if you went to a priest. This person admires me for not taking neuroleptics. But this was only the first step in my search for identity.

All my other relationships, except for the survivors, have nothing to do with psychiatry. People do not know about this episode in my past. And they would not understand.

When I was sixteen years old, I met a few people that came out of psychiatry. I found them a bit frightening and the world where they came out was very far and sinister to me. I am 38 years old now, as I write this and I have seen in psychiatry that the people behind those walls are not better or worse than the people from the outer world.

I have in this article not given practical advice to get off neuroleptics. Instead I have given some ideas, which might be useful. It was my intention to place the problem in a broader context. To understand yourself, you need to understand the society you live in. To discover yourself, declarations of the doctor about disease can be meaningless. The invention of the disease of schizophrenia is the answer of society to large numbers of people in great mental distress. This answer includes dangerous treatments.

For those who want to hear it, I would like to say that the whole problem changes if it is looked upon with other eyes. There is no absolute truth. What the doctor tells you can be lies. The use of neuroleptics becomes senseless if you reject the idea of being ill. Maybe there is a sanity in your mind that others do not have. Neuroleptics do not heal anything; the best they can do is stabilize. It is like taking morphine when you are in great pain. The cause remains, the pain will return.

May many of us not only draw attention on the violation of human rights in psychiatry, as it is reported world-wide, but also abandon the idea of being mentally ill and as a consequence stop the use of neuroleptics. Because they might kill something of great worth in you.

Leo P. Koehne

"Now I Give You Imap. This Will Also Help with Social Integration!"

Neuroleptics: Imap, Fluanxol, Melleril, Truxal / Antidepressants: Anafranil, Equilibrin / Tranquilizer: Diazepam

This report of my experiences does not provide a description of a classic psychiatric "career," including forced inpatient treatment and years of high-dose neuroleptics, as experienced and suffered by many others. My story is more an example of the ever-growing number of people who, because of unclear physical and mental symptoms, are referred by general practitioners to psychiatrics and who then become trapped in the vicious circle of treatment with psychiatric drugs.

It all began in 1991 when I went from doctor to doctor following the sudden occurrence of symptoms such as nausea, cardiac symptoms and a decrease in my capabilities, without any organic cause being found for the symptoms. In the end, I was given a referral to a psychiatrist: "He'll have to take a look at you." Without any feeling of unease, I subjected myself to his examination. After an hour, the diagnosis was clear: "reactive depression with anxiety attacks." Without discussing any alternatives such as psychotherapy, he prescribed Equilibrin *(active ingredient amitriptylinoxide)*, an antidepressant with sedative properties. "In modern psychiatry we now use this treatment, so take two tablets every day for six months and we'll get on top of this."

My initial doubts about this type of treatment were quickly dispelled in the face of the rapid success. The symptoms did in fact disappear within a few days and because I was finally feeling more or less well I began to look to the future with some optimism. Unfortunately, this phase only lasted a few weeks before the symptoms returned even more intensely and longer-lasting than before. I went back to the doctor, who I still trusted at this time, looking for advice and became a regular visitor to his practice: a double dose of Equilibrin, and when that did not help, weekly injections of Imap *(neuroleptic, active ingredient fluspirilene)*. "Then we'll meet once a week, that will help with social integration." It wasn't until later that I learned that Imap is not simply a mild depot neuroleptic. Almost a year had gone by—with completely discouraging results: ever increasing medication, ever decreasing quality of life. In the meantime, my anxiety had become so severe that I could barely leave the house and had to find another doctor because the practice of the previous doctor was more than 50 km away, a distance I could no longer manage. ("If you can't manage it then you will have to be hospitalized!") Furthermore, I had begun to read about psychiatric drugs and had begun to understand the wide variety of side-effects. But I was afraid that I had become dependent and I couldn't simply stop on my own, and anyway, I finally wanted to discover the cause of my problems and to find an effective treatment. So I tried another doctor, somewhat more skeptical this time but still hopeful. The only interest he showed in my story was in the medication I had received ("Hmm, what can I do for you?"). When he noticed that I was critical of the colorful variety of psychiatric drugs, he visibly lost interest. Unsure of myself and indecisive, I agreed to another pharmaceutical attempt: instead of Equilibrin I was now given Anafranil and on top of that Truxal *(neuroleptic, active ingredient chlorprothixene)* and Melleril. When I pointed out that in emergency situations I had found that tranquilizers had helped best, the doctor gave me a lecture ("not with me," "highly dangerous," "addictive" etc.)

Strangely, neither this psychiatrist nor the previous one wanted to know anything about the risks of antidepressants and neuroleptics: "when someone in Greenland has had a problem, then it has to be included in the package insert, that's the rules, but it's all rubbish." But when things still did not get better—in contrast, by now I was spending almost all my days in bed—and I told the doctor, he put me under extreme pressure: I was not suffering from an anxiety state but from a psychosis and: "either you take my (literally!) medication or I will have to send you to the hospital!"

Viewed ironically, this was in fact "a gentle" form of forced treatment which brought me to an unforgettable period in my life. My permanent companion was called Fluanxol, and in no small dosage. Today, I still remember those weeks as the worst of my life: I was only aware of my surroundings as through a veil, leaden tiredness accompanied by an inability to sit still, along with an inexplicable urge to keep moving. This meant that I literally wandered around in confusion and could find no rest. With the last of my strength I decided to stop this treatment. I would rather die in my bed than go through that again.

I managed to get the worst side-effects of Fluanxol more or less under control with the tranquilizers which I still had at home. With the help of some advice, which I had previously read somewhere, I stopped taking my medication: the low-potency neuroleptics immediately and the antidepressants bit by bit. Tranquilizers also initially helped me get over the physical withdrawal symptoms (agitation, outbreaks of sweating, increased anxiety). Precisely those tranquilizers—those dangerous drugs, as my psychiatrist tried to convince me? Not in my experience. In acute emergencies, these can be a blessing: if they are used responsibly and one is aware of the risk of addiction.

Through an acquaintance, who had been dependent on benzodiazepines for years, I knew about this danger and was careful not to take this tranquilizer regularly but only to use it as I needed it. I was lucky: I needed it less and less until it was enough to know that I had it in the house to be able to get through the most difficult situation.

By now I was freed from the strongest psychiatric drugs, but I had still not dealt with the symptoms which had started the whole thing. The doubt still remained, after having had it so continuously drilled into me, that I still needed the medication: what if the psychiatrists were right after all? What would happen next? Fortunately, at this time I got to know a general practitioner who showed no reservations on this score and who was the first doctor who approached my case in an unprejudiced manner and didn't insist on delving too deeply into my life. Unburdened by any traditional medical dogmas and, in particular, without making any claims to infallibility, he took on my case. He spoke frequently—and seriously—of "we" and "our common effort," and most importantly he sensed the pressure I was still under and gave me that most important of things—time. Finally, I had found someone who saw me as an equal partner and who was not trapped in medical or psychiatric patterns of thinking. I immediately had the feeling with him that he saw me as a person and not as a "case."

Together with this doctor I worked out small steps in learning to live again. In particular, the regular house calls (a rarity these days, unfortunately) gave me sense of security and support I needed to be able to take my first steps without medication. Since my body had been under the influence of psychiatric drugs for almost two years, it naturally took some time for everything to fall into place. But without the fear of being forced to take any medication, it was easier to put up with my symptoms. On the other hand, the doctor was also prepared to prescribe me the medication of my choice should I need it and in the dose that I needed. This regained freedom to make my own decisions also gradually freed me from my psychological dependence on the medication, and small successes encouraged me to continue down this route.

I am writing this report today, almost five years later. It was only during the interim period that many things about the start of my symptoms have become clear to me: it was the beginning of one of the many forms of anxiety which have come to affect an estimated ten million Germans today. I probably never suffered from a depression as my first psychiatrist believed. Bit by bit, I started my own behavioral therapy, the form of treatment which at present is still the most effective in dealing with anxiety. Not a two-week crash course, but slowly, step by step I confronted myself with situations I had long avoided. The fears and anxieties have not completely vanished, but much is livable and can be experienced, and the relapses continue to be more seldom. The one bottle of diazepam which I keep at home for security is still there in the cupboard, but untouched.

After I had got over the worst I began in earnest to research psychiatric drugs and psychiatry, a subject which I have not been able to put aside since. Of course my experience is not a universal prescription for withdrawing from psychiatric drugs, but there are two things I consider decisive: to be informed in time about the risks of psychiatric drugs and to have the self-confidence to risk withdrawal despite fears, even if many psychiatrists still maintain that it is too dangerous. Is the prescription of these drugs not itself dangerous? I have personally known many people who have been prescribed psychiatric drugs outside of the clinic and who have then not found the courage to manage without them because they have been persuaded of the opposite. But equally necessary for success are people around you whom they can trust—unfortunately not everyone is lucky enough to have the necessary support during crises. Overall, it appears that it is not just the withdrawal itself which is necessary for success but time and valuable experiences immediately after.

Translation from the German by Christina White

Closing Words

Karl Bach Jensen

Detoxification—in the Large and in the Small
Towards a Culture of Respect

When as a young man I went seriously out of my mind my family and I knew nothing else than the typical psychiatric response: different kinds of neuroleptic drugs in heavy dosages. Now I know psychiatry has nothing relevant to offer me. When I go crazy I stay far away from physicians to avoid any risk of being forced into psychiatric treatment. To defend oneself against psychiatric mistreatment in my country means to get no professional help at all when you go out of your mind.

In the psychiatric user/survivor movement nationally and internationally I have taken part in the fight for the right to drug free care and the right not to risk any treatment against your own will. But I have also felt a need to find and develop alternative knowledge and insight into the part of human life which psychiatry tries to control.

I have come to understand the phenomena which psychiatry deals with from a very different approach: to go out of your mind—whether you irrationally experience voices, visions, paranoia, euphoria, autism, depression or extreme anxiety or fright is a way to survive. Behind so-called mental illness you can discover a readiness of patterns of survival as a diversity built into humanity by nature and evolution. I—like other mental patients and psychiatric survivors—don't suffer from any brain disease, I or we don't carry any wrong genes. I might not be perfect, but I am a human being, my madness has a meaning, and I have the right to live as I am, without running any risk of having my brain and the rest of my body damaged by advanced psychiatric technology.

The psychotic person as a signpost in our culture

A good example of an alternative approach to the phenomena, which psychiatry labels as mental illness, is the Norwegian anthropologist and professor of philosophy—Jens-Ivar Nergård. In his book "Den vuxna barndomen. Den psykotiske personen som vaegvisare i vår kultur" *("The Adult Childhood. The Psychotic Person as a Signpost in Our Culture")* he draws parallels between the psychotic person in our modern culture and the traditional spiritual adviser, the shaman in the Samic or Lappish culture (the Samic or Lappish people are the indigenous population, who used to be reindeer-nomads, living in the northern part of Norway, Sweden, Finland and Russia):

> "The shaman is a person with special qualifications to see or feel what most of his people can't see or feel. So by the other members of the culture the shaman is looked upon as a person with a special gift or capability to get in touch with the 'extraordinary.' (…) He also was a person who could enter his own inner room and through that achieve a deeper contact with the members of his own society." (Nergård 1992, p. 94)

Nergård writes that the pain of a psychotic person in modern cultures comes from experiencing the culture. By isolating him/her the culture gets less and less insight into itself. Valuable knowledge is excluded from the community.

According to Nergård the shaman and the psychotic person are very much alike. But the shaman has an audience. He shares a perspective with his community, willing to listen to his experiences.

> "In our culture the psychotic person is an ill person. Therefore we do not count on any wisdom to get from him or her. Isolation and connected with that the lack of an 'audience' is the destiny of the psychotic person of our culture." (ibid., p. 96)

The condition called psychosis seems to be more a condition in the culture than of the individual person. A chronic state of psychosis reflects the chronic isolation of the psychotic person.

> "While the shaman is a guide in the Samic culture, the psychotic person is a carrier of a life-situation, which first of all in our culture is regarded as meaningless. (…) What makes the psychosis an illness in our culture might—just when it comes to the point—be the total isolation, the lack of an audience." (ibid., p. 97)

In cultures with no systematic forms to isolate or exclude extraordinary psychological phenomena, it seems as though they are not regarded as extraordinary or deviant. The one who in these cultures is different carries a pain, which everyone carries more or less. The pain is minimized when through rituals it is collectivized and becomes a common experience, where everyone recognizes him or her self.

The tragedy of the psychotic person is according to Nergård not that he sacrifices himself and his life, but that he is a part of a culture that doesn't understand, that his psychosis fundamentally should be recognized as an insight-based sacrificial act.

> "If the culture is unable to understand his and others situation like that, more and more people need to be sacrificed. The culture comes to miss it's own inner voice—a vital corrective to itself. In that way the lack of self-insight in the culture creates room for more and more psychotic patients. (…) Our rational culture of science is in lack of rituals and institutionalized patterns for collective acting and understanding, which could give the culture, in common, access to the experiences of the psychotic person. The foremost ritual of our culture consists in locking up the psychotic patient in an institution—and/or medicating him so that the living in the person slowly weakens and dies away." (ibid., pp. 98f.)

Patterns of mental exile as human diversity

It is a question of creative thinking and exploration to discover and imagine which patterns of psychological, emotional, behavioral and spiritual readiness could play a role for our ancestors to survive in conditions very different from modern "civilization."

Which diverse patterns of spiritual awareness, extraordinary perception and skills to communicate with spirits and ancestors meant life or dead for the survival of individuals, families, tribes and people in the childhood of human kind?

Which patterns of mental exile could play a lifesaving role for people living for generations under slave-conditions worse than for animals kept in farms and zoos, or individuals left behind and surviving amongst wild animals?

In the personal history of each individual there are reasons why this or that pattern of psycho-social survival belonging to the diversity of human beings comes into force.

If these patterns means a behavior that conflicts with the social context in which you are expected to function it turns into visible problems, a psycho-social distress which might be interpreted as symptoms of mental illness. Then you easily become an object of psychiatric theory and practice whether you want it or not.

If you accept the psychiatric approach your personal strategy to survive now turns into or is reinforced to something hostile to you, a "wrong" part of you, which has to be treated or from which you have to be cured. But the cure, building on a fundamentally wrong approach very often forces your patterns of survival to break through even stronger. Instead of helping you to leave your mental exile you are pushed to stay in it or even look for a further retreat.

I know this is not the whole story. Some people find that psychiatry helps a lot. But directly or indirectly to coerce other people into a system which obviously worsens their problems is not fair at all.

Against the inner nature of human kind

In my country more or less like in other industrialized countries agriculture has turned against nature. The wild herbs and animals have been defined as enemies against whom almost any kind of war has been legalized. But this war against the wild part of nature now has turned into a war against the human. Poisons spread all over the fields to fight and control the wild biological organisms and artificial fertilizers meant to maximize the profits, now more and more destroy the quality of our drinking water and the nutritional value of the food, which is produced. Consumers are turning against this way of treating the basis of our existence, mother earth and her nature.

If I am right about the nature of so-called mental illness, and I am quite sure that I am, a similar trend will show up against the technology of psychiatry which has turned itself against our inner nature—the "wild" part of humanity.

The answer in agriculture has been to change from fighting nature—from depending on the chemical industry to understand and co-operate. with nature according to organic, ecological principles and knowledge.

Similar to what happened to agriculture when industry and big business took over, the dominant part of psychiatry, more and more dependent on advanced technology, linking itself to industrial and financial giants, has become a serious threat against humanity.

To deal with madness in a proper manner means to discover or, if you do not understand its sense, at least accept the meaning of even the most weird and crazy attitudes. Why did nature develop a pattern to survive like that? Why does this certain individual have to survive by thinking, experiencing, behaving, feeling like he or she does? To discover the meaning of madness means to open your own mind, to create a dialogue with your human fellow and your inner self.

To co-operate with nature also means to be aware of the close connection, the dialectic relation between mind and body. Healthy nutrition means a lot when we try to balance our mind. To deal with strong emotions, to set free your spiritual self, to bring your consciousness from an inner mental exile back to social life you need a solid ground, a healthy body. Psychiatry has been little concerned with the body. Very often the methods that are used destroy the body instead. To cope with madness and to live a natural life means to live without synthetic psychopharmaceutical substances or to withdraw from such toxic drugs.

Alternatives and measures to encourage withdrawal

To disagree with the conventional concept of mental illness and the need for synthetic psychoactive drugs—especially when prescribed for long term daily use or even for life—doesn't mean to close your eyes or to deny the real problems many people experience. My point is not that we shouldn't care at all, that people should be locked up and left alone when they go crazy or out of their mind. A fundamental characteristic of alternative mental health services would be to help people to cope with their problems and to recover by use of mutual learning processes, advocacy, alternative medicine, proper nutrition, natural healing, spiritual practice, etc. (E.g. alternative pharmacy knows about herbs and homeopathic medicine which can help your body and mind to relax and regain it's balance.) There might not be that much profit in these things, but it is the future.

In this field ex-users/survivors can play an important role as staff-members and consultants, having the knowledge about what helped us to recover. Such services linked with a positive subcultural identity and dignity can be provided by the public or with public financial support by the user/survivor movement itself giving people the space to meet and create their own lives.

If people are locked up to save their life or to prevent them from doing serious damage to others, nobody should have the right to force upon us any kind of treatment. As a defense towards involuntary treatment psychiatric wills or advanced directives—describing the kind of treatment a person wants or doesn't want if it comes to involuntary commitment—should be legally adopted by all states and nations.

Alternative systems and decentralized services to meet the needs of people experiencing mental health problems would minimize and in the long run make the use of synthetic and toxic psychiatric drugs needless. Until the final abolition of these drugs a lot of people need help and support to withdraw from the drugs.

An integrated part of building a future ecological and humanistic oriented society system is the renunciation of toxic synthetic substances in the nature, the living area, nutrition and medicine. The renunciation of the deployment of chemical toxins in the psycho-social field could be developed under the following aspects: Raise awareness in the public, amongst professionals and consumers about the inhuman, dangerous and negative cost-benefit outcome of long term administration of synthetic psychiatric drugs.

• Oppose and fight international recommendations and national laws legitimating forced psychiatric treatment, especially legally protected conditions to long-term treatment.

- Collect and spread knowledge about withdrawal problems and how to solve them.
- Develop special services and institutions for people to overcome dependence on psychiatric drugs.
- Ensure that people are informed about risks of injury and dependence when psychiatric drugs are initially prescribed.
- Secure damages for pain and suffering, and compensation for disablement caused by prescribed psychiatric drugs.
- Develop methods, systems, services and institutions for acute, short term and long term help and support not depending on the use of synthetic psychiatric drugs at all.

Translation of Jens-Ivar Nergård's citations from the Swedish by Karl Bach Jensen

Closing Remarks by the Editor

Leading a fulfilling life means living without psychotropic drugs that act on your personality. It is for this reason that many users and survivors of psychiatry eventually decide to withdraw. They thus often come into conflict with those who prescribe psychoactive substances. In most cases, those who prescribe the drugs will dismiss their decision as unsound, they will not be willing to provide information on the effects of withdrawal from psychiatric drugs nor on how to minimize them.

Those who have gone through the process of withdrawal themselves and who have contact with others who have withdrawn are aware of the many factors that can ease the process. Publications that have in the past dealt with the subject of self-determined withdrawal from psychiatric drugs are very rare. In order to avoid the animosity of his colleagues, David Richman, a physician from Berkeley, California, published the first available guide in 1984 under the pseudonym "Dr. Caligari." He wrote:

> "The best way to minimize drug-withdrawal problems is to reduce drug intake gradually. This is especially important if the drug has been taken

for more than one or two months. If you have been taking small doses of psychiatric drugs, or have been taking such drugs for a brief time (i.e., a few days or weeks), then you may wish to try discontinuing 'cold turkey,' that is, just stop taking the drug." (Network 1984, p. 55)

A series of published statements were available in the context of a conference on "Alternatives to Psychiatry" in 1990 in East Berlin, where Marc Rufer spoke about the options available to doctors and therapists in supporting patients who wish to withdraw. He warned listeners about how difficult it is to withdraw despite one's own conviction because of the doubts and fears of others, and because of the hierarchical relationships in medicine and psychotherapy. He recommended the following to his colleagues:

> "As soon as an expert or a professional (or perhaps just a "reasonable person") is sitting across from another person who needs and is looking for help, a differential of power and powerlessness automatically develops. One of them makes the decision, the other must listen, accept and follow it, and must also be thankful. The only one who can really help is someone who refuses to accept such a position of power. Because out of this unequal distribution of power and out of a position of dependence within it, the one seeking help begins to live in the role of the patient who is ill. Out of gratitude, respect, fear—or whatever else—he forgets, that he can make his own decisions and live independently of this expert." (Rufer 1990)

At the same conference, Anna Ochsenknecht, a Berlin healing practitioner, described the natural healing effects of plants and the possibilities for combining their active substances in order to ward off undesired psychological states and to remain free of harmful psychoactive drugs. Three years later in the book "Statt Psychiatrie" *("Instead of Psychiatry")* she addressed in particular the effects of valerian, fenugreek seeds, fennel, oats, hops, jasmin blossoms, St. John's wort, kava-kava, lavender blossoms, marjoram, balm mint, orange blossoms, passion flowers, peppermint leaves, yarrow and whitethorn blossoms. She reported:

> "I do a lot of work with medicinal herbs. They regulate not only physical but also inner balance. This distinguishes them from chemical drugs that

only eliminate or suppress a specific symptom without activating the body's self-regulating forces. They thus also help to relieve or intercept severe withdrawal symptoms when psychiatric drugs are stopped. It is often the fear of withdrawal symptoms (such as sleep disorders, a racing heart beat, nausea, sweats, or inner restlessness, among others) that serves as a reason to continue taking the drugs that cause illness. It is a fear that is further spurred by many psychiatrists.

It is important to undertake a comprehensive search for possible ways of offering support. Not only to ease symptoms, but also to activate regulatory forces and thereby reestablish inner balance. (…)

The medicinal power of plants can be utilized in the form of teas, extracts (alcoholic/liquid or ether oils) or appropriate coated tablets. The prescriptions and tea mixtures I propose are meant as an inspiration to try them out, not as a long-term treatment for all and not according to the motto "a lot helps a lot." (Ochsenknecht 1993, pp. 83f.)

In 1991 Sylvia Caras from Santa Cruz, California published the brochure "Doing without drugs," in which she recorded recommendations from people who reported positive experiences with withdrawal (Caras 1991). And meanwhile, the American psychiatrist Peter Breggin and the psychologist David Cohen published their book "Your Drug May be Your Problem" (Breggin / Cohen 2000) with further tips. All these recommendations in addition to the personal experiences of the editors serve to complement the spectrum of supportive measures suggested by Richman. In summary, the following is recommended:

• Inform yourself about the risks and undesired effects of psychiatric drugs. Anticipate the withdrawal effects that may set in even after weeks:

"Withdrawal from psychiatric drugs can be a very trying experience. You should know that withdrawal can cause moderate to severe discomfort and outright misery at times. Being mentally prepared for this decreases the chance that you will become scared or discouraged. Patience and determination are needed." (Network 1984, pp. 56f.)

• Plan ahead. It may be wise to begin changing your situation (living arrangement, work, or social contacts) or your lifestyle before withdrawing. Consider changing your doctor or psychiatrist if you anticipate that yours may refuse to help support your withdrawal. Switch from injections to tablets or drops that you can dose yourself. Before withdrawing, inform yourself as to the risks of losing your apartment, welfare or other benefits if any of these are dependent upon your willingness to take psychiatric drugs. Look for the right season for change. Think about how long the process might take. Inform those close to you and whom you trust of your undertaking.

In 1985 Josef Schöpf from the University Clinic in Lucerne published an article about dependence on benzodiazepines in which he advised that withdrawal should be planned such that disruptive symptoms do not bring unpleasant social consequences. His advice can be applied to withdrawal from other drugs as well:

> "The choice of when to withdraw should be chosen to insure that a temporary lower level of productivity is compatible with the patient's responsibilities." (Schöpf 1985, p. 591)

- Get advice. Speak with those who have experienced withdrawal. Join a self-help group in which the individuality of each member is respected. Don't heed any sure-fire cures.
- Get legal protection. Contact independent patient spokespersons before you run the risk of being forced back into the psychiatric system. Or protect yourself with a Psychiatric Will (Lehmann 1993; Lehmann / Kempker 1993) before you are committed to a hospital (again). You should ask yourself: What do I need if I become anxious, depressive, suicidal, manic, or crazy? What will help me in that situation? What should I refuse? What will I accept? What am I risking? Who are the people who will support me?
- Create a quiet environment. Keep away from relatives who cannot be burdened. Avoid stress and aggressive places. Don't exhaust yourself in difficult social relationships. Don't answer the phone if telephoning is associated with stress. Go somewhere peaceful, for example to the seaside or the countryside, a meditation center or a church or library.
- Take care to get good nutrition. Eat well—regularly, but not excessively. Roughage, whole wheat foods, salad, fresh vegetables, fresh fruits, lots of liquids. Avoid drinks that make you nervous such as black tea and black

coffee. Avoid drugs such as alcohol, marijuana, cocaine, and other stimulants.

- Get enough exercise: go walking, hiking, jogging, dancing, swimming, cycling, gymnastics, aerobics. "Moderation is a key principle: as you increase your activities, do so gradually." (Network 1984, p. 56)
- Be sure to get enough sleep:

  > "If sleep does not come easily, it is better to rest in bed than to pursue some activity. Some people have found it helpful to drink an herbal tea (valerian and chamomile are good ones) to relax. Others have benefited from yoga and breathing exercises, warm baths and massages before sleep." (ibid.)

- Do something good for yourself. Listen to relaxing music, read pleasant literature. Keep in touch with people. Telephone with friends or visit them.
- Employ measures of affirmation, i.e. reaffirm yourself with effective words and images that make you feel strong and able to carry through with withdrawal.
- Seek out support. Have healing substances on hand to ease withdrawal. Take preparations that strengthen the organs and promote detoxification. Seek the company of people who understand what withdrawal entails. You may want to seek out doctors or therapists who are willing to forget their psychiatric knowledge and instead have understanding, sympathy and discretion.
- Live with awareness. Keep a diary, write things down.

No matter how many tips are on your list, remember: There is no patent recipe for excluding problems when coming off or withdrawing psychiatric drugs: the uniqueness of individuals, their problems and their possibilities mitigates against any hope of a generalized approach. The survey of factors described by the authors in this book as being essential for successfully withdrawing illustrates the diversity of strategies and needs.

If any problems are looming, the reduction of doses by degrees is the best way to decrease withdrawal risks. This is especially important if a psychiatric drug has been taken for more than one or two months. Optimally, all the necessary factors for successful withdrawal would be present simultaneously: a

responsible attitude, a pace of coming off which matches the dose and duration of drug treatment, supportive environments, appropriate assistance,
qualified specialists and a supporting self-help group.

As a rule you can assume that the circumstances while coming off are the
opposite of optimal. In the worst cases there is no other possibility than to
help oneself get out of the jungle of psychopharmacologic addiction. Ulrich
Lindner was taught by his brother who has experiences of withdrawal: "You
have to pull you yourself out of the swamp by the hair of your head—just like
Munchhausen." Gerda Wozart encourages:

> "We are on our own, called upon to live in a responsible way. We are not
> only sentenced by others, muzzled by others. We always have more forc-
> es (and self-helping forces, too) available than we might have thought in
> dark days."

Some authors argue that as a condition for success it is important to see
through the incompetence and the low probability of effective help from
medics prescribing psychiatric drugs, to give up illusions about their help and
to separate oneself from the doctor or psychiatrist as well as from an understanding of life-problems as illness. "I sacrificed twenty-one valuable years of
my life hoping pointlessly for an improvement or a cure," says Bert Gölden
and summarizes: "recognize your suffering and be your own therapist—help
yourself."

To make coming off successful in the long term, it is generally necessary to
refuse adjustment to unpleasant situations; this can mean leaving a burdensome environment as well as quitting an unsuitable relationship. Getting crazy is a signal showing the necessity of a change, says Maths Jesperson: "Madness is no illness to be cured. My madness came to call up a new life for me."

Those who learn to take feelings seriously, to follow their own intuition
and to take notice of and to react to warning signals of a developing crisis escape the danger to get psychiatric drugs prescribed for a second time. Thus
developing a calm response to burdensome circumstances in life, patience,
courage and determination and the understanding that harm and hurt are inherent to life was helpful for some authors. Now they admit their mistakes
and accept relapses without despairing immediately.

The authors have learned to live through fearful situations and to reduce deep-seated anxieties. Wilma Boevink reports:

> "During the years I developed the courage to face what I tried to cover with all my dependencies. I fought the monsters of my past, and to be able to do this, first I had to admit them and look into their eyes. (…) You have to find the courage to confess to yourself how things went so far."

The sooner (ex-)users and survivors of psychiatry developed understanding of the connection between violence or abuse and their difficulties, understood mad and troubling symptoms and reacted in alternative ways to crises, the easier it was for them to break off emotional involvement from life problems and deal with them. The hunt that is started after the end of an acute phase—madness or depression—has a preventing character, as Regina Bellion says: "Whoever gets to the bottom of his psychotic experiences afterwards obviously does not run into the next psychotic phase all too soon."

Some authors regard it as a fundamental condition to notice their own (co-)responsibility for their lives, their problem-burdened past and their responsibility for their future. Carola Bock says self-critically:

> "Today I know that I am partly to blame for the states of crisis because I acted wrong and was no angel at all. I often tried to solve my problems in a wrong way, too top-heavy, and I had not collected enough experience of life either."

The necessity to take care of healthy and regular sleeping habits is said to be a key component self-responsibility for some authors. First of all, a sensible and fulfilling occupation—a paid job or a leisure activity (especially writing)—as well as love and friendship add to the positive outlook on life which makes it much easier to come off psychiatric drugs. Not to lose the ground in argument, but to defend oneself and to be able to talk about delicate things is decisive, too. Friendships prove their value if the contact is continued during a crisis.

As long as they make an open non-invasive interchange of personal problems possible, self-help groups are as useful as friendship. Moreover, self-help groups build the scope for mutual advice and for the spread of information about possible damage caused by psychiatric drugs and problems with coming off, as Nada Rath reports:

> "Most important were the conversations with (ex-)users and survivors of psychiatry who had comparable experiences and a similar attitude towards the world."

For Una Parker co-counseling means the end of the danger of psychiatric drugs and electroshocks again:

> "It has made a very great difference to me, and I think that the support I have had from regular co-counseling sessions not only kept me out of the psychiatric system but also helped me be much more effective in my life."

Homeopathic decontamination, alleviation of withdrawal problems with naturopathic remedies (e.g. St. John's wort, valerian), body- and psychotherapy, conversations in groups or alone, sports, meditation, praying, and much more can additionally help with reducing problems of coming off and withdrawing.

Professional helpers note their human presence and their availability in the critical moments of coming off as a prerequisite for effective support. But the (ex-)users and survivors of psychiatry have to do their share in overcoming the problems that can appear when coming off, too. Constanze Meyer, psychologist and psychotherapist, knows that this is not always easy:

> "These solutions have in common that they normally need much time and an active confrontation with the own situation and the own attitudes and patterns of behavior."

The more afraid the (ex-)users and survivors of psychiatry are when coming off, the more important becomes the relationship based on trust with the professional helper and that, "the patient knows that he/she can rely on the therapist if there is any trouble" (healing practitioner Klaus John). His colleague Elke Laskowski indicates the interplay between specialist and human offerings: "Of course, conversation and offering the patient the opportunity to call at any time have an incomparable therapeutic effect."

Existing anxieties should be relativized and in that way reduced by accurate specialist information about risks of psychiatric drugs and coming off them. It is not very surprising that practices used during the withdrawal process, like acupuncture, are often recognized in reports of authors who have experiences with psychiatric drugs. Other measures, for example a complete change of diet or an considered use of other drugs, are, because of the frequent problems with getting on well without psychiatric drugs, surely worth trying by people who want to come off.

The experiences of the Berlin Runaway-House, as reported by Kerstin Kempker in her contribution, show how important and how successful intensively guided withdrawal is. Community, support, experienced staff (if possible with their own experience of withdrawal) and responsible doctors when they are needed—these are the conditions sought by (ex-)users and survivors of psychiatry who have long taken psychiatric drugs and want to quit. But centers offering help, and if necessary a place to live and 24-hour care, are very rare, not only in Germany.

(Ex-)users and survivors of psychiatry first experience that instead of receiving appropriate help for their psycho-social problems when they first develop, they are only offered psychiatric drugs. This experience of being denied appropriate help is repeated when they search for help in withdrawing from the drugs.

The current developments in the politics of psychiatry have shown no improvement; to the contrary, the lobbying of organized associations of relatives who are sponsored by the pharmaceutical industry has only led to the further consolidation of psychiatry into a coerced outpatient business.

Afterthoughts

As the editor of this book, I was struck by what seems to be an esoteric orientation among many of the contributing authors. For outsiders, this may seem strange, irrational and suspicious. The Munich psychologist Colin Goldner, for example, has warned of a number of charlatans and non-conventional forms of spiritual healing that in fact create and/or aggravate psychological problems and are often based on a very crude ideology (Goldner 2000). This book also addresses some unconventional forms of help for people wishing to withdraw from psychiatric drugs. It would be rather cheap and easy to discount the effectiveness of these alternative methods by labeling them mere placebo effects or figments of the imagination, while at the same time claiming that the risk of harm or dependency from such treatments is a lesser evil (compared, for example, to the toxicity of psychiatric drugs). It is not only my sense of fairness toward "my authors" that prevents me from doing this. I myself had quite a peculiar experience with unconventional methods in the early 1980s when I attended a reasonably costly weekend retreat organized by a Native American from Arizona. Given the mix of elements from Gestalt therapy to various kinds of unexplained, wondrous and hardly translatable methods offered there, it would be easy to denounce this kind of therapy as "humbug" if it weren't for the fact that it was a very positive experience for me. The insights I gained from the Native American's seminar had a lasting impact that influenced the course of my life. My own right to define what is good for me and what is not is a right that must be granted all the contributing authors of this book. (After all, it is the reader who must ultimately decide how useful any one of these contributions are in helping them find their own method for withdrawing from psychiatric drugs.)

Without a doubt it is important to keep an eye not only on therapists, doctors and in particular psychiatrists, but also on all those who are involved in the recent psycho-boom and particularly those who—not unlike the psychiatrists who prescribe drugs— charge too much for false claims to infallibly cure psychological and social problems. It should not be forgotten that psychotherapy or psychoanalysis may also be abused and/or create situations of dependency—as the book "Therapieschäden—Risiken und Nebenwirkungen von Psychotherapie" *("The Harms of Therapy—Risks and Side-Effects of Psychotherapy,"* 2002) by psychologists Michael Märtens and Hilarion Petzold have impressively demonstrated). Nor is the self-help sector free of people who wish to profit at the cost of those who are earnestly seeking help. In his contribution to this book, David Webb takes a critical look at the dark side of self-help groups.

"During times of struggle, one of the most annoying things was all those people who believe that what had worked for them could also work for me. The path to peace and freedom is unique for each individual and very personal."

Beyond health, nothing is more valuable than freedom and independence.

I would like to express my respect for and appreciation of the authors who have offered to tell their very personal stories of how they were able to withdraw from psychiatric drugs without winding up under the care of a doctor or in a clinic again, and how they were able to lead a life free of psychiatric drugs despite the diagnoses of doctors and psychiatrists. My respect and appreciation also extends to the professionals who help and support those who wish to stop taking psychiatric drugs. It is not always easy to help someone through this process, and they do so against the rules of their profession and thus often in renunciation of a life of relative comfort and leisure that would otherwise await them.

Translation from the German by Christina White

Appendix

Psychiatric Drugs' Active Ingredients and Trade Names

This table includes trade names and active ingredients of neuroleptics, antidepressants, tranquilizers and lithium preparations marketed in Australia, Canada, Great Britain, New Zealand and the USA at the time of its publication in 2003. It also lists carbamazepine and other substances chemically familiar with this antiepileptic drug. These substances, administered in the psychosocial field as so-called mood-stabilizers, are also able to provoke withdrawal problems.

The space in this book is far too limited to show every international trade name for the psychotropic active ingredients. These names are available on one of the web sites of Peter Lehmann Publishing, see

www.p.lehmann.berlinet.de/psychodrugs.htm

As far as the psychiatric drugs mentioned in this book, the reader may trust in the care given by the editor in making correct statements. On the other hand, there is a lot of confusion world wide referring to the classification of psychiatric drugs.

- No standard criteria exist for the assignment of a single psychiatric drug to a group of substances. For example, loxapine is classified in the USA as a (minor) tranquilizer, in Canada and Great Britain as a neuroleptic. Oxypertine is marketed in the USA as an antidepressant, in Great Britain as a neuroleptic, Flupent(h)ixol is marketed in Great Britain as a neuroleptic and antidepressant. Some drugs like tiapride are classified as a neuroleptic in one country and as an anti-Parkinson in another. Sometimes anti-Parkinson drugs like amantadine are indicated in the treatment of drug-caused parkinsonism in one country (USA), but in another country (GB) drug-induced symptoms are an excluded indication. Similarly, hydroxyzine is considered a tranquilizer in one country and an antihistamine in another. And sometimes a drug's status as a tranquilizer or neuroleptic is based on the dosages given.

- The classification of a drug can depend on its pharmaceutical basic schedule, biochemical mechanism, produced effects or the administrator's subjective intention. Some trade names are used differently in individual countries.
- In pharmaceutical lists you can find a lot of orthographical deviations. Active ingredients are written differently and often there are several indications for one ingredient. These variations must be considered when consulting this table.

Therefore no responsibility is accepted for the accuracy of this table of psychiatric drugs.

Active ingredient   Trade names

NEUROLEPTICS

Active ingredient	Trade names
alimemazine	Vallergan
amisulpride	Solian
aripiprazole	Abilify
benperidol	Benquil
chlorpromazine	Chloractil, Chlorpromazine, Largactil, Thorazine
clozapine	Clopine, Clozapine, Clozaril
dapiprazole	Rev-Eyes
deserpidine	component of Enduronyl, Oreticyl
droperidol	Droleptan, Inapsine; component of Innovar
flupent(h)ixol	Depixol, Fluanxol
fluphenazine	Anatensol, Fluphenazine, Modecate, Moditen, Permitil, Prolixin
haloperidol	Dozic, Haldol, Haloperidol, Peridol, Serenace
levomepromazine	see methotrimeprazine

loxapine	Daxolin, Loxapac, Loxapine, Loxitane
mesoridazine	Serentil
methotrimeprazine	Levoprome, Nozinan
molindone	Moban
olanzapine	Zyprexa
oxypertine	Forit, Oxypertine
pericyazine	Neulactil
perphenazine	Fentazin, Perphenazine, Trilafon; component of Etrafon, Triavil
pimozide	Orap
pipotiazine	Piportil
prochlorperazine	Antinaus, Buccastem, Compazine, Prochlorperazine, Stemetil, Stemzine
promazine	Promazine, Sparine
promethazine	Anergan, Avomine, Insomn-Eze, Pentazine, Phenergan, Promethazine; component of Mepergan, Phenergan VC
quetiapine	Seroquel
reserpine	Arcum R-S, Broserpine, De Serpa, Elserpine, Novoresperine, Raurine, Reserfia, Reserpaneed, Serpalan, Serpasil, Serpazide, Sertabs, T-Serp, Zepine; component of Demi-Regroton, Diupres, Diurese-R, Diutensen, Harbolin, Hydromox, Hydropine, Hydropres, Hydroserp, Hydroserpine, Hydrosine, Hydrotensin, Mallopres, Metatensin, Naquival, Regroton, Renese-R, Salutensin, Ser-A-Gen, Ser-Ap-Es, Serathide, Serpazide, Unipres, Tri-Hydroserpine
risperidone	Risperdal, Risperidone
sertindole	Serdolect
sulpiride	Dolmatil, Dogmatyl, Sulpiride, Sulpitil, Sulpor
tetrabenazine	Tetrabenazine, Xenazine
thioridazine	Aldazine, Mellaril, Melleril, Rideril, Thioridazine
tiotixene	Navane, Thiothixene, Thixit
trifluoperazine	Stelazine, Suprazine, Trifluoper, Trifluoperazine
triflupromazine	Vesprin
ziprasidone	Geodon, Zeldox
zotepine	Zoleptil
zuclopenthixol	Clopixol

MOOD STABILIZERS

carbamazepine	Atretol, Carbamazepine, Carbatrol, Epitol, Tegretol, Teril, Timonil
divalproex	see valproate
lithium	Camcolit, Camcolith, Cibalith, Eskalith, Li-Liquid, Liskonum, Lithicarb, Lithium, Lithobid, Lithonathe, Lithotabs, Priadel, Quilonum
oxcarbazepine	Trileptal
valproate	Convulex, Depacon, Depakene, Depakote, Epilim, Sodium Valproate, Valpro, Valproic Acid

ANTIDEPRESSANTS

amfebutamone	see bupropion
amitriptyline	Amitrip, Amitriptyline, Elavil, Emitrip, Endep, Enovil, Lentizol, Serotex, Triptafen, Tryptanol, Tryptizol; component of Etrafon, Limbitrol, Triavil
amoxapine	Amoxapine, Asenden, Asendin, Asendis
bupropion	Amfebutamone, Bupropion, Wellbutrin, Zyban
citalopram	Apertia, Celepram, Celexa, Cipram, Cipramil, Citalopram, Elopram, Lupram, Prisdal, Sepram, Seropram, Talohexal
clomipramine	Anafranil, Clobram, Clomipramine, Clopress, Placil
desipramine	Desipramine, Norpramin, Pertofran, Pertofrane
dosulepin	see dothiepin
dothiepin	Dopress, Dosulepin/Dothiepin, Dothapax, Dothep, Prothiaden
doxepin	Adapin, Anten, Deptran, Doxepin, Sinequan; component of Prudoxin Cream, Zonalon Cream Cream
escitalopram	Lexapro
fluoxetine	Auscap, Deprax, Eufor, Felicium, Fluohexal, Fluox, Fluoxetine, Lovan, Oxactin, Prozac, Psyquial, Sarafem, Veritina, Zactin
flupent(h)ixol	see chapter "Neuroleptics"
fluphenazine	see chapter "Neuroleptics"
fluvoxamine	Faverin, Fevarin, Fluvoxamine, Luvox
imipramine	Imipramine, Melipramine, Tofranil
isocarboxazid	Isocarboxazid, Marplan
lofepramine	Feprapax, Gamanil, Lofepramine, Lomont
maprotiline	Ludiomil, Maprotiline

mianserin	Mianserin, Tolvon
mirtazapine	Avanza, Mirtazon, Remeron, Zispin
moclobemide	Arima, Aurorix, Clobemix, Manerix, Maosig, Moclobemide, Mohexal
nefazodone	Dutonin, Nefadar, Serzone
nortriptyline	Allegron, Aventyl, Motipress, Motival, Norpress, Nortrilen, Nortriptyline, Pamelor
oxypertine	see chapter "Neuroleptics"
paroxetine	Aropax, Aroxat, Oxetine, Paroxetine, Paxil, Paxtine, Seroxat
phenelzine	Nardil, Phenelzine
protriptyline	Concordin, Vivactil
reboxetine	Edronax, Vestral
sertraline	Altruline, Lustral, Sercerin, Tolrest, Zoloft
thiethylperazine	Norzine, Torecan
tranylcypromine	Parnate
trazodone	Desyrel, Molipaxin, Trazodone
trimipramine	Surmontil, Tripress
tryptophan	Optimax, Tryptophan
venlafaxine	Dobupal, Efexor, Effexor

TRANQUILIZERS

alprazolam	Alprax, Alprazolam, Helix, Kalma, Xanax
bromazepam	Lectopam, Lexotan
buspirone	Biron, Buspar, Buspirone
chlordiazepoxide	Chlordiazepoxide, Librelease, Libritabs, Librium, Nova-Pam, Sereen, Tropium; component of Clindex, Clinoxide, Clipoxide, Librax, Lidox, Lidoxide, Limbitrol, Menrium
clobazam	Clobazam, Frisium
clonazepam	Clonazepam, Klonopin, Paxam, Rivotril
clorazepate dipotassium	Clorazepate Dipotassium, Gen-Xene, Tranxene, Tranxilene
diazepam	Antenex, Dialar, Diazemuls, Diazepam, Ducene, Pro-Pam, Rimapam, Stesolid, Tensium, Valclair, Valium, Valpam, Valrelease, Vazepam
estazolam	Estalozam, ProSom
flunitrazepam	Hypnodorm, Rohypnol

flurazepam	Dalmane, Durapam, Flurazepam
halazepam	Paxipam
hydroxyzine	Anxanil, Apo-Hydroxyzine, Atarax, Hydroxyzine, Hy-Pam, Hyzine-50, Ucerax, Vistaril
loprazolam	Dormonoct
lorazepam	Alzapam, Ativan, Lorapam, Lorazepam, Temesta
lormetazepam	Noctamid, Lormetazepam
loxapine	see chapter "Neuroleptics"
meprobamate	Equanil, Meprobamate, Meprospan, Miltown; component of Equagesic, Meprogese, Meprogesic, Micrainin, Milprem, PMB-200, PMB-400, Q-Gesic
midazolam	Hypnovel, Midazolam, Rocam, Versed
nitrazepam	Alodorm, Insoma, Mogadon, Nitrados, Somnite
oxazepam	Alepam, Murelax, Oxazepam, Ox-Pam, Serax, Serepax
prazepam	Centrax
quazepam	Doral
temazepam	Euhypnos, Nocturne, Normison, Razepam, Restoril, Somapam, Temaz, Temaze, Temazepam, Temtabs
triazolam	Halcion, Triazolam
zaleplon	Sonata, Zaleplon
zolpidem	Ambien, Stilnoct, Stilnox, Zolpidem
zopiclone	Imovane, Zileze, Zimovane, Zopiclone, Zo-Tab

ANTI-PARKINSON DRUGS (administered to conceal neuroleptic-induced muscle disorders)

amantadine	Amantadine, Symadine, Symmetrel
benz(a)tropine	Benztropine, Cogentin
biperiden	Akineton
orphenadrine	Banflex, Biorphen, Disipal, Marflex, Noradex, Norflex, Orphenadrine; component of Norgesic, Orphengesic
procyclidine	Arpicolin, Kemadrin, Mucinil, Procyclidine
tetrabenazine	see chapter "Neuroleptics"
trihexyphenidyl	Artane, Broflex, Pipanol, Trihexane, Trihexy, Trihexyphenidyl, Trihexyphenidyl/Benzhexol

Sources

Albrecht, Harro: "Null Wirkstoff—grosse Wirkung," in: Sonntagszeitung (Zurich) from November 30, 1997, pp. 99 –101

American Psychiatric Association: "Diagnostic and Statistical Manual of Mental Disorders DSM-IV-TR," 4. edit., text revision, Washington 2000

Andrews, P. / Hall, J. N. / Snaith, R. P.: "A controlled trial of phenothiazine withdrawal in chronic schizophrenic patients," in: British Journal of Psychiatry, Vol. 128 (1976), pp. 451–455

Arieti, Silvano: "Understanding and Helping the Schizophrenic: a Guide for Family and Friends," New York 1979

Ashton, Heather: "Benzodiazepine outcome in 50 patients," in: British Journal of Addiction, Vol. 82 (1987), pp. 665–671

Ashton, Heather: "The treatment of benzodiazepine dependence," in: Addiction, Vol. 89 (1994), pp. 1535–1541

Barnes, Mary / Berke, Joseph: "Two Accounts of a Fourney through Madness," New York 2002

Benkert, Otto: "Psychopharmaka," Munich 1995

Benkert, Otto / Hippius, Hanns: "Psychiatrische Pharmakotherapie," 3. edit., Berlin / Heidelberg / New York 1980

Bish, Alison / Golombok, Susan: "The role of coping strategies in protecting individuals against long-term tranquilizer use," in: British Journal of Medical Psychology, Vol. 69 (1996), pp. 101–115

Borison, Richard L. et al.: "Clozapine withdrawal rebound psychosis," in: Psychopharmacology Bulletin, Vol. 24 (1988), pp. 260–263

Boyesen, Gerda: "Über den Körper die Seele heilen. Biodynamische Psychologie und Psychotherapie," Munich 1987

Boyesen, Gerda: "Von der Lust am Heilen," Munich 1995

Bragdon, Emma: "The Call of Spiritual Emergency: from Personal Crisis to Personal Transformation," New York 1990

Boyesen, Gerda / Boyesen, Mona Lisa: "Biodynamik des Lebens. Grundlagen der Biodynamischen Psychologie," Essen 1987

Breggin, Peter R.: "Psychiatric Drugs: Hazards to the Brain," New York 1983

Breggin, Peter R.: "Toxic Psychiatry," New York 1991

Breggin, Peter R. / Cohen, David: "Your Drug may be your Problem," Cambridge 2000

Brooks, George W.: "Withdrawal from neuroleptic drugs," in: American Journal of Psychiatry, Vol. 115 (1959), pp. 931–932

Burgerstein, Lothar: "Burgersteins Handbuch der Nährstoffe," 10., revised and expanded edit., Heidelberg 2002

Calatin, Anne (ed.): "Ernährung und Psyche. Erkenntnisse der klinischen Ökologie und der orthomolekularen Psychiatrie," 6. edit., Heidelberg 1995

Caras, Sylvia: "Doing without Drugs," Santa Cruz 1991

Carpenter, William T. / Tamminga, Carol A.: "Why neuroleptical withdrawal in schizophrenia?," in: Archives of General Psychiatry, Vol. 52 (1995), pp. 192–193

Charney, Dennis S. et al.: "Abrupt discontinuation of tricyclic antidepressant drugs," in: British Journal of Psychiatry, Vol. 141 (1982), pp. 377–386

Chouinard, Guy / Jones, Barry D.: "Neuroleptic-induced supersensitivity psychosis," in: American Journal of Psychiatry, Vol. 137 (1980), pp. 16–21

Chouinard, Guy / Jones, Barry D.: "Neuroleptic-induced supersensitivity psychosis, the 'Hump Course,' and tardive dyskinesia," in: Journal of Clinical Psychopharmacology, Vol. 2 (1982), pp. 143–144

Chouinard, Guy et al.: "Factors related to tardive dyskinesia," in: American Journal of Psychiatry, Vol. 136 (1979), pp. 79–83

Chouinard, Guy et al.: "Withdrawal symptoms after long-term treatment with low-potency neuroleptics," in: Journal of Clinical Psychiatry, Vol. 45 (1984), pp. 500–502

Cook, Brian L. et al.: "Unipolar depression in the elderly: reoccurrence on discontinuation of tricyclic antidepressants," in: Journal of Affective Disorders, Vol. 10 (1986), pp. 91–94

Cooperstock, R.: "Women and psychotropic drug use," in: A. MacLennan (ed.): "Women, their Use of Alcohol and Other Legal Drugs," Toronto 1976

Crouch, G. / Robson, M. / Hallstrom, C.: "Benzodiazepine dependent patients and their psychological treatment," in: Progress in Neuropsychopharmacology and Biological Psychiatry, Vol. 12 (1988), pp. 503–510

Curran, Valerie / Golombok, Susan: "Bottling it up," London 1985

Degkwitz, Rudolf / Luxenburger, Otto: "Das terminale extrapyramidale Insuf-fizienz- bzw. Defektsyndrom infolge chronischer Anwendung von Neurolepticis," in: Nervenarzt, Vol. 36 (1965), pp. 173–175

Degkwitz, Rudolf: "Leitfaden der Psychopharmakologie," Stuttgart 1967

Demers-Desrosiers, L. A. / Nestoros, J. N. / Vaillancourt, P.: "Acute psychosis precipitated by withdrawal of anticonvulsant medication," in: American Journal of Psychiatry, Vol. 135 (1978), pp. 981–982

Dieterich, Michael: "Wir brauchen Entspannung," 6. edit., Gießen 1997

Dietl, Hans / Ohlenschläger, Gerhard: "Handbuch der Orthomolekularen Medizin," 2., corrected edit., Heidelberg 1998

Dilsaver, Steven C. / Greden, John F.: "Antidepressant withdrawal phenomena," in: Biological Psychiatry, Vol. 19 (1984), pp. 237–256

Dörner, Klaus / Plog, Ursula: "Irren ist menschlich," Rehburg-Loccum 1978

Duncan, John S. / Shorvon, Simon D. / Trimble, Michael R.: "Withdrawal symptoms from phenytoin, carbamazepine and sodium valproate," in: Journal of Neurology, Neurosurgery and Psychiatry, Vol. 51 (1988), pp. 924–928

Ekblom, B. / Eriksson, K. / Lindstroem, L. H.: "Supersensitivity psychosis in schizophrenic patients after sudden clozapine withdrawal," in: Psychopharmacology, Vol. 83 (1984), pp. 293–294

Epstein, Leon J. / Morgan, Richard D. / Reynolds, Lynn: "An approach to the effect of ataraxic drugs on hospital release rates," in: American Journal of Psychiatry, Vol. 119 (1962), pp. 36–47

Ernst, Klaus: "Psychopathologische Wirkungen des Phenothiazinderivates 'Largactil' (= 'Megaphen') im Selbstversuch und bei Kranken," in: Archiv für Psychiatrie und

Nervenkrankheiten, Vol. 192 (1954), pp. 573–590

Faedda, Gianni L. et al.: "Outcome after rapid vs gradual discontinuation of lithium treatment in bipolar disorders," in: Archives of General Psychiatry, Vol. 50 (1993), pp. 448–455

Faust, Volker: "Medikament und Psyche," Vol. 1: "Neuroleptics—Antidepressants—Beruhigungsmittel—Lithiumsalze," Stuttgart 1995

Fisch, Hans-Ulrich: "Die Wirkung von Neuroleptics auf das Erleben der Zeit," in: Luc Ciompi (ed.): "Zeit und Psychiatrie," Berne 1990, pp. 155–157

Fisher, Seymour / Greenberg, Roger P.: "How sound is the double-blind design for evaluating psychotropic drugs?" in: Journal of Nervous and Mental Disease, Vol. 181 (1993), pp. 345–350

Gadsby, Joan E.: "Addiction by Prescription: One Woman's Triumph and Fight for Change," Toronto 2000

Gardos, George / Cole, Jonathan O.: "Maintenance antipsychotic therapy: is the cure worse than the disease," in: American Journal of Psychiatry, Vol. 133 (1976), pp. 32–36

Gilbert, Patricia et al.: "Neuroleptic withdrawal in schizophrenic patients: a review of the literature," in: Archives of General Psychiatry, Vol. 52 (1995), pp. 173–188

Glaeske, Gerd: "Psychotrope und andere Arzneimittel mit Mißbrauchs- und Abhängigkeitspotential," in: Deutsche Hauptstelle gegen die Suchtgefahren (ed.): "Jahrbuch Sucht '98," Hamm 1997, pp. 43–66

Glick, Burton / Margolis, Reuben: "A study of the influence of experimental design on clinical outcome in drug research," in: American Journal of Psychiatry, Vol. 118 (1962), pp. 1087–1096

Goldberg, Solomon C. / Klerman, Gerald L. / Cole, Jonathan O.: "Changes in schizophrenic psychopathology and ward behaviour as a function of phenothiazine treatment," in: British Journal of Psychiatry, Vol. 111 (1965), pp. 120–133

Goldner, Colin: "Die Psycho-Szene," Aschaffenburg 2000

Golombok, Susan et al.: "A follow-up study of patients treated for benzodiazepine dependence," in: British Journal of Medical Psychology, Vol. 60 (1987), pp. 141–149

Green, Hannah: "I Never Promised you a Rose Garden," New York 1964

Greenberg, Roger P. / Fisher, Seymour: "Examining antidepressant effectiveness: findings, ambiguities, and some vexing puzzles," in: Seymour Fisher / Roger P. Greenberg (eds.): "The Limits of Biological Treatments for Psychological Distress," Hillsdale / Hove / London 1989, pp. 1–37

Greil, Waldemar / Schmidt, Stephan: "Absetzsyndrome bei Antidepressiva, Neuroleptika und Lithium," in: Hanfried Helmchen / Hanns Hippius (eds.): "Psychiatrie für die Praxis," Vol. 9, Munich 1989, pp. 272–281

Greil, Waldemar / Schmidt, Stephan: "Absetzsyndrome bei Antidepressiva, Neuroleptika und Lithium," in: Münchener Medizinische Wochenschrift, Vol. 130 (1988), pp. 704–707

Grof, Christina: "The Thirst for Wholeness. Attachment, Addiction, and the Spiritual Path," New York 1993

Grof, Stanislav: "The Adventure of Self-Discovery," Albany 1988

Grof, Stanislav / Bennett, Hal Zina: "The Holotropic Mind: the Three Levels of Human Consciousness and how They Shape Our Lives," San Francisco 1992

Grof, Stanislav / Grof, Christina: "Spiritual Emergency: when Personal Transformation Becomes a Crisis," Los Angeles 1989

Grof, Stanislav / Grof, Christina: "The Stormy Search for the Self: a Guide to Personal Qrowth through Transformational Crisis," Los Angeles 1992

Grohmann, Renate / Rüther, E ckart / Schmidt, Lutz G. (eds.): "Unerwünschte Wirkungen von Psychopharmaka," Heidelberg etc. 1994

Haley, Jay: "The effect of long-term outcome studies on the therapy of schizophrenia," in: Journal of Marital and Family Therapy, Vol. 15 (1989), pp. 127–132

Harding, Courtenay M. / Zubin, Joseph / Strauss, John S.: "Chronicity in schizophrenia: fact, partial fact or artefact," in: Hospital and Community Psychiatry, Vol. 38 (1987), pp. 477– 484

Hartlage, Lawrence C.: "Effects of chlorpromazine on learning," in: Psychological Bulletin, Vol. 64 (1965), pp. 235 –245

Hautzinger, M. / Janssen, P. L.: "Das chronische Schmerzsyndrom," in: Psychotherapeut, Vol. 39 (1994), pp. 177–194

Heinrichs, Douglas W. / Carpenter, William T.: "Experience with a drug-free month in schizophrenic outpatients," in: Psychopharmacology Bulletin, Vol. 21 (1985), pp. 117–119

Helmchen, Hanfried: Diskussionsbemerkung, in: Hanns Hippius / Helmfried E. Klein (eds.): "Therapie mit Neuroleptics," Erlangen 1983, p. 171

Hofmann, G. / Kryspin-Exner, Kornelius: "Klinische Erfahrungen mit einem neuen Neuroleptikum (TP 21, Melleril)," in: Wiener Medizinische Wochenschrift, Vol. 110 (1960), pp. 897– 901

Hogarty, Gerard E. / Goldberg, Solomon C. / Baltimore Collaborative Study Group: "Drug and sociotherapy

in the aftercare of schizophrenic patients," in: Archives of General Psychiatry, Vol. 31 (1974), pp. 609–618

Hüllinghorst, Rolf: "Zur Versorgung Suchtkranker in Deutschland," in: Deutsche Hauptstelle gegen die Suchtgefahren (ed.): "Jahrbuch Sucht '98," Hamm 1997, pp. 123–141

Hunt, Neil / Bruce-Jones, William / Silverstone, Trevor: "Life events and relapse in bipolar affective disorder," in: Journal of Affective Disorders, Vol. 25 (1992), pp. 13–20

Huxley, Aldous: "Brave New World," New York 2000

Irle, Gerhard: "Depressionen," Stuttgart 1974

Jamison, Kay: "An Unquiet Mind," New York 1995

Jesperson, Maths: "Was hilft mir, wenn ich verrückt werde?," in: Kerstin Kempker / Peter Lehmann (eds.): "Statt Psychiatrie," Berlin 1993, pp. 38–40

Kändler, S. H. / Volk, S. / Pflug, B.: "Benzodiazepinentzug mit Carbamazepin," in: Nervenarzt, Vol. 67 (1996), pp. 381– 386

Karon, Bertram P.: "Psychotherapy versus medication for schizophrenia," in: Seymour Fisher / Roger P. Greenberg (eds.): "The Limits of Biological Treatments for Psychological Distress," Hillsdale / Hove / London 1989, pp. 105–150

King, J. R. / Hullin, R. P.: "Withdrawal symptoms from lithium," in: British Journal of Psychiatry, Vol. 143 (1983), pp. 30–35

Kirsch, Irving / Sapirstein, Guy: "Listening to Prozac but hearing placebo: a meta-analysis of antidepressant medication," in: Prevention & Treatment, Vol. 1 (1998), article 0002a

Klein, Ehud et al.: "Alprazolam withdrawal in patients with panic disorder and generalized anxiety disorder," in:

American Journal of Psychiatry, Vol. 151 (1994), pp. 1760–1766

Klein, Ehud et al.: "Discontinuation of lithium treatment in remitted bipolar patients: relationship between clinical outcome and changes in sleep-wake cycles," in: Journal of Nervous and Mental Disease, Vol. 179 (1991), pp. 499–501

Konz, Franz: "Der große Gesundheits-Konz. UrMedizin. Besiegt Krebs, Rheuma, Fettsucht, Allergie und chronische Leiden... und hält immer fit, schlank und gesund," revised edit., Munich 1995

Krämer, Dietmar / Wild, Helmut: "Neue Therapien mit Bach-Blüten 1–3," Interlaken 1989

Kuhn, Roland: "Probleme der praktischen Durchführung der Tofranil-Behandlung," in: Wiener Medizinische Wochenschrift, Vol. 110 (1960), pp. 245–250

Kuschinsky, Gustav / Lüllmann, Heinz / Mohr, Klaus: "Kurzes Lehrbuch der Pharmakologie und Toxikologie," Stuttgart / New York 1993

Lapierre, Y. D. / Gagnon, A. / Kokkinidis, L.: "Rapid recurrence of mania following lithium withdrawal," in: Biological Psychiatry, Vol. 15 (1980), pp. 859–864

Larcoursiere, Roy B. / Spohn, Herbert E. / Thompson, Karen: "Medical effects of abrupt neuroleptic withdrawal," in: Comprehensive Psychiatry, Vol. 17 (1976), pp. 285–294

Latta, Doris: "Frauen und Medikamente. Besonderheiten in der Arbeit mit medikamentengefährdeten / -abhängigen Frauen," in: Deutsche Hauptstelle gegen die Suchtgefahren (ed.): "Jahrbuch Sucht '95," Hamm 1994, pp. 79–92

Lawrence, Janet M.: "Reactions to withdrawal of antidepressants, antiparkinsonian drugs, and lithium," in: Psychosomatics, Vol. 26 (1985), pp. 869–877

Lehmann, Peter: "Schöne neue Psychiatrie," Vol. 1: "Wie Chemie und Strom auf Geist und Psyche wirken," Berlin 1996 (a)

Lehmann, Peter: "Schöne neue Psychiatrie," Vol. 2: "Wie Psychopharmaka den Körper verändern," Berlin 1996 (b)

Lehmann, Peter: "Theorie und Praxis des Psychiatrischen Testaments," in: Kerstin Kempker / Peter Lehmann (eds.): "Statt Psychiatrie," Berlin 1993, pp. 253–281

Lehmann, Peter / Kempker, Kerstin: "Unconventional approaches to psychiatry," in: Clinical Psychology Forum, 1993, No. 1, pp. 28–29

Leonhard, Karl: "Aufteilung der endogenen Psychosen," 5., revised edit., Berlin 1980

Lerer, Bernard et al.: "Carbamazepine and lithium," in: Psychopharmacology Bulletin, Vol. 21 (1985), pp. 18–22

"Lithium," in: Lancet, 1969, pp. 709–710

Lundbeck AG: "Prelapse, Preventing Relapse in Schizophrenia," Opfikon-Glattbrugg 1998

Lusznat, R. M. / Murphy, D. P. / Nunn, C. M. H.: "Carbamazepine vs. lithium in the treatment and prophylaxis of mania," in: British Journal of Psychiatry, Vol. 153 (1988), pp. 198–204

Mander, A. J.: "Is there a lithium withdrawal syndrome?," in: British Journal of Psychiatry, Vol. 149 (1986), pp. 498–501

Mander, A. J. / Loudon, J. B.: "Rapid recurrence of mania following abrupt discontinuation of lithium," in: Lancet, 1988, pp. 15–17

May, Philip R. A.: "Treatment of Schizophrenia: a Comparative Study of Five Treatment Methods," New York 1968

May, Philip R. A. / Goldberg, Solomon C.: "Prediction of schizophrenic patients' response to pharmacotherapy," in: Morris A. Lipton / Alberto DiMascio / Keith F. Killam (eds.): "Psychopharmacology," New York 1978, pp. 1139–1153

Meltzer, Herbert Y.: "Novel Antipsychotic Drugs," New York 1992

Misri, P. / Sivertz, K.: "Tricyclic drugs in pregnancy and lactation," in: International Journal of Psychiatry in Medicine, Vol. 21 (1991), pp. 157–171

Müller, Peter / Günther, U. / Lohmeyer, J.: "Behandlung und Verlauf schizophrener Psychosen über ein Jahrzehnt," in: Nervenarzt, Vol. 57 (1986), pp. 332–341

Neild, Larry: "Escape from Tranquillisers and Sleeping Pills: a Proven DIY Withdrawal Plan," London 1990

Nergård, Jens-Ivar: "Den vuxna barndomen. Den psykotiske personen som vægvisare i vår kultur," Dualis 1992

Network Against Psychiatric Assault (ed.): "Dr. Caligari's Psychiatric Drugs," Berkeley 1984

Niskanen, Pekka / Achté, Kalle A.: "The Course and Prognosis of Schizophrenic Psychoses in Helsinki," Helsinki 1972

Ochsenknecht, Anna: "Die seelische Balance—Pflanzenheilkundliche Unterstützung bei psychischen Problemen und beim Entzug von Psychopharmaka," in: Kerstin Kempker / Peter Lehmann (eds.): "Statt Psychiatrie," Berlin 1993, pp. 82–94

Otto, Michael W. et al.: "Discontinuation of benzodiazepine treatment: efficacy of cognitive-behavioral therapy for patients with panic disorder," in: American Journal of Psychiatry, Vol. 150 (1993), pp. 1485–1490

Pauling, Linus: "Das Vitamin-Programm," Munich 1990; English edition: "How to Live Longer and Feel Better," New York 1986

Pfeiffer, Carl Curt: "Nutrition and Mental Illness: An Orthomolecular Approach to Balancing Body Chemistry," Rochester 1988

Prien, Robert F. / Kupfer, David J.: "Continuation drug therapy for major depressive episodes: how long should it be maintained?," in: American Journal of Psychiatry, Vol. 143 (1986), pp. 18–23

Prien, Robert F. et al.: "Drug therapy in the prevention of recurrences in unipolar and bipolar affective disorders," in: Archives of General Psychiatry, Vol. 41 (1984), pp. 1096–1104

Randolph, Theron G. / Moss, Ralph W.: "An Alternative Approach to Allergies," New York 1980

Reimer, Fritz: "Das 'Absetzungs'-Delir," in: Nervenarzt, Vol. 34 (1965), pp. 446–447

Remien, Jörg: "Bestimmung der Arzneimittelabhängigkeit durch eine quantitative Analyse des individuellen Verbrauchs aller ärztlich verordneten Arzneimittel," Munich 1994

Rickels, Karl et al.: "Benzodiazepine dependence, withdrawal severity, and clinical outcome," in: Psychopharmacology Bulletin, Vol. 24 (1988), pp. 415–420

Rufer, Marc: "Glückspillen: Ecstasy, Prozac und das Comeback der Psychopharmaka," Munich 1995

Rufer, Marc: "Irrsinn Psychiatrie," 3., revised edit., Berne 1997

Rufer, Marc: "Unterstützung bei Verrücktheitszuständen und beim Entzug psychiatrischer Psychopharmaka," lecture at the congress "Alternativen zur Psychiatrie," organized by the Forum Anti-Psychiatrischer Initiativen and by Netzwerk Arche, Berlin, October 19–21, 1990

Sashidharan, S. P. / McGuire, R. J.: "Recurrence of affective illness after withdrawal of long-term treatment," in: Acta

Psychiatrica Scandinavica, Vol. 68 (1983), pp. 126–133

Schöpf, Josef: "Physische Abhängigkeit bei Benzodiazepin-Langzeitbehandlungen," in: Nervenarzt, Vol. 56 (1985), pp. 585–592

Schooler, Nina R. et al.: "One year after discharge," in: American Journal of Psychiatry, Vol. 123 (1967), pp. 986–995

Schou, Mogens: "Is there a lithium withdrawal syndrome? An examination of the evidence," in: British Journal of Psychiatry, Vol. 163 (1993), pp. 514–518

Schou, Mogens / Weeke, A.: "Did manic-depressive patients who committed suicide receive prophylactic or continuation treatment at the time?," in: British Journal of Psychiatry, Vol. 153 (1988), pp. 324–327

Simpson, George M.: "Neurotoxicity of major tranquilizers," in: Leon Roizin / Hirotsugu Shiraki / Nenad Grcevic (eds.): "Neurotoxicology," New York 1977, pp. 1–7

Solyom, Leslie / Solyom, Carol / Ledwidge, Barry "Fluoxetine treatment of obsessive-compulsive disorder," in: Canadian Journal of Psychiatry, Vol. 36 (1991), pp. 723–727

Sommer, Helma / Quandt, Jochen: "Langzeitbehandlung mit Chlorpromazin im Tierexperiment," in: Fortschritte der Neurologie—Psychiatrie und ihrer Grenzgebiete, Vol. 38 (1970), pp. 466–491

Stierlin, Helm / Wynne, Lyman C. / Wirsching, Michael: "Vorwort," in: Helm Stierlin / Lyman C. Wynne / Michael Wirsching (eds.): "Psychotherapie und Sozialtherapie der Schizophrenie," Berlin etc. 1985, pp. XIII–XIV

Suppes, T. et al.: "Discontinuation of maintenance treatment in bipolar disorder: risks and implications," in: Harvard Review of Psychiatry, Vol. 1 (1993), pp. 131–144

Tattersall, Mark L. / Hallstrom, Cosmo: "Self-help and benzodiazepine withdrawal," in: Journal of Affective Disorders, Vol. 24 (1992), pp. 193–198

Tausch, Reinhard: "Hilfen bei Streß und Belastung," Reinbek 1996

Tegeler, J. / Lehmann, E. / Stockschläder, M.: "Zur Wirksamkeit der langfristigen ambulanten Behandlung Schizophrener mit Depot- und Langzeit-Neuroleptics," in: Nervenarzt, Vol. 51 (1980), pp. 654–661

Tornatore, Frank L. et al.: "Reactions to Psychotropic Medication," New York / London 1987

Tornatore, Frank L. et al.: "Unerwünschte Wirkungen von Psychopharmaka," Stuttgart / New York 1991

Trickett, Shirley: "Coming off Tranquilizers and Sleeping Pills," London 1991

Tune, Larry E.: "Neurological side effects of psychotropic medications in the elderly," in: Charles A. Shamoian (ed.): "Psychopharmacological Treatment Complications in the Elderly," Washington / London 1992, pp. 45–62

Ungerstedt, Urban / Ljungberg, Tomas: "Behavioral patterns related to dopamine neurotransmission," in: Advances in Biochemical Psychopharmacology, Vol. 16 (1977), pp. 193–199

Watzlawick, Paul: "Self-fulfilling prophecies," in: Paul Watzlawick (ed.): "The Invented Reality: how do we Know What we Believe we Know?," New York 1984, pp. 95–116

Weekes, Claire: "Peace from Nervous Suffering," New York 1972

Wehde, Uta: "Das Weglaufhaus—Zufluchtsort für Psychiatrie-Betroffene. Erfahrungen, Konzeptionen, Probleme," Berlin 1991

Wilkinson, D. G.: "Difficulty in stopping lithium prophylaxis?," in: British Medical Journal, 1979, pp. 235–236

Woggon, Brigitte: "Neuroleptics-Absetzversuche bei chronisch schizophrenen Patienten. 1. Literaturzusammenfassung," in: International Pharmacopsychiatry, Vol. 14 (1979), pp. 34–56

Young, Michael A. / Meltzer, Herbert Y.: "The relationship of demographic, clinical, and outcome variables to neuroleptic treatment requirements," in: Schizophrenia Bulletin, Vol. 6 (1980), pp. 88–101

Zehentbauer, Josef: "Chemie für die Seele. Psyche, Psychopharmaka und alternative Heilmethoden," 8., actual. new edit., Munich 1997 (b)

Zehentbauer, Josef: "Körpereigene Drogen. Die ungenutzten Fähigkeiten unseres Gehirns," 5. edit., Düsseldorf 1997 (a)

Zehentbauer, Josef: "Psycho-Pillen. Wirkungen, Gefahren und Alternativen," 4. edit., Munich 1998

Zehentbauer, Josef: "Die Seele zerstören. Neuroleptics, der größte Arzneimittelskandal des Jahrhunderts," Video documentary, Munich 1989

About the Authors

Karl Bach Jensen. Born 1951 in Denmark. During 1973 and '74 locked up in a state mental hospital. Forcibly drugged with heavy dosages of neuroleptic drugs and electroshocked. Voluntary psychiatric patient in '75, '80 and '85. Since then, no personal contact with psychiatry. Get help from personal network and from natural remedies when madness appears. Since 1980 taken part in the national user-/survivor-movement in Denmark. Co-founder of the European Network of (ex-)Users and Survivors of Psychiatry in 1991. Chair of the Network 1994– 1996. Co-founder and board-member of Landsforeningen af Nuværende og Tidligere Psykiatribrugere (LAP), the Danish Association of Users and Ex-users of Psychiatry. Since 2001, one of two European members of the board of WNUSP. Worked for many years as a teacher in public school. For seven years employed as the manager of a drop-in and activity centre in Kolding, Denmark. These years employed as a consultant in a social development center doing evaluations, research and courses. Edited a couple books critical towards psychiatry and wrote a number of articles in Danish magazines.

Regina Bellion, born 1941, in the Federal Republic of Germany (FRG), cleaning-woman, factory-worker, haute-couture sales-woman, teacher, waitress etc. Today living in early retirement.

Carola Bock (FRG), pseudonym, born 1949, industrial accountant, in early retirement since 1991.

Wilma Boevink, born 1963, social scientist on psychiatric care, an active member of the Dutch usermovement in psychiatry. Being a longterm user herself now working in Utrecht at the Trimbos-Institute (the Dutch Institute for Mental Health and Addiction). She works in the research department, integrating her personal experiences in her work. Author (together with José van Beuzekom, Erna Gaal et al.) of "Samen werken aan herstel. Van ervaringen delen naar kennis overdragen" *("Working Together on Recovery: from Sharing Experiences to Implementing Knowledge")*, Utrecht: Trimbos-Institute 2002.

Michael Chmela: Born 1958, in Vorarlberg, Austria. From 1976 to 1983 studied medicine in Graz. From 1997 to 1999 Chair of the information and contact-center for self-help-groups "Club Antenne" in Vorarlberg. 1999, co-founder of the so-called trialogue in Vorarlberg. Active preparation and participation of the First Austrian Conference of people who have experiences with psychiatry, held in Linz 1999. Co-founder of the Austrian Network of (ex-)users and survivors of psychiatry, chair since 2001. 2000, co-founder of the registered organization <omnibus> and chair. Since July 2001, leader of the peer-conseling-center "Gleiche beraten Gleiche" *("Peers advice Peers")* in Bregenz, Vorarlberg. Since 2000 lecturer at the Klagenfurt University for social professions, main foci: self-help, movement of (ex-) users and survivors of psychiatry, empowerment, salutogenesis. Publications in different specialist journals about patients' rights and dangers of the anti-stigma-campaign.

Bert Gölden, born 1955, in FRG. Educated as type-setter in 1969, further education as film-setter. From 1985 to 1987 independent work as film-setter. A handicap led to an early retirement from working life. Since 1996, active working in the self-help and public relations work of the Deutschen Gesellschaft Zwangserkrankungen e.V. (DGZ; *German Society for Obsession Diseases*). In 1996 he founded a self-help group for people with obsession diseases and their relatives. Since 1996, too, participant in a "Psychosis-Seminar." Since 2000 regional representative of Nordrhein der DGZ e.V. *(North-Rhine Society for Obsession Diseases)* as well as contact for personal advice. From autumn 2001, actively working in the committees of DGZ e.V.

Ilse Gold (FRG), born 1949. She was committed to a closed ward by a specialist for internal diseases for two weeks in 1991; secretly and by her own decision she quit taking Haldol and never took any psychiatric drugs again. Ilse Gold tragically lost her fight against breast cancer, which developed after the psychiatric treatment, on September 7, 1998.

Gábor Gombos, born 1961, is a physicist. He is engaged with the survivor-of-psychiatry-movement, since 1993. Since 1996 he is the chair of a Hungarian self-help association, Voice of Soul. He is the East European board member of the European Network of (ex-)Users and Survivors of Psychiatry, member of the International Panel of the World Network of Users and Survivors of Psychiatry, board member of the Hungarian Branch of the World Association of Psychosocial Rehabilitation.

Katalin Gombos, Hungary, born 1954, computer expert, has more than ten years of experience with psychiatry and neuroleptics. She is one of the founders and board-member of Voice of Soul Association of (ex-)Users and Survivors of Psychiatry.

Maths Jesperson. Born 1954. From 1980 to 1981 inmate of a psychiatric institution. From 1982 to 1988 producer of the actors' group Mercuriustheatre as well as local politician of the Green Party in Lund, Sweden. Converted 1984 to Catholicism. Since 1988 regional secretary of RSMH (Riksförbundet før Social och Mental Hælsa; *Swedish national organization of [ex-]users and survivors of psychiatry)*. Founding member of the European Network of (ex-)Users and Survivors of Psychiatry 1991. From 1991 to 2000 editor of the *European Newsletter of (ex-)Users and Survivors of Psychiatry*. Since 1999, writer of cultural articles in a daily newspaper. Parallel research at the University of Lund (faculty of theatre). Since 2000, actor in the Stumpen-Ensemble, a theatre group with psychiatric survivors, drug addicts and homeless people as actors.

Klaus John, born in 1958, in West-Germany, married, father of two children, healing practitioner since 1985 with main focus on: acupuncture, electro-acupuncture according to Voll, homeopathy, guided affective imagery, hypnosis, transpersonal psychology and colortherapy. Three year training in transpersonal psychology with Stanislav Grof, USA. Workshops in this field since 1988. Teacher for autogenic training at adults education centers since 1990. Certified Holotropic Breathwork™ practitioner since 1991.

Manuela Kälin (Switzerland), pseudonym. 1969, education as nurse. Practical work in different wards, abroad, too. 1983/84 education as medical masseuse. Three years physiotherapy in a hospital. Further education in complementary medicine. Since 1990 working in her own office in Switzerland.

Kerstin Kempker, born 1958 in Wuppertal (FRG), two daughters, lives in Berlin. From 1996–2001 she worked as leading social worker at the Runaway-House Berlin. Co-founder of the association "Für alle Fälle e.V." *("In Any Case")*, which works on the creation of a peer-counseling project. Now self-employed as author and project-advisor. Last book publications: "Mitgift. Notizen vom Verschwinden" *("Dowry: Notes of Vanishing,"* Berlin 2000); "Flucht in die Wirklichkeit. Das Berliner Weglaufhaus" *("Escape into Reality: the Berlin Runaway-House,"* ed. Berlin 1998).

Leo P. Koehne, pseudonym, born in 1970, in FRG, studied politics and works as a freelance journalist. Since 1994 member of the German Association of (ex-) Users and Survivors of Psychiatry.

Jan Kuypers, born in 1942, in Flanders/ Belgium. Chemist. Former teacher of mathematics and researcher for process engineering. 1983, non-intended founder of the psychiatry-critical Ombudscenter Kisjot, named after Don Quixote. 1993 project leader for the setting of a Flemish representative union for (ex-)users and survivors of psychiatry. 1990 and 2001 co-founder of the European resp. the World Network of Users and Survivors of Psychiatry. Further academic education in philosophy, criminology, play-theory, ethics, semiotics, churches' history, anthropology, brain-biology, health economics and forensic psychiatry. Hobbies since the middle of the 80ies: Co-founder of the authors' circle Littera and of a school for high talents als well as board-member for the science-philosophic working-group De Ronde Tafel *(The Round Table).*

Elke Laskowski, born in 1958, in FRG, mother of a daughter, wife. Studied social work and decided to become a nature cure therapist after working with so-called mentally ill people and find another way. She has become a healing practitioner. Since 1991, she works in her own office in Langenhagen near Hannover with hypnosis, Bach flowers, stones, colors and biodynamic body- and aura-work.

Peter Lehmann (FRG). Author and publisher. Education as a social-pedagogist. Living in Berlin. Author and editor since 1986, then foundation of Peter Lehmann Publishing and Mail-Order Bookstore. Different publications. From 1994 to 2000, board-member of the German organization of (ex-)Users and Survivors of Psychiatry. From 1997 to 2000, member of the Executive Committee of Mental Health Europe, the European section of the World Federation for Mental Health. From 1997 to 1999, Chair of the European Network of (ex-)Users and Survivors of Psychiatry (ENUSP), since 1999, board member for the countries of Austria, Belgium, Germany, Luxembourg and Switzerland. Since 2002, ENUSP secretary. 2002, co-founder of "Für alle Fälle e.V."

("In Any Case") and board-member in this organisation.

Ulrich Lindner, born in Lübeck, FRG in 1936, living in Unterreichenbach near Pforzheim (Southern Germany). Retired theologian, philologist and historian. Member of the German organization of (ex-) users and survivors of psychiatry, leader of Selbsthilfe für seelische Gesundheit Nordschwarzwald e.V. *(Self-Help for Mental Health in the Northern Part of the Black Forest)*.

Iris Marmotte (pseudonym, FRG), studied German, arts and pedagogic in the German Democratic Republic (GDR), but was removed from the university and put into prison because of political reasons shortly before finishing her studies ("not a socialist personality"). Nurse job in a children's and adolescents' psychiatric ward of a regional hospital. 1983 imprisonment with political reasons, 1984 release from prison and GDR-nationality because of "special efforts of the Federal Republic of Germany (FRG)" and move to FRG. 1986 registration at the University of Bremen and continuation of her studies. 1990 phase of examination and interruption of the studies, because of illness, "revolving-door-patient," from 1992 to 1995 in sheltered living. 1994, "Die blaue Karawane" *("The Blue Caravan")*, in Bremen co-founder of the "Nachtschwärmer"-*("Nocturnal-Reveler"-)*projects and work as board-member, founding-member of the music-band "Die Therapie-Resistenten" *("The Therapy-Resistant")*. 1995 job as neighbourly helper and reestablishment of the studies. 1997 job as night watch in a hospital and pedagogical worker in a home for mentally ill persons. 2000, finished her studies, since then, grammar school teacher.

Constanze Meyer, born in 1959, in FRG, psychologist and psychotherapist. Since the beginning, her studies dealt intensively with women-specific health-issues. Many years of full-time work at "Schwindel-Frei" *("Head-for-Heights")*, an information and counseling center for drug-dependent women in Berlin-Tempelhof, Reinhardtstr. 5, D–12103 Berlin, phone +49 30 7528034. "Schwindel-Frei" has a women-specific starting point that equally takes psychosomatics and addiction into account. Since 2001, exclusively working in independent psychotherapeutic office in Berlin-Spandau.

Harald Müller (FRG), pseudonym.

Eiko Nagano (pseudonym), born 1953, in Japan. From 1968 until 1999, she was a psychiatric user. She graduated from Waseda University, Tokyo, in 1979 in sociology. Since 1981, she has been a member of the Zenkoku "Seishinbyou" sha Shudan, the Japanese National Group of Mental Disabled People. Publications: "Seishin Iryou" *("Psychiatric Treatments,"* Tokyo: Gendaishokan 1990); "Seishin Iryou User no Mezasumono—Oubei no self-help katsudo" *("About the Interests of Users of Psychiatry—Self-Help Activities in Europe and the USA,"* Osaka: Buraku kaihour syupansha 1999).

Mary Nettle (England). Having obtained a Higher National Diploma in Business Studies and a Diploma in Advanced Marketing from Bristol Polytechnic, she worked for several years in marketing research with Audits of Great Britain and with Quaker Oats Ltd. In December 1992, she became self employed as a mental health user consultant. Involved in presenting the user perspective in all aspects of mental health. She is an Honorary Fellow of Brunel University and has been appointed by the United Kingdom's government to work part time for the Mental Health Act Commission mainly in South West England. She is an active member of MindLink, the service user voice within Mind, the mental health charity covering England and Wales, and its chair person from 1995 to 2000.

Una M. Parker, Yorkshire, England, born 1935. Retired school teacher. Quaker. Lives with black cat in a flat in Leeds since 2001, leaving behind the large village where she had lived for 33 years. Still friends with husband who lives in Australia, since 1993. Two adult daughters. Appointed in 1996 as governor (voluntary) of the mental hospital in which she was a patient 30 years ago. Co-counselor (Re-evaluation Counseling) since 1974. Now speaks to groups and runs workshops on mental health. Belongs to local, national and international groups of psychiatry survivors, particularly Mindlink and ECT Anonymous. Attended the Forum that met in Bejing alongside the UN Fourth World conference on Women in 1995. Enjoys singing, circle dancing, T'ai-Chi, co-counseling, visiting family and friends, reading, writing, using computer, knitting, sewing, gardening, stroking her cat…

Nada Rath, née Dmitrasinovic 1940 in Yugoslavia, industrial chemist, now living in Germany, early retirement 1995, co-founded the German organization of (ex-)users and survivors of psychiatry in 1992, board-member of this organization from 1996 to 1998. 1997 initiator of the foundation of the Hessian regional organization of (ex-)users and survivors of psychiatry.

Erwin Redig (Belgium). Spent several years in psychiatry. Living as a free man now in Antwerp, Belgium, and have connections with the national and international survivor movements. The work is essentially humanistic; it is about human rights and human dignity. *Erwin Redig died on June 14, 1999.*

Hannelore Reetz (FRG), pseudonym, born 1943, accountant, today part-time working as a dentist assistant, married, clean since 1990.

Roland A. Richter, born in 1963, in FRG, worked as a social worker in state institutions until 1995, since then he is working as a case worker for people in custodial care and sheltered living, for people who are regarded to be chronical mentally ill. Since 1995, has lived in Bad Münstereifel/Nordrhein-Westfalen, works self-employed as judicially appointed guide and advices stationary institutions as advisor for organizations in the management of quality.

Marc Rufer (Switzerland), Dr med, psychotherapist. After finishing studies of medicine worked as a junior doctor in a big psychiatric state hospital. From the beginning had big difficulties with the psychiatric "diagnostic" and "therapy" of psychic "disorders." The step to criticize psychiatry as a whole, was made after a time of intensive debates. With books and many articles in magazines and newspapers he tries to make critical thoughts about the psychiatric system public. Book publications: "Irrsinn Psychiatrie" *("Insane Psychiatry,"* Berne 1988); "Wer ist irr?" *("Who's Crazy?,"* Berne 1991); "Glückspillen. Ecstasy, Prozac und das Comeback der Psychopharmaka" *("Happy Pills. Ecstasy, Prozac and* *the Comeback of Psychotropic Drugs,"* Munich 1995).

Jasna Russo, born in Belgrade, in 1964. Member of the Berlin Association for Protection against Psychiatric Violence (running the Runaway-House Berlin). Publications in: Kerstin Kempker / Peter Lehmann (eds.): "Statt Psychiatrie" *("Instead of Psychiatry,"* Berlin 1993); Wildwasser Bielefeld e.V. (ed.): "Der aufgestörte Blick—Multiple Persönlichkeiten, Frauenbewegung und Gewalt" *("The Disturbed Look: Multiple Personalities, Trauma and the Women's Movement,"* Bielefeld 1997); Kerstin Kempker (ed.): "Flucht in die Wirklichkeit—Das Berliner Weglaufhaus" *("Escape into Reality: the Berlin Runaway-House,"* Berlin 1998); Claudia Brügge (ed.): "Frauen in ver-rückten Lebenswelten" *("Women in Crazy Worlds,"* Berne 1999); Jim Read (ed.): "Something Inside so Strong," London 2001.

Lynne Setter, country of origin New Zealand, born 1963, no children, divorced. Occupation—International Marketing Consultant. First suicide attempt aged 9, hospitalized a number of times from early teenage to recent years. Lived in Asia, Europe, the Middle East and the United States. After ten years abroad, now living in New Zealand.

Martin Urban (FRG), born 1939, psychologist and psychotherapist, worked for seven years in a psychiatric and for six years in a hospital for psychosomatic medicine, now working in his own office near Stuttgart. As a member of the association of German psychologists, he is the head of the section "Clinical psychologists in psychiatry." He edited the book "Psychotherapie der Psychosen—Konzentrische Annäherungen an den Weg

der Heilung" *("Psychotherapy of Psychoses: Concentric Approaches to the Way of Healing,"* Lengerich 2000).

Wolfgang Voelzke (FRG), academically qualified economist, employed since 1975 by the town administration in Bielefeld. Beginning 2000, he works as co-ordinator for psychiatry and addiction. He co-founded the national organization of (ex-)users and survivors of psychiatry in Germany and the local organization of (ex-)users and survivors of psychiatry in Bielefeld.

David Webb is a white, middle-class man, born in 1955, who lives in Melbourne, Australia. Studied and worked as a computer software developer and university lecturer until 1994. Surviving suicidality, heroin, Methadone, antidepressants and neuroleptics, he has returned to part-time lecturing. He is a dedicated activist against the abuses of psychiatry and has recently commenced research into suicide and spirituality.

Gerda Wozart (pseudonym), born in 1946, in Bavaria. Longer stays in England and France. Studied in Perpignan, married twice, loads of kids (her own others'). For some time she has been living in the Black Forest. Lecturer in an adult education center, founded her own office for writing and translation, publishes poems and short stories. Since 2001, first chairwoman of the Independent German Authors' Organization (FDA) in Baden-Württemberg.

Josef Zehentbauer, born in 1945, in FRG, married, four children. Doctor, psychotherapist and author. Several years' work in neurology (University of Würzburg), different psychiatric clinics and the emergency ward of a mental hospital. Worked as a doctor in Nigeria and India.

Initiated projects with Franco Basaglia and other exponents of Italian "Critical Psychiatry." Publications including among others: "Die Auflösung der Irrenhäuser oder: Die Neue Psychiatrie in Italien" *("The Resolution of the Madhouses or: the New Psychiatry in Italy,"* 1983; Munich, 4. edition 1997); "Chemie für die Seele. Psyche, Psychopharmaka und alternative Heilmethoden" *("Chemistry for the Soul: Psyche, Psychotropic Drugs and Alternatives Methods of Cure,"* Königstein 1986; 9. edition Munich 2002); "Die Seele zerstören. Neuroleptika, der größte Arzneimittelskandal des Jahrhunderts" *("To Destroy the Soul. Neuroleptics: the Biggest Drug Scandal of the Century,"* video documentary, Munich 1989); "Körpereigene Drogen. Die ungenutzten Fähigkeiten unseres Gehirns" *("The Body's Own Drugs: the Unused Capabilities of Our Brain,"* Munich 1993, 11. edition 2001); "Psycho-Pillen. Wirkungen, Gefahren und Alternativen" *("Psycho-Pills: Effects, Risks and Alternatives,"* Munich, 4. edition 1998); "Abenteuer Seele. Psychische Krisen als Chance nutzen" *("Adventure Soul: to Use Psychic Crises as a Chance,"* Düsseldorf 2000); "Melancholie—Die traurige Leichtigkeit des Seins" *("Melancholy: the Sad Lightness of Being,"* Stuttgart 2000; 2. edition 2002).

Katherine Zurcher. Born in the USA, lives in Switzerland. She was diagnosed with fibromyalgia *(chronic illness which causes muscular pain, headache, fatigue and many other symptoms)* in 1999. She regrets having tried so hard to adapt to society. She enjoys writing and poetry, taking photographs, riding her bike, communing with nature, philosophic discussions and much more. She still searches for the person her younger self wanted to become before she got lost.

Index

Peter Lehmann Publishing

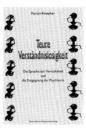

Publications in German

▶ Kerstin Kempker: Teure Verständnislosigkeit. Die Sprache der Verrücktheit und die Entgegnung der Psychiatrie · 1991 · ISBN 3-925931-04-X

▶ Uta Wehde: Das Weglaufhaus. Zufluchtsort für Psychiatrie-Betroffene · Vorwort von Jeffrey M. Masson · 1991 · ISBN 3-925931-05-8

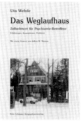

▶ Peter Lehmann: Schöne Neue Psychiatrie. Band 1: Wie Chemie und Strom auf Geist und Psyche wirken · Mit dem Artikel "Elektroschock" von Leonard Roy Frank · 1996 · ISBN 3-925931-09-0

▶ Peter Lehmann: Schöne Neue Psychiatrie. Band 2: Wie Psychopharmaka den Körper verändern · 1996 · ISBN 3-925931-10-4

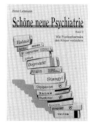

▶ Kerstin Kempker (Hg.): Flucht in die Wirklichkeit – Das Berliner Weglaufhaus · 1998 · ISBN 3-925931-13-9

▶ Kerstin Kempker: Mitgift – Notizen vom Verschwinden · 2000 · ISBN 3-925931-15-5

▶ Bernd Kempker, "Dem eigenen Ableben emotionslos zusehen" – Psychopharmaka in Altenheimen · Hörkassette 2000 · ISBN 3-925931-16-3

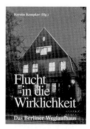

▶ Peter Lehmann (Hg.): Psychopharmaka absetzen – Erfolgreiches Absetzen von Neuroleptika, Antidepressiva, Lithium, Carbamazepin und Tranquilizern · Vorworte von Loren R. Mosher und Pirkko Lahti · 2. Auflage 2002 · ISBN 3-925931-27-9

▶ Claudia Brügge: Wohin mit dem Wahnsinn? Ausgewählte Aspekte der Kontroverse um Anstaltspsychiatrie und mögliche Alternativen. Kritischer Überblick über psychiatrische, antipsychiatrische und feministische Positionen – am Beispiel der Konzeptionen von Soteria (Bern), vom Weglaufhaus-projekt Berlin und vom Therapieansatz Polina Hilsenbecks · 2004 · ISBN 3-925931-29-5

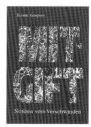

▶ Birgit Heuer / Renate Schön: Lebensqualität und Krankheitsverständnis. Die Auswirkung des medizinischen Krankheitsmodells auf die Lebensqualität von chronisch psychisch Kranken · 2004 · ISBN 3-925931-30-9

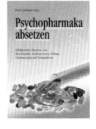

▶ Susanne Spieker: Bedarf oder Bedürfnis?! Alternative (zur) Psychiatrie · 2004 · ISBN 3-925931-32-5

▶ Therese Walther: Die "Insulin-Koma-Behandlung" – Erfindung und Einführung des ersten modernen psychiatrischen Schockverfahrens · 2004 · ISBN 3-925931-34-1

▶ Karin Roth: Geschichte und Entwicklung des Europäischen Netzwerks von Psychiatriebetroffenen · 2004 · ISBN 3-925931-35-X

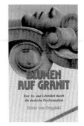

▶ Dörte von Drigalski: Blumen auf Granit. Eine Irr- und Lehrfahrt durch die deutsche Psychoanalyse · Geleitwort von Gaby Sohl · Neuausgabe 2003 · ISBN 3-925931-37-6

▶ Heinz Kampmann / Jeanette Wenzel: Psychiatrische und antipsychiatrische Vorstellungen von Hilfe im Wandel der Zeit · 2004 · ISBN 3-925931-39-2

▶ Elisabeth Reuter: Der Missbrauch der Hilflosigkeit und das therapeutische Glaubensbekenntnis des Bert Hellinger · Vorwort von Wolfram Pfreundschuh · Nachwort von Klaus Weber · 2004 · ISBN 3-925931-40-6

Peter Lehmann Mail-Order Bookstore

▶ About 300 specialist titles in (mostly) German and English language edition by Artaud, Basaglia, Breggin, Foucault, Frame, Goffman, Gruen, Illich, Laing, Masson, Rufer, Watzlawick, Zehentbauer and many more. Moderate delivery charges. Plus the convenience of paying via our bank accounts in Austria, Belgium, Germany, Great Britain, Netherlands, Spain, Switzerland, USA or via PayPal.

Peter Lehmann Publishing & Mail-Order Bookstore

Zabel-Krüger-Damm 183 · D-13469 Berlin · Germany
Tel. +49 30 8596 3706 · Fax +49 30 4039 8752
E-mail: pl@peter-lehmann-publishing.com
www.peter-lehmann-publishing.com

Peter Lehmann's international internet-portal on self-help & alternatives to psychiatry:
www.p.lehmann.berlinet.de/alternatives.htm